CLINICAL
HEMATOLOGY

*A Problem-Oriented
Approach*

CLINICAL HEMATOLOGY

A Problem-Oriented Approach

James P. Isbister, M.D.

Head, Department of Hematology
Royal North Shore Hospital of Sydney
Sydney, New South Wales, Australia

D. Harmening Pittiglio, Ph.D., MT(ASCP)

Chairman and Professor
Department of Laboratory Sciences
Thomas Jefferson University
Philadelphia, Pennsylvania

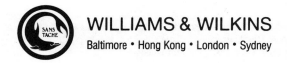

WILLIAMS & WILKINS
Baltimore • Hong Kong • London • Sydney

Editor: Nancy Collins
Associate Editor: Carol Eckhart
Copy Editor: Stephen Siegforth
Design: Alice Sellers/Johnson
Illustration Planning: Lorraine Wrzosek
Production: Raymond E. Reter
Cover Design: Bets. Ltd.

Accurate indications, adverse reactions, and dosage schedules for drugs are provided in this
book, but it is possible that they may change. The reader is urged to review the package information data of the manufacturers of the medications mentioned.

Printed in the United States of America

Library of Congress Cataloging-in-Publication Data

Isbister, James P.
  Clinical hematology.
  Bibliography: p.
  Includes index.
  1. Blood—Diseases. 2. Hematology. I. Pittiglio,
D. Harmening (Denise Harmening) II. Title.
[DNLM: 1. Hematologic Diseases. 2. Hemostasis.
WH 100 I76c]
RC636.I76 1988   616.1′5   87-16067
ISBN 0-683-04349-8

88 89 90 91   10 9 8 7 6 5 4 3 2 1

Preface

Why would one want to add yet another basic text on clinical hematology to the plethora already available? The reason I give is that most of the currently available books describe hematological diseases or laboratory abnormalities rather than address problems as they confront the clinician. Various terms have been used for a problem solving approach to clinical medicine, including decision analysis, clinical algorithms and the diagnostic process and it is hoped that this book will present such an approach for clinical hematology.

The "Catch 22" which confronts all medical students during their undergraduate training is that they cannot learn medicine unless they see patients, and they cannot learn from patients unless they have the knowledge. One of the aims of medical education should be to resolve this apparent dilemma. The learning of facts in relation to specific diseases out of context of the patient is almost a certain recipe for failure. If individual diseases can be learned in the context of patient-oriented clinical problem solving, the knowledge and practice components of clinical medicine hopefully will be integrated.

It is the hope of the author that this book presents an integrated approach to clinical hematological problems as they are likely to present to the clinician, or indeed, to any specialty of clinical medicine. A patient or a family physician is unlikely to spontaneously say "I need a hematologist," as most hematological disorders manifest in other systems of the body and it is not until investigations are initiated that the true nature becomes apparent.

Clinical hematology is one of the few disciplines in which the specialist is able to closely integrate clinical and laboratory medicine within the one speciality. It is hoped that the reader will be able to perceive the close relationship that there should be between clinical and laboratory medicine. It is only with the correct approach to a clinical problem that diagnostic and laboratory services will be appropriately and effectively utilized. Unfortunately, few clinicians are now able to spend sufficient undergraduate or postgraduate education time in laboratory medicine where the scientific basis of medicine originated during the 19th century. Unless the basic pathophysiological mechanisms of disease are understood, diagnosis and therapy are unlikely to be logical.

It is inevitable that the vast range of hematological disorders are likely to present in a variety of different ways. In this book, the author has discussed the disease in relation to the problem where it is most likely to present. However, extensive cross referencing will be necessary and the reader will be directed appropriately during his or her investigations. If the primary need of the reader is to find information about a particular disease, this is best approached by using the index.

The author is indebted to many friends, colleagues, mentors and students for help in the preparation of this book. Sir John Dacie, the late Sheila Worlledge, Professor David Galton, Professor Robert Pitney, James Biggs and

Fred Gunz have all had a considerable influence on my training and think-ing. David Ma, K. S. Lau, Roger Scurr, Richard Hollis, Fred Gunz and Christopher Arthur have critically read much of the manuscript and offered numerous helpful suggestions. Undergraduate and postgraduate students remain among my greatest stimuli to continued learning. In preparation of the manuscript I am particularly grateful to Mrs. Arechea Hounsell for her enthusiastic help with diagrams and proofreading. Lastly, I owe Rod Laird and David More a special thanks for nursing me up the learning curve of computing, for introducing me to all the software which makes writing a pleasure and for continued tolerance and assistance when the inevitable hardware and software "bugs" threatened progress. Without computers this book would never have been started. The technology of word processors, reference systems and graphics allow busy clinicians the opportunity to put some of their experience down on paper.

James P. Isbister

This book provides a comprehensive and concise overview of clinical hema-tology. An integrated and problem solving approach has been provided for hematological diseases as they relate to the clinical manifestations in each patient population. Each disease process is discussed utilizing laboratory parameters and general treatment protocols. Basic concepts of hemato-poiesis, including red cell function, hemostasis, and cells of the host defense system, serve as an introduction to the pathogenesis of hematological dis-orders. Organomegalies, including lymphadenopathy and disorders of the spleen and thymus, followed by a discussion of malignancy and hematolog-ical aspects of infection and systemic disease, complete the scope of this text. The interpretation and investigation of abnormal laboratory results facili-tate the practical application of the material presented. An entire chapter devoted to the preventive aspects of hematology represents a unique con-tribution. Dr. Isbister's innovative approach precisely blends the theoretical and practical aspects of clinical hematology into a well-balanced, easy to use textbook.

Denise H. Pittiglio

Contents

Chapter 10

Hematological Aspects of Infection and Systemic Disease 205

Chapter 11

The Interpretation and Investigation of Abnormal Laboratory Results 217

Chapter 12

Preventive Medicine Aspects of Hematology 225

Index 239

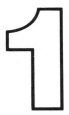

Basic Concepts of the Hematopoietic System

How can I possibly have come so far, and yet still have so far to go?
Ashleigh Brilliant (1933–   )

The very first step towards success in any occupation is to become interested in it.
Sir William Osler

Blood has always fascinated man, being regarded as the essence of life. Much of the humoral theory of disease was probably based on the ancients' observations of shed blood in various disease states. William Harvey was well attuned to the "Admirable faculties of the blood." Harvey wrote: "Blood acts above all the powers of the elements and is endowed with notable virtues and is also the instrument of the Omnipotent Creator, no man can sufficiently extol its admirable and divine faculties." The heart, Harvey wrote "is the mere organ for its circulation and it clearly appears that the blood is the generative part, the fountain of life, the first to live, the last to die and the primary seat to the soul." There are several concepts central to an understanding of the normal hematopoietic system which allow a logical analysis of the various disorders which may affect the blood and its associated organs. The study of disorders of the blood is unique among medical specialties as it offers the hematologist the opportunity to relate the normal to the disordered in a way which is not readily possible in other systems. It is simple to study the blood in the laboratory, with ready access via venipuncture, bone marrow by aspiration or lymphoid tissue examination by biopsy. Most of these samples can be obtained on a regular basis without significant risk to the patient. Because of this ready availability of hematological tissue more has been learned about disease mechanisms in hematology than any other area of medicine. It has been possible to extrapolate many of the principles learned in hematology to other systems of the body, especially in malignant disease and autoimmune disorders.

Functions of the Hematopoietic System

In the hematopoietic system nature has created a most diverse, adaptable, coordinated, and efficient machinery to achieve numerous essential bodily functions, with servocontrol mechanisms which would be the envy of any Apollo mission engineer (Fig. 1.1).

PRINCIPAL FUNCTIONS

Transport System

Supply oxygen for aerobic metabolism
Nutrients
Carrier proteins: specific and nonspecific
Immune globulins
Host defense systems
Remove products of metabolism

Host Defense System

Hemostasis
Nonspecific inflammatory response
Phagocytic system
Specific immune defense

Body Homeostasis ("Miliéu Interieur")

Temperature regulation
Electrolytes and water

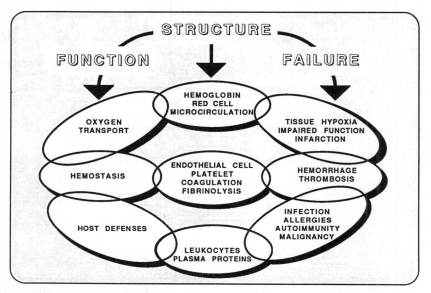

Figure 1.1. The hematopoietic system

Communications between organs and tissues

Until recently, each of the components of the hematopoietic system have been studied in isolation and the overall integration of the system is only now becoming increasingly apparent. What is seen in the specialized hematopoietic organs is only part of the story, and the highly specialized hematopoietic components present in individual nonhematopoietic organs are now becoming apparent. The central role of the liver in producing the majority of plasma proteins is well accepted and this organ must be accredited with an equal place with the bone marrow when considering the body's overall defense system.

One of the most remarkable developments in hematology over the past few years has been the way that different areas of the subject have come together. Although our knowledge has been expanding and splintering into an ever-increasing number of isolated areas of study, unexpected connections are emerging between apparently distinct components of the body's systems. This more holistic integration of knowledge is allowing an unfolding of a more logical and understandable hematopoietic system.

Basic Biological Principles

The hematopoietic system (Fig. 1.2) has the following biological characteristics:

The system is normally disseminated throughout the body.

The system derives from a single pluripotent stem cell deriving from the bone marrow, each cell line developing under the influence of a specific humoral factor responsible for maturation.

The system has one of the highest rates of continuous replication with all components having a limited lifespan.

Although each component of the system has its specific functions there is close, coordinated cooperation.

Each component has an immediate reserve for increased demands of stress, but a much larger potential regenerative reserve if adequate time is available for activation.

The defense component of the system can react both in a nonspecific and a specific (adaptive) manner.

Inappropriate or excessive activation of the defense system may be responsible for tissue damage.

For active components of the defense system there are inhibitors, inactivators and control mechanisms.

From these biological characteristics it can be seen that the system has enormous reserve

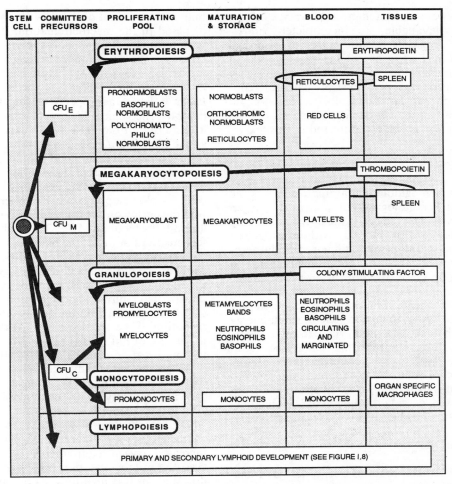

Figure 1.2. Development of the hematopoietic components—CFU = colony forming units; E = erythroid; M = megakaryocyte; C = granulocytes and monocytes

and replacement capacity due to its disseminated nature and that disease may present anywhere in the body. The system is not only able to delicately control potent cellular and humoral reactions, but also is able, with appropriate education, to evolve an efficient and well-directed immune attack.

Oxygen Transport

Of all the systems of the body which have been dissected by subspecialties into their individual parts to be analyzed in isolation, the oxygen transport chain must be the classical

example. The dangers of such a fragmented subspecialty approach would also be best illustrated by this system. The "numbers game" has been played by each subspecialty in its attempt to quantify its link in the oxygen transport chain, and attempts to correct defects have been seen in isolation from the rest of the system and frequently to the detriment of other links in the transport chain and, ultimately, the patient. Oxygen transport has to adapt to a wide range of circumstances and has a remarkable ability to ensure the adequate delivery of oxygen to essential tissues. Endeavors such as mountain climbing, marathon running and sprinting all place different stresses on the system and the various adaptations available are incompletely understood. There is a wide range of disorders which may affect any of the various links in oxygen transport. This flexibility and reserve in oxygen transport allows the patient to continue normal functions, albeit with lower reserve. Only the hematological aspects of oxygen transport will be addressed in this text.

THE RED CELL

The hemoglobin-containing red cell is the central hematological component of oxygen transport. The red cell is the only functionally complete cell in the body without a nucleus and is also unique in that it has minimal aerobic metabolism (i.e., no mitochondria). In giving up these structures to improve its primary functional capacity, the red cell is unable to replicate structural and functional proteins as well as unable to generate high-energy phosphate compounds via oxidative phosphorylation. On the other hand the "enucleated" red cell is endowed with unique properties of flexibility and fluidity in order to carry out its role in gas exchange to and from the tissue, passing through vessels which may be as small as half its own size. In spite of its metabolic limitations the red cell is able to sustain vital functions for an average of 120 days.

The red cell requires energy for gas transport, maintenance of membrane integrity and flexibility, functioning of the sodium/potassium pump and protection of hemoglobin against peroxidation. Some 90% of energy is supplied via the anaerobic Embden-Myerhoff glycolytic pathway, with the other 10% of energy from the hexose monophosphate shunt. However, the main function of this shunt is the production of nicotinamide adenine dinucleotide phosphate (NADPH) which is required for generation of reduced glutathione (GSH) which is essential for the protection of hemoglobin, red cell enzymes and membrane components against oxidation.

HEMORHEOLOGY

The fluidity of the red cell is not only important for each individual cell to negotiate the vast network of capillaries, but also is a major determinant of the flow characteristics of blood in the macrocirculation. Blood is a nonnewtonian fluid in that the viscosity decreases as the shear rate increases, a property known as thyxotropy. This characteristic means that blood becomes more fluid the faster it flows, a property arising from the complex rheological behavior of the red cell. The fluidity of blood decreases exponentially as the hematocrit rises above 45% and it has been calculated that blood would have the consistency of concrete above a hematocrit of 65% if it were not for the flexibility of the red cell. As blood approaches the microcirculation the perfusion pressure falls and the blood autodilutes by about 50%. This Fahraeus effect ensures fluidity of the blood in the microcirculation under low shear conditions, especially as the red cells will tend to aggregate if the normal large vessels' hematocrit is maintained. This physiological hemodilution is closely connected with the autoregulatory vasomotion of the arteriolar bed. At rest maximum flux of red cells (i.e., oxygen availability) occurs at hematocrit of 30% (Hb 10g/dL or 10 gm %); above this the rising viscosity/reducing perfusion offsets the greater oxygen-carrying capacity. The hemoglobin above 10g/dL or 10gm % is reserve for exercise when the rheological and oxygen delivery characteristics are different. During times of increased oxygen requirements (such as exercise) the microcirculation dilates to increase flow and, in this high-flow setting, permits a rise in the hematocrit and thus greater oxygen availability. As will be discussed in relation to hyperviscosity and vascular disease this ability to control hemodilution in the microcirculation may be lost. The distal hypoxic microcirculatory bed behaves in the expected physiological manner, but this occurs in a low perfusion, low pressure setting.

HEMOGLOBIN FUNCTION

Barcroft, the oxygen physiologist, suggested that without the evolution of hemoglobin, "Man might never have achieved any activity which the lobster does not possess." The evolutionary movement of hemoglobin from the plasma into a unique protective cellular environment of its own was a major step. Not only did it prolong the life of the hemoglobin molecule, it provided an environment allowing efficient and flexible operation of the molecule in its interaction with oxygen and carbon dioxide. A complex "bath" of enzymes, proteins and electrolytes allows ideal functioning of the hemoglobin molecule, protecting it from irreversible oxidation and its surrounding cell from destruction. The relationship of the partial pressure of oxygen to oxygen saturation of hemoglobin is expressed in the oxygen dissociation curve. Hemoglobin is a unique oxygen binding molecule for the efficient uptake of oxygen in the high partial pressure environment of the lungs, avidly retaining it while circulating in the arterial vasculature and releasing it when the appropriate partial pressures are reached in the capillary bed. Hemoglobin exists in a low oxygen affinity deoxygenated form which switches to a high affinity oxygenated form as the partial pressure rises. The partial pressure at which this switch occurs determines its affinity, a characteristic crudely measured in the P_{50} estimation (the partial pressure at which the hemoglobin molecule is 50% saturated). Hemoglobin affinity is affected by temperature, pH, 2,3-DPG, carbon dioxide and carbon monoxide levels.

THE OPTIMAL HEMOGLOBIN LEVEL

The hemoglobin level is one of the oldest measurements in laboratory medicine and the most frequently performed blood test. However, debate continues as to the optimal level, and as with any long-lasting controversy, there is probably no ideal level for all conditions. The normal range for hemoglobin is affected by the following variables and the level must be interpreted in the light of these factors.

Pregnancy Despite a rise in red cell mass during pregnancy there is a greater increase in the plasma volume. Blood is hemodiluted to ensure microcirculatory flow to the placenta. Rises in various plasma proteins, neutrophils and platelets may also make it necessary for a lower hematocrit to ensure blood fluidity.

High altitude dwellers A compensatory polycythemia occurs due to the reduced inspired oxygen tension.

Acute hypoxia Rapid ascent to altitude causes a rise in hematocrit due to plasma volume contraction. This short-term adaptive response increases oxygen-carrying capacity.

Smoking Chronic carbon monoxide exposure has the same effect as hypoxia in reducing plasma volume or increasing the red cell mass.

Physical fitness The effects of physical fitness remain unclear. The lower hemoglobin levels reported in some athletes is probably due to the absence of the effects of smoking and stress, but the question of "sports" anemia is still unresolved.

Associated disease Any condition which affects oxygen transport or plasma volume may alter the hemoglobin level.

HEMATOLOGICAL FAILURE OF OXYGEN TRANSPORT

Oxygen delivery to the tissues may fail as a result of a variety of hematological defects (Fig. 1.3) which include:

Quantitative red cell deficiency Anemia from any cause results in reduced oxygen-carrying capacity of the blood.

Qualitative red cell defects Various red cell membrane defects will reduce the flexibility of red cells, thus impairing their ability to negotiate the microcirculation.

Quantitative excess of red cells Polycythemia, whatever the cause, will impair microcirculatory perfusion.

Quantitative excess of other cells An excess of leukocytes or platelets may impair microcirculatory flow.

Disorders of hemoglobin function Decreased or increased O_2 affinity of hemoglobin will impair oxygen uptake or tissue release respectively.

Platelet aggregation Essential thrombocythemia and other conditions in which hyperaggregability may occlude the microcirculation.

Leukocyte aggregation Leukemic blast cells or normal granulocytes may aggregate in the microcirculation resulting in occlusion.

Microvascular thrombosis This may be seen as a feature of disseminated intravascular coagulation or secondary to primary microvascular disease (e.g., thrombotic thrombocytopenic purpura, hemolytic uremic syndrome).

Plasma hyperviscosity Monoclonal or polyclonal hypergammaglobulinemia, cryoglobulins or cryofibrinogen cause hyperviscosity.

Hemostasis

THE TRIAD OF HEMOSTASIS

The body has a sophisticated system for plugging and repairing breaches of the circulatory system. Hemostasis is achieved by an integrated and regulated vascular, cellular

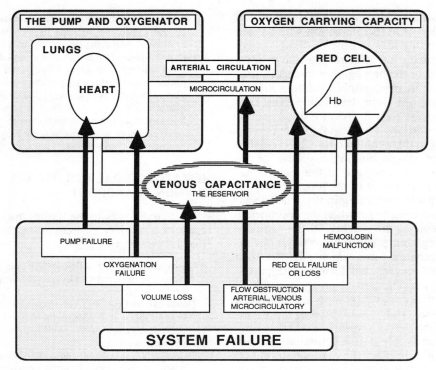

Figure 1.3. Oxygen transport

and humoral system providing hemostatic plugs when and where they are required. The triad of vascular constriction, platelet plugging and fibrin clot formation provides the framework around which hemostasis operates.

Until recently the vascular system and its lining endothelial cells has been generally regarded as an inert conduit for the transportation of blood and its role in hemostasis was seen as essentially a mechanical one of vasoconstriction. Nothing could be further from the truth as is now becoming apparent. The vascular system is a dynamic organ of the body with the endothelial cell fulfilling a pivotal role in blood/tissue interactions. Its role in the control of hemostasis is a fascinating story and has been alluded to by workers for many decades. Early investigations of hemostatic mechanisms emphasized the "action" components of the system in an attempt to answer this question: Why does blood clot? However, many of the recent advances have come about by readdressing the problem in the inverse: How does blood remain fluid? This approach places a different emphasis on the mysteries of hemostasis. Of necessity, he-

mostasis has been studied in vitro under nonphysiological conditions. It has been possible to dissect the individual components of the system and, dare one say, it is unlikely that many more individual factors or components will be discovered. It is simplistic and fraught with difficulties to attempt to analyze different components of the hemostatic system in isolation. The challenge at present is to understand the interrelationships between these components and to evolve a holistic understanding of this essential component of the host defense system (see Fig. 1.4).

ACTIVATION OF THE HEMOSTATIC MECHANISM

Until recently there has been a rather simplistic view of the initiation phase of hemostasis. Platelets adhere to damaged endothelium to form the platelet plug, at the same time the contact phase of the platelet-dependent intrinsic coagulation system is activated. Alongside this is an independent extrinsic fast coagulation system requiring the release of tissue thromboplastin for its activation. Although a triad of hemostasis provides a con-

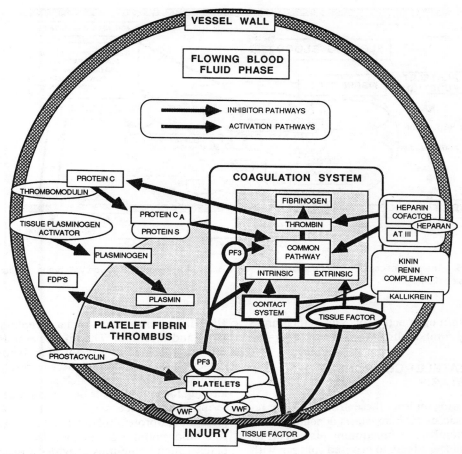

Figure 1.4. Overview of the hemostatic system—PF3 = Platelet factor 3; VWF = von Willebrand's factor; FDPs = fibrin degradation products; AT III = antithrombin III

ceptual framework, these hallowed subdivisions are artificial, and do not explain the observed facts. Positive and negative interactions between all the components allow the initiation and amplification of hemostasis to be an integrated and closely regulated host defense. The potential for damage to the host from overactivity or underactivity is considerable. Congenital deficiencies of individual components has lead to some of our understanding of the role of these components in the overall hemostatic plan.

THE VASCULAR COMPONENT OF HEMOSTASIS

Following injury, vascular constriction occurs controlling the initial rate and volume of bleeding. With large volume losses from the circulation this vascular reaction is systemically mediated via the sympathetic nervous system. With the more frequent smaller injuries the local breaching of vascular integrity and tissue disruption contribute to the initial stages of hemostasis in which the vasoconstrictor component is mediated by thromboxane A_2 released in association with platelet aggregation. The intact endothelial cell's interaction with normal blood components is aimed at ensuring the fluidity of blood in the normal state or limiting the hemostatic reaction to the site of injury. Vascular endothelial cells play an active part by synthesizing a range of substances which act at the membrane surface or are released, having negative interactions with platelets and the coagulation system (e.g., prostacyclin, antithrombin

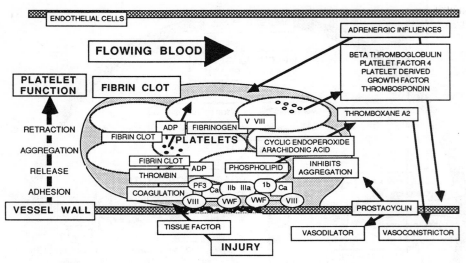

Figure 1.5. The platelet component of hemostasis—PF3 = platelet factor 3; VWF = von Willebrand's factor; ADP = adenosine diphosphate

III, plasminogen activator, von Willebrand's factor, thrombodulin).

THE PLATELET COMPONENT OF HEMOSTASIS

Following on from these initial vascular reactions successful hemostasis depends on adequate numbers of functioning platelets (Fig. 1.5). Platelets adhere to exposed collagen with the assistance of von Willebrand's factor and platelet membrane glycoproteins. The exact mechanisms are unclear, but platelet membrane receptors for intrinsic platelet proteins and vessel wall proteins are involved. Central to this sequence of adhesion is von Willebrand's factor which is the large multimeric component of factor VIII which is essential for normal platelet adhesion, but which also serves as the carrier for the coagulent portion which is essential in the intrinsic coagulation cascade.

Once platelet adhesion has occurred, platelets undergo a series of morphological and biochemical changes which climax in the release reaction and aggregation. This aggregation process recruits more platelets in order to form the definitive platelet plug. There are numerous agents which will initiate platelet aggregation, of which the important physiological ones include: adenosine diphosphate (ADP) binding to membrane glycoproteins

IIb/IIIa, adrenaline via alpha receptors, collagen and thrombin. The minute amounts of thrombin formed as a result of activation of the extrinsic coagulation cascade result in a positive feedback loop which promotes platelet plug formation while at the same time altering the platelet membrane to expose a phospholipoprotein (platelet factor 3) causing it to bind modified coagulation factor V. The platelet membrane thus provides a phospholipid surface on which the vitamin K dependent coagulation factors, with the aid of calcium, can bind to form a multimolecular complex.

Most of the platelet agonists, alluded to above, activate platelet arachidonic acid pathways to produce thromboxane A_2, a potent platelet aggregator and vasoconstrictor. Important enzymes in this pathway include phospholipase, cyclooxygenase (inhibited by aspirin) and thromboxane synthetase. Prostacyclin, with its reciprocal actions to thromboxane A_2, is the counterpart of arachidonic acid metabolism from the endothelial cell, except the final enzyme is prostacyclin synthetase.

During this release reaction numerous platelet activator and vasoactive substances are released, including adenosine diphosphate, serotonin, platelet factor IV (a heparin neutralizing protein), beta-thromboglobulin (function unknown) and platelet-derived growth factor (stimulates smooth muscle and fibroblast proliferation).

THE COAGULATION PHASE OF HEMOSTASIS

The soluble plasma coagulation proteins constitute the component of the hemostatic system which is activated following the primary phase of hemostasis when the platelet plug has been formed (Fig. 1.6). This complex group of plasma proteins is responsible for the formation of the fibrin clot. Fibrin is the end product of this cascade of proteolytic activity where precursor coagulation proteins are activated to potent proteolytic enzymes which, with the aid of cofactors, activate precursors further down the coagulation "amplifier."

Most reactions in the sequence result from the assembly of a reaction complex of an activated factor (serine protease), a precursor (substrate) and an accelerator (factor V or VIII) on a specific lipid surface (platelet or damaged endothelium) with the complex bound together by calcium.

Pathways for Factor X Activation

The activation of factor X is regarded as the focal point of the 2 pathways to activation of the coagulation cascade. Factor Xa can be produced via 2 different routes—the intrinsic and extrinsic pathways. The division is rather artificial and in recent years the separation between the pathways is becoming blurred. However, it remains helpful from the diag-

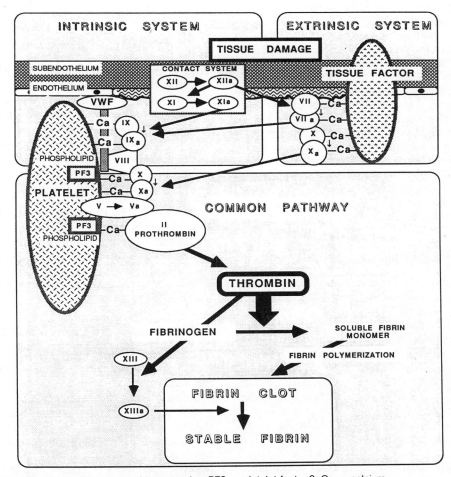

Figure 1.6. The coagulation phase of hemostasis—PF3 = platelet factor 3; Ca = calcium

nostic point of view and does assist in understanding the system's complexities.

The Extrinsic Coagulation System

Direct rapid activation of the common pathway occurs via the extrinsic pathway by which damaged tissue releases tissue thromboplastin which activates factor VII, a potent converter of factor X, and thus the common pathway. It is activation of this extrinsic system which leads to rapid clotting of blood in a syringe following a difficult venipuncture. Thromboplastin is a lipid-protein complex of which the protein component (apoprotein III) is probably an integral plasma membrane protein of most cells. When endothelial cells are damaged it is likely that membrane thromboplastin interaction with factor VII is the initial activation of coagulation.

Although the traditional view is that factor X is the main site of action for factor VII and tissue thromboplastin, it has now been established that the VII/tissue thromboplastin complex can activate factor IX of the intrinsic system, leading to a bypass of the slower contact phase. The small amounts of thrombin locally generated potentiate platelet aggregation. It would thus appear that the extrinsic pathway is intimately involved in the primary platelet/vessel phase of hemostasis, as the activity of factor VII on Factor IX is thromboplastin dependent and coagulation is localized to the injured tissue and does not occur in the fluid phase.

The Intrinsic Coagulation System

The intrinsic coagulation system is initiated by activation of the contact phase, involving factors XI, XII, high molecular weight kininogen and prekallikrein. The other plasma proteolytic systems, fibrinolytic, kinin and complement systems, may be activated in parallel with coagulation. Paradoxically, the contact system's role in coagulation activation may be the lesser of its functions. After this contact (and probably extrinsic pathway) activation of factor IX, IXa, VIIIc, X and calcium interact on the platelet phospholipid surface to produce activated factor X which enters the common pathway of coagulation. Factor VIII is discussed in detail in chapter 6.

The Common Pathway of Coagulation

Thrombin Generation

Activated factor X is at the center of the coagulation sequence as it is the entry point into the final common pathway to fibrin formation. The critical enzyme resulting from common pathway activation is thrombin. Close control of thrombin activation is crucial to the success of hemostasis. Intricate mechanisms are present to regulate the generation and localization of action of this potentially lethal enzyme. Thrombin results from the prothrombinase complex which includes prothrombin, factor Xa, lipid surface (platelet), factor Va and calcium. Thrombin is the final proteolytic enzyme of the coagulation sequence which converts fibrinogen to fibrin.

Fibrinogen Conversion

Fibrinogen is a relatively large, sparingly soluble and high blood level plasma protein, from which is formed the bulk matrix (fibrin) of the hemostatic plug. Fibrin may covalently bind to proteins produced by fibroblasts indicating that fibrin formation may be important for wound healing. Thrombin acts on fibrinogen by releasing two fibrinopeptides—A and B—constituting 3% of the molecule. The fibrin monomers resulting from this thrombin cleavage are able to polymerize and enter the solid phase as a fibrin gel. This relatively fragile fibrin gel is subsequently stabilized by the action of factor XIII. Factor XIII is initially activated by thrombin to XIIIa which is then able to form covalent cross linkages between the alpha and gamma chain of neighboring fibrin monomers. The resultant cross-linked fibrin clot is chemically and mechanically reinforced and thus more stable and insoluble.

THE REGULATORS OF HEMOSTASIS

The ultimate aim of the hemostatic system in arresting hemorrhage is achieved by ensuring hemostatic plugs are placed in the correct location, at the right time and in sufficient quantity (Fig. 1.7). To achieve this localization of hemostasis requires an intricate regulatory system. Parallel to and within the hemostatic system are complex positive and negative feedbacks to ensure fine tuning and protection against inappropriate and exces-

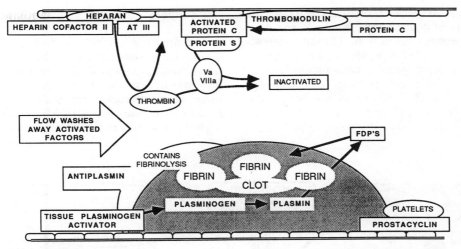

Figure 1.7. Regulators of hemostasis—ATIII = antithrombin III; FDPs = fibrin degeneration products

sive activation. It is thus not surprising that perturbations in this complex defense system can produce a wide range of clinical disorders from excessive thrombosis, microvascular obstruction and atheroma to hemostatic failure.

Blood Flow

The aphorism "if you want blood to remain fluid keep it flowing" highlights the central role of blood flow in limiting excessive activation of hemostasis. With adequate flow the local concentration of activated coagulation factors is continuously decreased with the influx of fresh blood. The activated factors which are washed away are selectively metabolized by the liver.

Regulation of Platelet Function

As already mentioned, arachidonic acid metabolism in the endothelial cell produces prostacyclin which has diametrically opposite actions on vessel wall tone and platelet aggregation to thromboxane A_2, the end product of arachidonic acid metabolism in the platelet. It is likely that these differences are indicative of a delicate balance existing between blood fluidity and thrombosis.

Biochemical Inhibitors

The generation of thrombin itself has feedback actions on factors V and VIII to assist in

the aborting of excessive coagulation. However, the main control of hemostasis appears to be via specific inhibitors of activated coagulation factors. These inhibitors limit the diffusion of activated coagulation factors from the site of clot formation.

Protease Inhibitors

There is a family of plasma proteins whose function is to control the action of proteolytic enzymes which contain serine at their active site. The complex formed by a one to one interaction of enzyme and inhibitor is cleared from the circulation. The affinity of the inhibitors varies depending on which system they are predominantly destined to mediate. The four host defense proteolytic systems of the plasma (coagulation, fibrinolysis, complement and kinin) all have their own biochemical inhibitors, but there is a considerable degree of cross reactivity (Antithrombin III can inhibit thrombin, factors Xa, IXa, XIa and XIIa, as well as plasmin, trypsin and chymotrypsin.) This action is markedly potentiated by heparin, or by heparin from endothelial cells. Other plasma proteins with inhibitory action include alpha$_2$ macroglobulin, alpha$_1$ antitrypsin (inactivates XIa), C1-esterase inhibitor (inhibits XIa, XIIa and kallikrein).

Protein C

Protein C is a vitamin K dependent zymogen which is activated to a protease by thrombin. Activated protein C inactivates the cofactors of coagulation, factors V and VIII and stimulates fibrinolysis. Thrombin activation of protein C is mediated in conjunction with a specific protein thrombomodulin at the endothelial cell surface. The activated protein C in conjunction with another vitamin K dependent protein, protein S, cleaves factors V and VIII to inactive fragments.

Fibrinolysis

The final regulation system of hemostasis is directed towards lysing excess fibrin and also ultimately removing the clot in order that flow may be restored. With contact activation there is a parallel activation of the fibrinolytic system with conversion of plasminogen to plasmin. Plasmin is a relatively non-specific

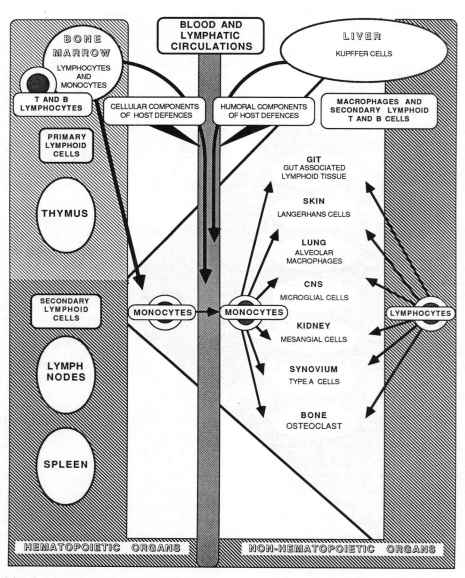

Figure 1.8. Structure of the host defense system

endopeptidase which can lyse fibrin, but also cleaves fibrinogen, factors V and VIII and complement components. Plasminogen has a high affinity binding for fibrin as a clot is formed. This mechanism ensures that the protective fibrinolytic system is incorporated in the final hemostatic plug. Plasminogen activators (serine proteases) are released from endothelial cells and other tissues activating this plasminogen in the clot. To prevent systemic fibrinolytic activation, circulating alpha$_2$, antiplasmin inactivates any plasmin released into the fluid phase. The fragments of fibrin released are termed fibrin degradation products (FDPs) and the larger initial fragments resulting may have some inhibitor action on further fibrin polymerization.

FAILURE OF THE HEMOSTATIC SYSTEM

Underactivity or overactivity of the hemostatic system may be responsible for disease and are addressed in chapters 5 and 6. In mechanistic terms the disorders can be summarized as follows:

Congenital deficiencies of coagulation factors, platelet function or regulation proteins may occur due to genetic defects, resulting in under or overactivity of the hemostatic system.
Acquired deficiencies or overactivity may occur in platelet or coagulation function.
Inappropriate activation may occur as seen in disseminated intravascular coagulation.
Excessive activation may be responsible for venous thrombosis and pulmonary embolism and other forms of venoocclusive disease.

Host Defense System

The body has a highly coordinated host defense system for combating invasion by microorganisms, trauma and foreign substances (Figs. 1.8 and 1.9). This system maintains an equilibrium with the environment, preventing spontaneous infection, but under stress has a remarkable reserve for both an imme-

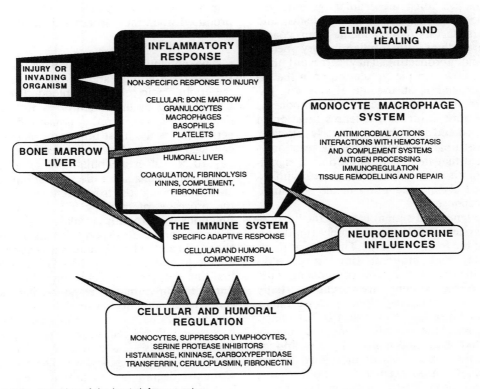

Figure 1.9. Function of the host defense system

diate response and a reactive potential, which can be brought into action in times of need. The mechanistic analysis of the body's defense mechanisms has resulted in study of individual components in isolation and as a result it is possible to lose sight of the holistic functioning of the system, with its complex interactions between cellular and humoral components. There are finely tuned positive and negative feedback controls and excessive or inappropriate activation may result in host tissue damage or consumption of the individual components.

Local protective barriers, such as skin and mucous membranes, are important physical barriers which are kept intact with cooperation from the cellular and humoral components of the host defense system. There is also a close relationship between the host defense system and the hemostatic system and infection is less likely if hemorrhage is prevented, thus reducing the likelihood of there being nidus for infection.

The bone marrow and liver produce most of the components of the nonspecific defense system, providing the cellular (granulocyte, monocytes-macrophages, and platelets) and humoral factors (complement, kinin, coagulation proteins, other inflammatory mediators and fibronectin). They carry out their functions within the circulation or in the tissues, depending on the site of invasion. Except for the macrophages, most components of the nonspecific host defenses function in the blood and at the blood-capillary interface; it is not unless an inflammatory reaction is initiated that there is mobilization of significant numbers of cells into the tissues with associated plasma exudation in the inflammatory response.

The lymphoid system is a specific host defense system which can accurately aim the attack at the foreign invader. The cellular (lymphocyte) and humoral (immunoglobulin) components of this specific component of the host-defense system are found partially within the circulating blood, but the major component of the cellular arm is distributed throughout the specific lymphoid organs (lymph nodes, spleen and thymus) and as lymphoid components of individual organs (especially gut-associated lymphoid tissue, skin and liver). The lymphoid system is programmed to react in a predetermined fashion which depends on the nature of the antigen and the site of stimulation. A specific cellular and humoral antibody response is produced after the antigen has been processed. At this point the hematopoietic and hepatic components have to be called on again to provide the final attack mediators to effect the specific inflammatory destruction of the invading organism.

THE COMPONENTS OF THE HOST DEFENSE SYSTEM

The Effector and Phagocytic Cells

The granulocytes and macrophages are the dedicated professional effector cells of the host defense system. These cells have been likened to "Attila the Hun" in that they deploy a wide range of biological weapons which tend to be nonselective in their attack on invading microorganisms and may produce surrounding host tissue damage as a result of the inflammatory response. The most powerful of these weapons in the phagocytic armamentarium is a group of oxidizing agents produced when the cells are activated.

Granulocytes

The polymorphonuclear leukocytes (neutrophils), eosinophils and basophils make up the granulocytic cells of the blood. The neutrophil makes up the "infantry" of the body's defense forces and is rather nonspecific in its action, but is the most important phagocytic cell against acute bacterial infections. Each day 10×10^{10} neutrophils (100 g) are produced and have a short life span of only several days, being lost from the circulation in the processes of carrying out their normal functions. Neutrophils circulate in the blood (5% of the granulocyte pool) and are normally shed from all the body's mucosal surfaces and adhere to endothelial surfaces as the cells of first-line defense. The cells enter the tissues during the inflammatory response. Signals are generated from infected or damaged tissues which causes neutrophils to migrate and adhere to endothelial cells near the site of injury. The neutrophils are able to ingest organisms by the process of phagocytosis. The cells subsequently degranulate to initiate the microbial killing action of these professional defense cells.

The functions of eosinophil and basophil granulocytes are less well defined than those of the neutrophil and in some ways their roles in host defense remain rather enigmatic. The eosinophils are specifically active against the larvae of parasites and play a role in the body's reaction against parasitic infections. They also work in concert with the basophil and lymphocyte in specific immune reactions of the body, but their functions have not been fully elucidated. The basophil and its tissue equivalent, the mast cell, contain potent vasoactive substances (histamine, serotonin and slow-reacting substance) and anticoagulant (heparin). The basophil clearly has a crucial role as an effector cell of the immune system, but at present more is known about malfunction of the systems than normal function, as seen in immediate anaphylactic reactions.

The Monocyte/Macrophage System

The monocyte/macrophage system is a longer lived and more developed defense system. The monocytes originate from the bone marrow, but undergo further development in individual tissues of the body to become organ-specific macrophages. The monocyte/macrophage cells are central in the host defenses and arguably provide the pivot around which the whole system operates, in particular providing the link between the nonspecific and specific host defenses. Each tissue has its specialized macrophage whose structural and functional development is uniquely suited to the organ in question and within organs there appears to be further heterogeneity of macrophage function. The ubiquitous functions of this system are summarized in Figure 1.9.

THE PLASMA FACTORS

The plasma contains a plethora of proteins involved in the mediation of host defenses. Of the soluble factors involved in the inflammatory and immune responses their origins are from local cellular release at the site of reaction or via localization and activation of circulating inactive plasma proteins. The potent biochemical components of the host defense arsenal are thus kept in check as inactive plasma proteins requiring local detonators, manufactured locally by cells or contained as functionally active components in isolated sealed packages (granules and lysosomes).

THE IMMUNE SYSTEM

In contrast to the nonselective defense components outlined above the immune system has the potential to be highly specific and has been likened to the intelligence corps and strategic operations of the military. Specific information is meticulously collected from the sites of invasion, sifted for clues to identity (antigen processing), strategic plans appropriate to the insult are activated and carried out by the defense forces outlined above. The military analogy can be carried further when one considers the means by which the immune system is made specific. The development of computers during the second world war for code breaking was a major advance for intelligence collection. The immune system, like a computer, has basic hardware and an operating system which determines the mode of functioning of the various cellular components. This programming of the system allows heterogeneity in the immune response (humoral versus cell mediated) to the wide variety of insults to which the body may be exposed. The immunological computer has an enormous potential memory for antigens, but the system requires initial primary education in order to fill this antigenic memory bank. This educational process (immunization) allows the immune system to respond rapidly to identical or similar future insults and provide a well orchestrated and specific plan of attack before the invading organism or antigen is able to progress into the tissues. The unique capabiltiy of lymphocytes to "dedifferentiate" (i.e., blast transform) allows amplification to occur. The responding lymphoid cells reproduce themselves to increase the numbers of specific effector cells and lay down memory cells.

Antigen processing and immune induction are complex when one considers the awesome responsibility of the immune system to distinguish self from not-self, but at the same time to interact with the host environment in a symbiotic manner. Clearly, tolerance of common environmental antigens (e.g., food and airborn antigens), skin and gut bacteria and self antigens is essential. The balance between normal immune function, allergy, autoimmunity and invasion of pathogens or tumors is a complex and delicate one. The major histocompatibility antigens (MHC) have a central function in determining and controlling the response to individual antigens, and thus their association with a wide spectrum of diseases. Inciting antigens need to be presented by monocytes to T-cells in association with MHC antigens. Cytotoxic killer T-lymphocytes react to viral antigens presented to them in association with the class I MHC antigens (HLA-A, B and C), whereas the T-lymphocytes (e.g., helper cells) which cooperate with other host-defense cells, as seen in the delayed hypersensitivity response, require class II MHC antigens (HLA D and DR).

THE CELLULAR COMPONENTS OF THE IMMUNE SYSTEM

Macrophages

The role of these cells has been summarized above. Their central function in the immune system involves initiation of the immune response, antigen processing, immune modulation and effector actions in the inflammatory response.

Lymphocytes

Our expansion in knowledge of the functioning of lymphocytes is one of the success stories of modern biology for which a number of Nobel prizes have been awarded. During the first hundred years of modern scientific medicine the lymphocyte was thought to be an unimportant end cell. This initial impression has been shattered with the unfolding of a remarkable story of complexity, adaptability, homeostasis and vital functionings within the immune system. The system is broadly divided into cell-mediate (T-lymphocytes) and humoral antibody (B-lymphocytes) arms for the effecting of specific immune action. However, within and alongside the immune system there are intricate modulator servocontrol mechanisms for upregulating and downregulating the system. All cellular components of the immune system have their origin in the bone marrow. Further development for their programming occurs in the primary lymphoid tissues—in the case of T-

lymphocytes, the thymus and the B-lymphocytes, the bone marrow. The subsequent stimulation, education and effector functions of the immune system occur in the secondary lymphoid tissue. These tissues are the specialized hematopoietic organs, the lymph nodes, spleen and bone marrow or the specialized host defense components of individual organs. These components are found in most tissues, but in high concentration in the gastrointestinal tract (gut-associated lymphiod tissues), liver, skin (especially T-lymphocytes) and lung. Figure 1.10 outlines in schematic form the immune system and its various cellular and humoral components.

T-Lymphocytes

These thymus-derived lymphocytes can be characterized by 4 distinct attributes—their specificity, function, cell surface antigenic profile and state of activation. A wide range of techniques is available for in vitro study of these cells. The T-lymphocytes are divided into the cytotoxic T-cells, T-helper cells and T-suppressor cells. The cytotoxic T-cells mediate their attack sequence via the process known as delayed hypersensitivity. In this reaction antigen-specific T-lymphocytes localize at the site of immune action and secrete lymphokines which localize the inflammatory response to the invaded site. This reaction is particularly important in defense against parasitic and intracellular microorganisms and is central to graft rejection reactions.

B-Lymphocytes

These bone marrow derived lymphocytes differentiate into plasma cells which are responsible for antibody production. Under most circumstances B-lymphocytes require cooperation from T-lymphocytes in order to develop and ultimately produce antibody. The most primitive antibody response and also the antibody produced during the primary immune response is IgM, which is a low affinity antibody. As the humoral immune response evolves and matures higher affinity antibody is produced. The circulating antibody in the plasma is IgG and that produced in secretions is IgA. In the case of IgA a secretory piece is inserted into the dimeric mole-

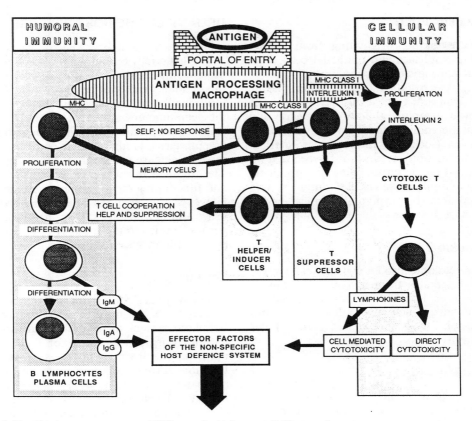

Figure 1.10. The immune response—MHC = major histocompatibility complex

cule at the time of mucosal secretion, and this prevents enzyme digestion of the molecule before it is able to interact with antigen.

After antibody has "marked" the foreign substance or microorganism for destruction the phagocytic cells or "killer" mononuclear cells move in for action. The complement system may be an intermediary in this process. The effector cells have receptors on their surfaces for immunoglobulin and complement components.

Natural Killer Lymphocytes (NK Cells)

These are lymphoid cells which have spontaneous cytotoxic activity, but do not require prior sensitization. This activity can be against a wide range of targets, including virally infected cells, tumor cells and normal hematopoietic cells and is probably also important in host defenses against protozoal and fungal infections. Interferon and interleukin-2 will potentiate the acticity of NK cells.

CHEMICAL MEDIATORS OF THE IMMUNE SYSTEM

The complexity of chemical mediators in the immune system is far beyond the scope of this book. The unravelling of connections between neuroendocrinology and immunology is opening up new vistas in our appreciation of the body's response to various insults whether they be infectious, toxic or psychological. However, within the immune system there are a family of substances which go under the broad title of cytokines. These soluble chemicals act as second signals between cells for activating, regulating and expressing the system. The interleukins and interferons are central in both the afferent and efferent limbs of the immune reaction.

Interleukin-1 (ILI)

This cytokine, originating from monocytes/macrophages and epithelial cells is responsible for fever induction, initiation of the acute phase response, alteration in plasma metal (iron and zinc) levels, release of bone marrow neutrophils, alterations in energy and protein metabolism and T and B lymphocyte activation (including induction of interleukin-2 production). It can thus be seen that interleukin-1 has activities in the nonspecific response to injury as well as the immune system and appears to be the pivotal chemical mediator in host defenses.

Interleukin-2 (IL2)

This cytokine, also known as T-cell growth factor, originates from activated mature T-lymphocytes. Interleukin-2 induces proliferation of antigen-activated killer, helper and suppressor T-lymphocytes and natural killer cell activity.

Interleukin-3 (IL3)

Studies in mice have shown this cytokine to be the second messenger to "wind up" the whole defense arm of the hematopoietic system. IL3 has a colony stimulating and hematopoietic regulatory action to initiate recruitment of stem cells to proliferate and differentiate. A similar cytokine in humans remains to be identified.

Interferons

The interferons are peptides which have nonspecific antiviral, antiproliferative and immunoregulatory activities. There are three classes—α-interferon from lymphocytes, β-interferon from fibroblasts, macrophages and epithelial cells, and γ-interferon from T-lymphocytes.

B-Lymphocyte Growth and Differentiation Factors

Most humoral antibody immune responses require cooperation from T-lymphocytes for proliferation and differentiation into plasma cells. These factors are products of stimulated T-lymphocytes.

ORGANS OF THE HOST DEFENSE SYSTEM

Having briefly outlined the cellular and humoral components of the host defense system this chapter would not be complete without a thumbnail sketch of the organ distribution of the hematopoietic system. The term reticuloendothelial system (RES) is used as an all-embracing term for the cellular components of the host defense system throughout the body. The title is a misnomer now that the origin and functioning of the system is understood. However, the term has become hallowed by usage and is generally still applied when one wishes to refer to the monocyte/macrophage and lymphoid systems together.

Thymus

The thymus gland originates from both the epithelium of the third branchial pouch and lymphoid system to form the vital primary lymphoid organ responsible for T-cell development. The thymus subserves most of its function during intrauterine life and in the postnatal period. Lymphoid stem cells committed to T-cell differentiation migrate to the gland via the circulation where they proliferate and mature under the influence of thymosin. The thymus involutes after puberty. The thymus produces a variety of hormones, e.g., thymosin. The precise role of these hormones in T-cell differentiation is currently under investigation.

Lymph Nodes

The lymph nodes provide the bulk of secondary lymphoid tissue where filtration, phagocytosis and immune functions take place. Foreign material arrives via the afferent lymphatics and is filtered in the cortex of the node, which is composed of macrophages and B-lymphocytes (the follicles). Antigenic stimulation occurs with the formation within the follicles to form germinal centers. If the stimulus provokes a T-lymphocyte response, proliferation of cells in the paracortical areas is seen. Lymphocyte traffic may enter the node via the lymphatics of the blood vessels, leaving via the efferent lymphatic to finally reenter the circulation through the thoracic duct. Information from this initial immune response can thus be transmitted throughout the immune system.

Spleen

The spleen has been colloquially known as the "lymph node of the blood" or the blood filter. These titles are not inappropriate, but one of the most remarkable facts about the spleen is that despite its wide range of extraordinary functions (Table 1.1) most of them can be bypassed with minimal ill-effects. The spleen receives 500 to 700 ml blood per minute. The 100-year debate on the open and closed theories of circulation has been resolved with both mechanisms applying. The smaller volume of blood slowly migrates through the splenic cords (open circulation). With disorders in which there is increased red cell traffic through the splenic cords (e.g., spherocytic red cells or venous obstruction) intense red pulp congestion occurs. Closed direct fast circulation occurs through the Malpighian bodies. This is increased during immunostimulation. Plasma skimming is the process by which plasma and the leukocytes preferentially pass to the white pulp while blood of high hematocrit remains in the axial stream of the splenic artery and goes to the red pulp. The red pulp is the vascular bed which filters the cellular components of the blood.

In the faster closed circulation which takes 90% of the blood there is a conventional vascular arrangement in which there is mural (including endothelial) continuity from artery to vein (venous sinuses). In the slow open circulation which takes 10% of the blood supply there is a vascular arrangement in which continuity is broken in the vascular wall between the artery and vein. This slow open circulation allows the spleen to sort, store, differentiate or remove cells. Blood cells may need to go through the spleen several times before they achieve the appropriate localization.

Pooling is the term which has come to be applied to the phenomenon where any cellular component of the blood is concentrated in the spleen to a level above that of its level in the circulating blood. The normal human spleen is not a significant red cell reservoir (20 to 60 ml) as it is in some other species, however, there is a selective removal and matur-

Table 1.1
Functions of the Spleen

Hematological Functions
  Commando course for reticulocytes
    Red blood cell membrane smoothing
    Red blood cell surface pits and craters
    Howell-Jolly bodies
    Heinz bodies
    Pappenheimer bodies   } pitting
    Acanthocytes
  Senescent damaged red blood cell removal

  Disease states
    Spherocytes (HS)
    Sickle cells, HbC cells
    Antibody-coated blood cells of any type

Immune Function
  Immune surveillance
    Delivery of antigenic information
    Focus for lymphocyte traffic
  Immune clearance
    Opsonization: Initiation of specific antibody
               production
               Recruitment of nonspecific
                opsonins
    Phagocytosis: Removal of
               intravascular pathogens
          Uptake of immune complexes
          Disposal of senescent cells
  Immune regulation
    Development of B- and T-cell memory
    Maturation of T-suppressor cells
    Control of autoimmunity
    Regulation of immune network

ing of reticulocytes which occurs in the splenic sinuses. The reticulocyte when it leaves the bone marrow still has remnants of aerobic metabolism and must undergo a final maturing process in the spleen. Mitochondria cluster at the edge of the erythrocyte where they are surrounded by a thin layer of cytoplasm. They are extruded in the splenic sinusoids and picked up by the cordal macrophages. Nuclear remnants (Howell-Jolly bodies) and cytoplasmic iron granules (Pappenheimer bodies) are removed by the process of pitting by macrophages at the sinus wall. The reticulocyte also has excess membrane removed resulting in reduction in surface to volume ratio. In relation to platelets the spleen is a reservoir for over 25% of the platelet mass. The platelets can be mobilized in times of stress (e.g., hemorrhage) and an elevated count is seen after splenectomy. The spleen also accumulates certain lymphocytes in the white pulp.

Hematopoiesis occurs in the spleen from the 12th week of gestation until birth (lymphopoiesis continues after birth). Pluripotent stem cells are in the spleen and splenic irradiation causes leukopenia. The potential for hematopoiesis in the spleen continues throughout life and may occur under stress (e.g., thalassemia, pernicious anemia and hemolytic anemia). Reactive hematopoiesis in the spleen should be distinguished from myeloid metaplasia which is seen in relation to certain hematological malignancies (myeloproliferative disease, some leukemias) or occasionally in secondary carcinoma. The phagocytic cells of the spleen are also adept at removing iron from ingested red cells and transferring it into the plasma for return to the bone marrow. The question of humoral factors from the spleen affecting bone marrow function is still debated and the role of the spleen in plasma volume control is also unclear.

FAILURE OF HOST DEFENSE SYSTEM

Quantitative or qualitative deficiencies in the host defense system are probably responsible for a wider range of disorders than any other pathophysiological mechanism.

Infection Recurrent, overwhelming or opportunistic.

Allergies Failure of immunoregulation appears to have a role in the body reacting inappropriately with antigens it would either tolerate or contain locally at the portal of entry.

Autoimmunity Transient or chronic immunoregulatory failure results in a wide range of clinical disorders.

Malignancy Failure of immune surveillance may be one of the factors involved in malignancy.

Further Reading

Alberts, B, Bray, D, Lewis, JM, Roff, M, Roberts, K, and Watson, J: *Molecular biology of the cell.* New York: Garland Publishing, Inc., 1983.

Babiar, BM, Stossel, TP *Hematology: a pathophysiological approach.* New York: Churchill Livingstone, 1984.

Cawley, JC, ed. *Integrated clinical science: hematology.* London: William Heinemann, Medical Books Limited, 1983.

Dickerson, RE, Irving, G. *Hemoglobin: structure, function, evolution and pathology.* California: The Benjamin Crimmings Publishing Company, Inc., 1983.

Jaffe, ES, ed. *Biology of endothelial cells.* Boston: Martinus Nijhoff Publishers, 1984.

King, DW, Fenoglio, CM, Lefkowitch, JH *General pathology: principles and dynamics.* Philadelphia, Lea & Febiger, 1983.

Trubowitz, S, and Davis, S. *The human bone marrow: anatomy, physiology, and pathophysiology.* Vol. 1 and 2. Florida, C. R. Press, Inc., 1982.

Weiss, L. *The blood cells and haemopoietic tissues.* 2nd ed. New York: Elsevier, 1984.

Wintrobe, MM. ed. *Blood, pure and eloquent: a story of discovery, of people and ideas.* New York: McGraw-Hill Book Company, 1980.

Woolf, N ed. Biology and pathology of the vessel wall: a modern appraisal. Eastbourn, UK, Praeger, 1983.

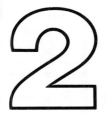

The Diagnostic Process

He is a great physician who, above all other men understands diagnosis.

Jacob Bigelow (1786–1879)

A sick man may wear a wrong diagnosis around his neck like a millstone, and the doctor's task may be first to undiagnose him so recovery can begin

John L. McClenahan (1915–)

Your reasoning is excellent, It's only your basic assumptions that are wrong.

Ashleigh Brilliant (1933–)

Just when I nearly had the answer, I forgot the question.

Ashleigh Brilliant (1933–)

The hematologist involved in both clinical (Table 2.1) and laboratory (Table 2.2) medicine is constantly reminded of the inseparable relationship between the clinical findings on a patient and the subsequent ordering and interpretation of laboratory investigations. During the last decade, there have been spectacular developments in medical science which have resulted in clinicians relying less on their own abilities and more on technology. The traditional dictum in the diagnostic process of history, physical examination and special investigations has been under continuing threat in recent years. In the past, the clinician personally collected both the clinical and laboratory information on a patient in order to establish a diagnosis. However, in recent years, there has been an increasing gap between clinical and laboratory medicine, leading not only to poor communication, but also inappropriate utilization of laboratory services and incorrect interpretation of laboratory data.

Clinical pathologists for many years have attempted to bridge the gap between clinical and laboratory medicine with such approaches as interpretive reporting and utilization review. The aim has been to give the requesting clinician some guidelines to further investigations. However, this approach has tended to create more problems than it

has solved. With only limited clinical information in hand, pathologists have frequently been guilty of biasing diagnostic possibilities and leading the clinician "down the garden path."

Despite the technological information explosion in medicine, methods must be found to achieve an effective diagnostic process. Unfortunately, the cost spiral in medicine has tended to direct how and when diagnostic services should be used. As the ultimate aim should be to produce cost-effective medicine for the greatest number of patients, it is inappropriate that cost considerations should be the prime mover. It has generally been the author's experience that the effective use of laboratory investigations in the diagnosis and management of patients has ultimately led to significant cost savings. As it is no longer possible for clinicians to spend a significant part of their training in laboratory medicine, it is essential that appropriate, problem-oriented approaches to clinical investigation be developed in utilization of these services.

Since the days of William Osler, the diagnostic paradigm has centered on this sequence: history, physical examination and special tests. Medical students for decades have been instructed in the objective documentation of clinical history and subsequent clinical findings. From this information, a

Table 2.1
Clinical Presentations of Hematological Diseases

System and Clinical Syndrome	Pathophysiological Mechanisms *or* Hematological Disease Process
Hematological	
Lymphadenopathy and splenomegaly	Reactive or malignant
Plethora	Polycythemia
Pallor	Anemia
Pale sallow complexion	Anemia secondary to: Hemolysis
	Pernicious anemia
	Myxedema
	Severe anemia secondary to malignancy
Cardiovascular	
Congestive cardiac failure	Anemia, especially megaloblastic
	Volume overload with blood component therapy
Apparent CCF[a]	SVC obstruction from mediastinal lymphoma
	Hyperviscosity syndrome with hypervolemia
Pulmonary embolism	
Palpitations	Anemia
Peripheral edema	Venous or lymphatic obstruction
Reduced exercise tolerance	Anemia
Peripheral ischemia	Vasculitis
	Essential thrombocythemia
Raynaud's phenomenon	Cold agglutinins
	Cryoglobulins
	Cryofibrinogen
	Hyperviscosity syndromes
Shock syndrome	Septicemia: Postsplenectomy sepsis
	Neutropenia
	Hypogammaglobulinemia
	Anaphylaxis: C1 esterase deficiency
	IgA deficiency
	Cold urticaria
	Mastocytosis
	Acute hemorrhage from bleeding disorders
	Spontaneous splenic rupture
Hypertension	Hyperviscosity syndromes
	Hematological stress syndrome
Respiratory	
Airway obstruction	Angioneurotic edema due to C1 esterase deficiency
	Tonsillar enlargement: Infectious mononucleosis
	Lymphoma
Cyanosis	Methemoglobinemia
	Sulfhemoglobinemia
	Reduced O_2Sat from low affinity hemoglobins
Dyspnea	Anemia
	Pulmonary embolism
	Pneumonia with impaired host defenses
	Acute interstitial lung disease: Vasculitis
	Infective
	Leukostasis
Pneumonia classical or atypical	Impaired host defenses
Pneumonia	
Adult respiratory distress syndrome	Leukostasis
	DIC
	Blood transfusion: Incompatible transfusion

Table 2.1—*continued*

System and Clinical Syndrome	Pathophysiological Mechanisms *or* Hematological Disease Process
	Leukoagglutinins
	Incompatible transfusion
	Microaggregates
	Plasma reactions
Pleurisy	Splenic infarct
	Pulmonary infarct: Pulmonary embolism
	Vasculitis
Hemoptysis	Bleeding disorders
	Pulmonary infarct
Chest X-ray abnormality	Pulmonary or mediastinal lesion
	Rib and thoracic spine fractures
	Lytic bone lesions
Genitourinary	
Acute renal failure	Hypercalcemia from hematological malignancy
	Hyperuricemia
	DIC
	Renal vein thrombosis
Chronic renal failure	Autoimmune complication hematological malignancy
	Obstructive
Nephrotic syndrome	Amyloid
	Lymphoma
	Chronic malaria
Polyuria	Hypercalcemia from hematological malignancy
Dark urine	Hemolysis
	Hematuria associated with bleeding disorders
	Porphyria
Renal colic	Clot colic associated with bleeding disorders
	Ureteric obstruction from lymphadenopathy
	Hyperuricemia, hypercalcemia
Vaginal bleeding	Menorrhagia associated with bleeding disorders
Priapism	Thrombosis from microvascular obstruction
	Microvascular obstruction: Leukostasis
	Sickle cell disease
Abnormal urinalysis	Hemoglobinuria
	Bence-Jones proteinuria due to multiple myeloma
Gastrointestinal	
Glossitis	Vitamin deficiencies: Vitamin B12/folate
	Iron deficiency
Dysphagia	Pharyngeal webs: Iron deficiency
	Mediastinal mass
Jaundice	Hemolysis
	Liver disease secondary to hematological malignancy
	Obstruction from lymph nodes
Biliary colic	Pigment stones
Portal hypertension	Myeloproliferative disease
	Veno-occlusive disease
	Portal vein thrombosis
Chronic liver disease ± cirrhosis	Hemochromatosis
	Malignant infiltration
Abdominal masses, masses detected on organ imaging or laparotomy findings	Lymph nodes, spleen, or liver
	Malignant infiltration of kidneys
Intestinal obstruction	Hemostatic failure

Table 2.1—*continued*

System and Clinical Syndrome	Pathophysiological Mechanisms *or* Hematological Disease Process
Abdominal pain ± peritonitis	Lymphoma Vincristine therapy C1 esterase deficiency Hemolytic anemias Acute intermittent porphyria Bleeding disorders: Intramural hemorrhage Retroperitoneal hemorrhage Rectus hemorrhage Intrahepatic or splenic hemorrhage Infarcts: Thrombotic disease Vasculitis DIC Hyperviscosity syndromes Myeloproliferative disease Ruptured spleen: Glandular fever (spontaneous) Myeloproliferative disease Angioneurotic edema from C1 esterase deficiency
Melena and/or hematemesis	GIT lesion associated with hemostatic defect Vascular defects such as telangiectasia
Malabsorption	Vitamin B12, folate and iron deficiency
Anorectal problems	Infection in compromised host
Musculoskeletal	
Joint pains	Bleeding with hemostatic defects, e.g., hemophilia Immune complex disease Leukemic infiltrates
Gout	Hyperuricemia: Myeloproliferative and malignancy
Bone pain	Infarcts: Sickle cell disease DIC Leukemia Expanding bone lesions in leukemia or lymphoma
Myalgia	Bleeding in congenital and acquired disorders
Psoas pain spasm	Retroperitoneal hemorrhage in congenital and acquired bleeding disorders
Fractures	Bone pathology from hematological malignancy especially multiple myeloma
Bone deformities	Erythroid hyperplasia in the congenital anemias Congenital syndromes associated with thrombocytopenia or immunodeficiency
Neurological	
Coma, psychosis or localizing signs, or headaches	Hyperviscosity Leukostasis Bleeding in congenital and acquired bleeding disorders Microvascular obstruction in DIC, TTP, or arteritis Meningitis: opportunistic infections Malaria Acute intermittent porphyria Large vessel occlusions Paraneoplastic syndromes (e.g., inappropriate ADH)
Dementia	Vascular obstruction: Thrombocythemia Hyperviscosity Vasculitis SLE

Table 2.1—*continued*

System and Clinical Syndrome	Pathophysiological Mechanisms *or* Hematological Disease Process
Paralysis	Megaloblastosis due to B12 deficiency
	Spinal cord compression from plasmacytoma or lymphoma
	Peripheral neuropathy: Amyloid
	Monoclonal gammopathy
	Porphyria
	Nerve compression from hematoma
	Perineural leukemic/lymphomatous infiltration
Paresthesias	Peripheral neuropathy B12 deficiency
Ataxis	Ataxis telangiectasia
	Vitamin B12 deficiency
Dermatological	
Acute mucocutaneous bleeding	Bleeding defects due to thrombocytopenia or quantitative platelet defects
Palpable purpura	Vasculitis
Urticaria	Blood transfusion in IgA deficiency patients
Bullous erruptions	Porphyrias
Infection	Varicella
	Herpes simplex
	Bacterial infections
	Fungal infections
Skin necrosis	Microthrombosis due to vasculitis or anticoagulants
Livedo reticularis	Venular occlusion in hyperviscosity and cryoglobulinemia
Alopecia	Chemotherapy
	Autoimmune disease
Photosensitivity	Autoimmune disease
Vitiligo	Autoimmune disease
Erythroderma	Skin infiltration in T-cell malignancies
Palpable lesions	Infiltration: Leukemia and lymphoma
	Mast cell disease
Pigmentation	Hemochromatosis
	Busulphan, Bleomycin, Adriamycin
	Mastocytosis
Nail changes	Koilonychia in iron deficiency
	Paronychia in immunodeficiency
Warts	Immunological defect
Abnormal scar formation	Poor wound healing: Fibrinogen abnormalities
	Factor XIII deficiency
	Collagen disorders
Pruritus	Hodgkin's disease
	Mastocytosis
	Polycythemia rubra vera
	Iron deficiency
Leg ulcers	Microvascular occlusion: Hereditary spherocytosis
	Vasculitis
	Cryoglobulins
	Postphlebitic syndrome
ENT and Dental	
Acute mouth and throat ulceration	Agranulocytosis
Gum hypertrophy	Infiltration in acute monocytic leukemia
Tooth extraction bleeding	Bleeding disorders
Epistaxis	Bleeding disorders
Ocular	
Blindness or decreased acuity	Bleeding disorders

Table 2.1—*continued*

System and Clinical Syndrome	Pathophysiological Mechanisms *or* Hematological Disease Process
	Hyperviscosity
	Vasculitis
	Severe anemia
	Retinal vein or artery occlusion
General	
Fever	Infection in compromised hosts
	Blood transfusion
	Malignancy, especially Hodgkin's disease and histiocytic malignancies
Weight loss	Malignancy
Night sweats	Malignancy
Malaise and lethargy	Infectious, inflammatory, or malignant disease
Endocrine, Metabolic and Electrolyte	
Disturbances	
Hypercalcemia	
Hypokalemia	Hematological malignancies
Hyperuricemia	
Hyperglycemia	Corticosteroid therapy
Metabolic acidosis	Acute leukemia

[a]CCF, crystal-induced chemotactic factor; SVC, SVC, superior vena cava; DIC, disseminated intravascular coagulation; GIT, gastrointestinal tract; TTP, thrombotic thrombocytopenic purpura; ADH, antidiuretic hormone; SLE, systemic lupus erythematosus; ENT, ears, nose, throat.

provisional diagnosis is made with a series of possible differential diagnoses. Diagnostic investigations are then performed to either confirm or repudiate the provisional diagnosis. Unfortunately, this paradigm has been rigidly accepted into the modern era of technological medicine and this classical Oslerian approach to diagnosis tends to be a one-way road. With so many expensive and potentially hazardous investigations available, it is important that

the diagnostic process is seen as a continuing spiral rather than a one-way road (Fig. 2.1).

The author does not wish to deny the importance of history and physical examination, but rather to emphasize its reanalysis throughout the diagnostic process in the light of information which becomes available from further investigations. It may thus be necessary to reundertake a carefully directed history and physical examination in the light of

Table 2.2
Laboratory Presentations of Hematological Disease (See Chapter 11)

Elevated ESR[a]	Thrombocytosis	Abnormalities detected in the blood transfusion laboratory:
Cytopenias	Atypical mononuclear cells	Positive Coombs test
Anemia	Abnormal blood film	Autoagglutination
Neutropenia	Abnormal results on biochemical investigation:	Serum auto and alloantibodies
Lymphopenia		Plasma protein abnormalities
Thrombocytopenia	Hypercalcemia	Abnormally colored serum
Cytophilias	Hyperuricemia	Abnormal coagulation test results
Polycythemia	Elevated protein	
Neutrophilia	Elevated LDH	
Lymphocytosis	Abnormal liver function test results	
Eosinophilia		
Basophilia	Serum iron abnormalities	
Monocytosis	Reduced PaO_2	
	Uremia	

[a]ESR, erythrocyte sedimentation rate; LDH, lactic dehydrogenase.

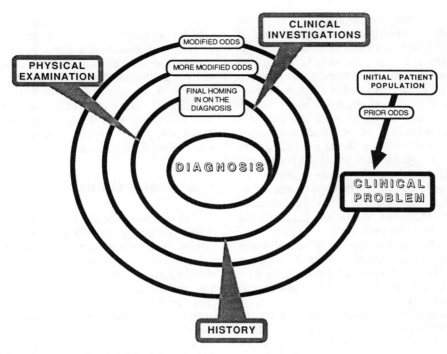

Figure 2.1. The diagnostic spiral "physician-oriented data processing."

information as it becomes available from the diagnostic investigations. The long-surviving aphorism that diagnosis is 70% history, 20% examination and 10% investigations probably still applies. Although more definitive and exact information can be obtained from investigations, they are still ordered and interpreted in the light of the clinical information. It is thus common that the final diagnosis comes from specific investigations, but the ordering and interpretation of investigations leading up to the ultimate diagnostic test is carefully directed by a problem-oriented clinician.

It is important to understand the philosophical differences between a clinician and a pathologist. A good clinician starting with a patient's problem is able to gradually collect historical and clinical information which will direct him further in his assessment. The clinician is progressively biased as he balances the probabilities during the information-collecting process. The diagnostic process moves towards the laboratory with appropriate tests being ordered as a result of this probability-oriented ("biased") assessment as to where the clinician is likely to find confirmation of

his clinical suspicions. This is in contrast to the pathologist whose responsibility is to accurately and objectively collect data and only interpret that information to the point where the clinician can then assimilate it into his problem-oriented data base. The contribution of the pathologist may range from typical "number crunching" where specific parameters can be objectively measured and interpreted in relation to statistical reference ranges, to the other end of the spectrum where the pathologist may be giving an objective interpretation of qualitative information, such as a histological biopsy. The pathologist must thus be objective in his assessment and, although he may find clinical information helpful to assist in interpretation, it should be emphasized that errors may occur when a pathologist overinterprets on the basis of minimal or incorrect clinical information.

The Diagnostic Spiral

Figure 2.1 illustrates the modern approach to diagnosis. The aim of the diagnostic spiral is not only to ensure accurate diagnosis, but also at the same time to achieve it with the minimum of investigations. On the basis of the initial history and findings on clinical examination, the clinician should order the minimum of high yield investigations which will subsequently direct the diagnostic process. On the basis of these initial investigations, the clinician can then incorporate this information into his patient data base, which will then be interpreted in the light of further clinical findings. Further detailed, specific and potentially more expensive investigations can then be ordered and from subsequent information it may be possible to make a definitive diagnosis. However, a further "trip around the spiral" may be necessary.

Using this approach, many unnecessary and expensive investigations can be avoided and only those having a high yield will be performed. This is in contrast to the "poker machine pathology" or "biochemical bingo" which tends to be practiced when tests are inappropriately ordered. There are many dangers along the diagnostic path of which the clinician must be constantly aware. With the high degree of automation in pathology, it is relatively simple and inexpensive now to produce numerous biochemical and hematological results as part of a profile type investigation. These profile investigations have been a major boon to medicine in alerting the clinician to important and potentially serious abnormalities which may or may not be related to the patient's basic problem. However, they have had a major disadvantage where incidental abnormalities are found when a profile was performed for another reason. If the clinician does not carefully assess the probabilities of the abnormality being related to the patient's original problem, he may fall victim to a "garden path" approach to diagnosis. Instead of carefully considering the likelihood of a laboratory abnormality being related to the patient's current problem, the doctor may initiate investigations on the basis of an abnormal finding which may be a "red herring" in relation to the patient's original problem.

In reaching a diagnosis, the clinician should know whether he has obtained a conclusive answer or merely a working hypothesis. In some cases, a diagnosis cannot be made, yet the patient requires therapy. In this circumstance, treating the symptoms, signs and "numbers" is acceptable medicine, provided access is left for the ultimate diagnosis which may emerge from continual assessment of information accruing during the course of the disease. The passage of time, colloquially known as "masterly inactivity" is underutilized as a diagnostic tool when there is no compelling reason to treat the patient. In our instant society, everybody expects an instant diagnostic label. A wrong label is worse than no label at all, for it stops doctors' thinking.

Diagnostic Categories

The ultimate aim of the diagnostic process is to arrive at the cause of a patient's problem in order to direct therapy. However, there are various levels of diagnosis and the clinician should have a clear idea as to the type of diagnosis which has been made. In some circumstances, the definitive disease is diagnosed and the underlying cause is known. For example, in most cases of vitamin B12 deficiency, not only can the effects of B12 deficiency be clearly diagnosed, but also the B12 deficiency itself can be specifically identified and subsequently the underlying cause elucidated. Unfortunately, this is not always the case and it may not be possible to establish such a complete diagnosis. For example, a patient may be diagnosed as suffering from autoimmune hemolytic anemia, but the underlying initiating process (e.g., lymphoma or viral infection) may not be apparent. At an even more superficial level, the clinician may only be able to identify individual pathological processes of the disease rather than basic mechanisms or underlying causes. For example, recurrent venous thrombosis and pulmonary embolism may be a major problem for the patient, but the underlying causal factors may not be identified.

Diagnosis is thus established at a particular mechanistic level. In classical reductionist medicine, students are taught to find the single underlying cause. This approach has been successful since the birth of scientific medicine in the 19th century, but is losing hold today. In some diseases the single defect in DNA can be identified, such as sickle cell disease, but unfortunately this classical reductionist approach is probably inappropriate for the majority of modern diseases afflicting man today as they are unlikely to have a sin-

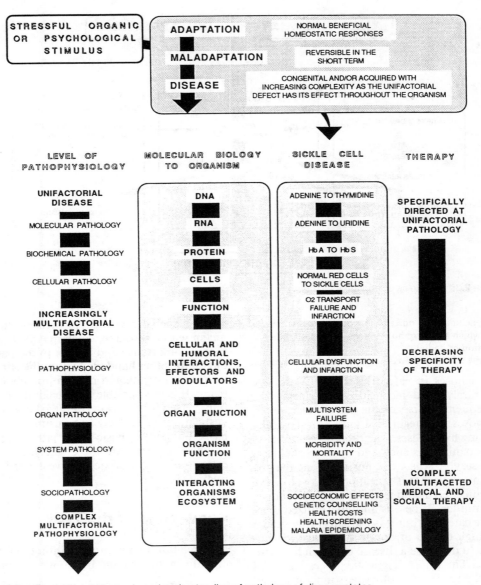

Figure 2.2. The levels of diagnosis and understanding of pathology of disease states

gle identifiable cause; rather, multiple factors interrelate on the background of multiple genetic predispositions. Figure 2.2 is an attempt to illustrate the depth of understanding of pathophysiology of disease and level of diagnosis. Sickle cell disease is used as an example.

Diagnoses may be classified as follows:

Type 1 The pathognomonic diagnosis where there is categorical, clinical or investigative proof.

Type 2 Diagnosis beyond reasonable doubt, where assessment of all the clinical and investigative information leads one to the conclusion of certainty, but where a pathognomonic test is not known or not available.

Type 3 Diagnosis on probabilities, where assessment of all the clinical and investigative information leads one to the conclusion that this is the most likely, but far from proven diagnosis.

Type 4 Diagnosis by exclusion, colloquially known as a "trash can" diagnosis, where all diseases likely to explain the clinical features have been

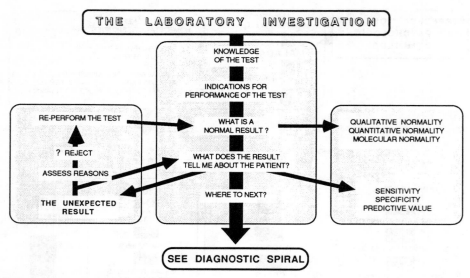

Figure 2.3. Principles of laboratory utilization

excluded and one possible diagnosis remains for which there are no methods either for confirmation or denial.

Type 5 Observation or therapy without a diagnosis.

Diagnoses in categories 1 and 2 are safe and rarely need reconsideration during the subsequent course of the disease. However, diagnoses in categories 3 and 4 are basically working hypotheses. They should continue to be recognized as such and open to change if necessary. A type 4 diagnosis has one big disadvantage in that it presupposes the clinician has considered, and is aware of, all diagnostic possibilities. Type 5 is an underutilized diagnostic category, but it is the safest when there is a high degree of doubt. A clinician is unlikely to diagnose a disease of which he is unaware. The whole diagnostic process assumes that the clinician or other personnel involved are aware of all diseases. This is unlikely, the degree of approximation depending on the resources and expertise available. The diagnostic personnel must be continually aware of their limitations, so that appropriate referral can be initiated when necessary.

Important Concepts in Laboratory Utilization

The range of laboratory investigations available to assist in investigation and treat-ment is ever increasing and presents the clinician with a resource which may be of paramount importance and benefit to the patient, but on the other hand may tempt the clinician to overinvestigate and inappropriately investigate. It is not possible for the clinician to be fully versed in all aspects of the laboratory investigations he is likely to be using on a daily basis, but certain basic information must be known if patients are to be safely, economically and appropriately investigated and treated (Fig. 2.3).

Knowledge of the Test

In relation to any investigation the following information should be known or sought:

- What are the sensitivity and specificity of the test?
- Will the test result provide further relevant information?
- Could the result of the test change the provisional diagnosis?
- Will the test give a better understanding of the disease?
- What is the cost of the test?
- What risk to the patient and staff is associated with the test?
- What intrinsic problems are there in the performance and interpretation of the test of which the clinician needs to be aware?

- What patient variables may alter interpretation of the result?
- How and where should the test be carried out, in particular, what are the collection, handling and transportation requirements?
- What is a "normal" result for the test in question? If the result can be quantified numerically, what is the reference range and how was it obtained?

Reasons for Performing the Test

There should be clearly defined reasons why an investigation is being performed as it is likely to effect the interpretation and subsequent clinical action. Investigations may be performed for the following reasons:

- To confirm or exclude the diagnosis of disease;
- Population screening for disease;
- Monitoring disease;
- Monitoring therapy;
- To assist in determining the prognosis of disease;
- To improve understanding of the disease, i.e., for education and research;
- Peer, patient or medicolegal pressure;
- Because the clinician wants it!

NORMALITY

The meaning of normal will depend on the nature of the investigation being performed. There are three levels of normality.

Qualitative Normality

When the parameter(s) in question cannot be quantified with any degree of accuracy the result is dependent on the observer's opinion. The result is a subjective analysis and highly observer dependent. The clinician is dependent on the experience and expertise of the pathologist. Histopathological interpretation is the classical example of qualitative normality.

Quantitative Normality

When the result of the investigation can be numerically quantitated the interpretation of normality depends on the use of statistics and the knowledge of a reference range which may or may not be appropriate to the patient in question. The use of statistics has been invaluable in laboratory medicine, but along with their introduction have been many problems which are illustrated in the following syndromes.

The Ulysses Syndrome

In order for a normal range to exist there will be 5% of patients who are "normal" but lie outside two standard deviations of the mean. Like Ulysses returning from Troy 5% of normal people may be subjected to potentially dangerous "clinical adventures" in an attempt to diagnose and treat nonexistent disease. To put it another way, it has been stated that: "If you go to your doctor make sure you are sick or else he will keep investigating you until something goes wrong, and then you will be sick."

The Ugly Duckling Syndrome

A patient may not be comparable to the reference range and it may be appropriate for the particular patient to be outside the reference range. A result thus appears to be abnormal when taken out of context, but is in fact an expected finding when taken in conjunction with the clinical findings (e.g., a fall in the serum iron as part of the acute phase response). Normal ranges are constructed using healthy people and then applied to diseased people.

The Clark Kent Syndrome (Alias Superman)

In this syndrome a seemingly normal laboratory parameter is in reality abnormal because it indicates absence of the "normal" response to the disease state, such as the absence of neutrophilia in sepsis which could be an important clue to host defense failure.

Wooden Horse Syndrome

The bell-shaped curve of the normal range may hide many abnormalities. A parameter may alter significantly but remain within the normal range, so that no clinical action is initiated. In contrast a change in the result from just below two standard deviations of the mean to just above may be of no clinical or statistical significance yet inappropriate clinical action may be initiated. The wooden horse syndrome may also be a problem when two variables are not independent and should be interpreted in association. Serum calcium must be interpreted in relation to the serum protein level, and although both parameters may be within the normal range a patient could have hypercalcemia if the protein is towards the lower limit of the normal range.

Molecular Normality

Molecular normality is absolute and statistical methods are not needed for interpretation. There may be an amino acid substitution resulting in an abnormal protein. With molecular biology being a clinical reality, it is likely that more diseases will be identified by their molecular abnormality, detectable by DNA probing techniques.

SENSITIVITY, SPECIFICITY, PREDICTIVE VALUE

The sensitivity, specificity and predictive value are all measurements of the usefulness of a test in separating patients who have a particular disease from patients who have other diseases or are healthy. Sensitivity measures the capacity of a test to identify patients with disease, i.e., the percentage of patients with disease who have a positive test result. The specificity measures the capacity of a test to identify people who do not have the disease, i.e., the percentage of patients without the disease having a negative test result. The ideal test would be 100% sensitive and 100% specific. Such a situation could only exist when molecular measurements are being made, but for quantitative normality such a test does not exist. Sensitivity is inversely related to specificity, i.e., the more likely a test is to detect patients with the disease, the more likely is it to yield false-positive results in patients without disease.

When a clinician requests a specific laboratory investigation in the process of investigating a patient he has already assigned the patient to a population which is likely to have a particular disease. The actual likelihood of the patient having the disease in question is known as the "prior odds" and will depend on the patient population with which the clinician deals and his ability as a diagnostician. Following the performance of the investigations the results will either support or refute the diagnosis and "revised odds" will be developed. The predictive value of a positive test result is the percentage of all positive results that are true positives. The predictive value of a test is determined by the sensitivity, the specificity and the frequency of the disease in the population tested. A good clinician is one who selects carefully the patients on which certain investigations are performed and as a result is more likely to come up with a positive result. Consideration of these facts clarifies why a test used for nonselective population screening must fulfill more rigorous criteria than a test used in clinical medicine for diagnosis when the prior odds have been established by selecting the patients on whom the test will be performed.

LABORATORY ERROR

Extreme caution should be exercised before the result of a laboratory test is attributed to laboratory error. If the result does not fit with the clinician's preconceived clinical impressions there is a tendency to attribute such results to laboratory error without carefully considering the possibilities. The following are possible explanations when a laboratory result appears to be at variance with that expected and if important clinical decisions rest on the result the investigation should be repeated.

- The result is correct, but the significance has been missed. It could thus be a clue to diagnosis that is being ignored.
- The result is correct, but has been affected by patient variables, e.g., therapy, drugs.
- The result is correct, but the patient is one of 5% of normal people who are outside two standard deviations of the mean.
- The result is correct, but it is the wrong patient. Such an error could be made at several points along the line. On the basis of probabilities it is unlikely to be a laboratory error, but rather a sample collection or labelling error.
- The result is incorrect. This could be due to: collection or transportation problems; clerical or computer error; technical error; problems with the sample, e.g., interference to the test from patient variables affecting the method used.

Clinical Presentations of Hematological Disease

Disorders of the hematopoietic system would have a broader spectrum of clinical presentations than disease of any other system. There are several explanations for this unique position of hematology in clinical medicine. First, there are few symptoms or signs of disease which would immediately direct the patient or the doctor of initial contact to consider a hematopoietic disorder. A patient is thus unlikely to think to himself "I need a hematologist," in contrast to the common situation today wherein patients and general practitioners may quickly assess the need for consultation with a particular specialist. Extensive unexplained bruising and bleeding, profound anemia, or lymphadenopathy and hepatosplenomegaly are the only clinical features which are likely to alert a patient or his doctor to the possibility of a blood disorder in the first instance. Secondly, the hematopoietic system is disseminated throughout the body and disease may present in any other system. Thirdly, the initial presentation of disease of the hematopoietic system may be manifest by hematopoietic failure, such as anemia, bleeding and infection, all of which may distract the clinician to the organ system of initial involvement. As discussed in the chapter on anemia, reduced oxygen-carrying capacity may present in several different ways. Infection may present in any organ system and an underlying host defense failure may not be suspected. The same applies to bleeding where there may or may not be a local lesion in another organ, but the hemorrhagic presentation directs the patient and the doctor towards that particular organ or specialty.

It is thus not surprising that neither patient nor the doctor of initial contact thinks in terms of disorders of the hematopoietic system or the need for a hematologist. The basic nature of hematological disease means that the clinician must always be alert to the classical "double bluff" in medicine. Whatever the clinical presentation of a patient's disease, the clinician must always keep an open mind to the possibility that an underlying disorder in the hematopoietic system could be responsible. This does not mean that extensive hematological investigations need to be performed on all patients. It is, however, the clinician's responsibility to consider the probabilities in any individual patient that the particular disease is likely or unlikely to have occurred in isolation.

The assessment of these probabilities is not always easy. If the patient presents with mul-

tiple problems, disseminated in time (e.g., recurrent infections or recurrent bleeding episodes) and/or place (e.g., different organs of the body), the threshold for considering an underlying hematopoietic disorder is lower. This is in contrast to the elderly patient who may present with an episode of pneumonia as the initial feature of multiple myeloma. As pneumonia is not uncommon in elderly patients, the likelihood of there being an underlying hematopoietic defect is relatively small. However, if the patient has been complaining of progressive lethargy and back pain and is found to have osteoporosis in association with a vertebral crush fracture, the possibility of myeloma would readily spring to mind.

Textbook presentation of disease is relatively easy to diagnose. The astute clinician is the one who "smells a rat" and asks further questions. As emphasized in the diagnostic process, the initial clinical and laboratory screening for hematopoietic disease is relatively simple and cost effective.

In simplistic terms, disorders of the hematopoietic system can be divided into 3 categories:

1. Quantitative deficiency.
2. Quantitative excess.
3. Qualitative defect.

Presentation of Hematopoietic Disease Due to Systemic Failure

FAILURE OF OXYGEN TRANSPORT (CHAPTERS 3 AND 4)

As the blood is an integral component of the oxygen transport system, it is not surprising that clinical features of systemic or local oxygen transport failure may be a manifestation of hematopoietic disease such as anemia, hyperviscosity syndromes, microvascular disease and interaction between a hematopoietic cause of oxygen transport failure and vascular, cardiac, or respiratory disease.

FAILURE OF HOST DEFENSES (CHAPTER 7)

Cellular or humoral defects in both the nonspecific hematopoietic defenses or the specific immunological defense system may present with typical or atypical infections. The specific defect will determine the nature and localization of infection.

HEMOSTATIC FAILURE (CHAPTERS 5 AND 6)

Underactivity (bleeding) or overactivity (thrombosis) may occur as a result of defects in the hemostatic system. As discussed in chapters 5 and 6, the delineation and investigation of excessive or inappropriate underactivity or overactivity of the hemostatic system can be difficult. However, initial clinical and laboratory assessment can, in the majority of cases, determine whether further specialist investigation is necessary. The main trap in the presentation of hemostatic failure is where it is not obvious that the underlying problem is in fact bleeding or thrombosis. Occult bleeding (e.g., retroperitoneal hemorrhage or intramural bowel bleed) may produce a clinical picture which would not lead the clinician to suspect that there was an underlying hemorrhage.

Presentation of Hematopoietic Diseases Due to Reactive or Malignant Organ Enlargement (Chapter 8)

Many reactive and malignant disorders of the hematopoietic system may present with organ enlargment. This is colloquially known as the "lumps and bumps" presentation. As emphasized, dissemination of the hematopoietic system means that such organomegaly may present overtly as palpable masses or after detailed investigations. Generalized lymphadenopathy and hepatosplenomegaly would obviously direct the clinician towards the hematopoietic system. In contrast, an extrahematopoietic mass presenting in the nervous system may take some time for its "true colors" to be revealed.

A Summary of the Presentations of Hematological Disease

Table 2.1 lists several clinical presentations of disease in different systems of the body where hematological disorders need to be considered. Fortunately the diagnostic process dictates initial localization of the pathology and subsequent tissue diagnosis. On this basis, if the diagnosis is pursued to its logical conclusion, the presence of an underlying hematological disorder will eventually be established. It has, however, been the author's experience that this diagnostic route can at times be excessively devious and treacherous. As there is definitive treatment for most hematological diseases presenting with a mass lesion (whether malignant, reactive or hemorrhagic) it is important that the underlying pathology be identified before irreparable end-organ damage has occurred. A classical example is the management of the acute onset of spinal cord compression. Although there may be many underlying causes for which little can be done, disorders of the hematopoietic system are the one group wherein effective therapy, and possible cure, may be available.

Conclusion

From the above considerations it can be seen that hematological disease may present in a plethora of guises or disguises. It is only with constant awareness of the probabilities, and the maintenance of an open mind for the subtle clues, that early diagnosis of hematological disease will be made. There are relatively inexpensive, simple investigations which will help "swing" probabilities towards or against hematological disorder.

Further Reading

Mendel, D. *Proper doctoring.* Berlin: Springer-Verlag, 1984.
Sullivan, MS, and Rawnsley, HM, eds. *Clinics in laboratory medicine: controversies in laboratory medicine.* Mar. 1984. Vol 4 No. 1. Philadelphia: W.B. Saunders Company Ltd.

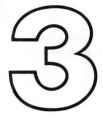

Anemia

The growth of observation consists in a continual analysis of facts of rough and general observation into groups of facts more precise and minute.

Walter Pater (1839–1894)

Observation runs sadly to waste when it is made upon cases piecemeal.

P. L. Latham (1789–1875)

Anemia is defined as a reduced hemoglobin level in the peripheral blood and is probably the commonest hematological problem to confront any branch of medicine. Despite hemoglobin measurement being one of the oldest measurements in medicine and one that can now be measured with a high degree of accuracy, the interpretation of results still remains controversial. Not only is the normal range still under debate, but the physiological mechanisms which control the peripheral blood hemoglobin level are only partially understood and the effects of lifestyle and habits are becoming increasingly apparent.

The Clinical Problem

Anemia may present with the classical symptoms and signs of pallor, lethargy, poor exercise tolerance, dyspnea, faintness, nausea and anorexia. On the other hand anemia may be compounding a defect elsewhere in the oxygen transport system and will not result in the classical clinical picture. Furthermore, one of the commonest entries into the diagnostic pathway of anemia is via a "routine" blood count. Whatever the mode of presentation, several important questions need to be addressed from the outset before too many conclusions are reached and these same questions may need to be readdressed throughout the patient's clinical course.

INITIAL QUESTIONS WHEN A REDUCED HEMOGLOBIN LEVEL IS FOUND

1. What is the lower limit of normal for hemoglobin in this patient? Consider age, sex, pregnancy, altitude dweller, smoking and alcohol status, physical fitness, associated disease.
2. Does this hemoglobin level explain the patient's symptoms? If not, why not?
3. Is anemia an expected or unexpected finding?
4. Does the degree of anemia require immediate intervention?
5. Is there likely to be any sudden stress on the status quo?
   For example, blood loss, surgery, fever, exercise or the development of complications in other components of oxygen transport.
6. Is the cause of anemia immediately apparent from the clinical findings or initial blood count report?
7. What appears to have been the rate of onset of the anemia?
8. Is the anemia interacting with other defects in oxygen transport to produce or accentuate the clinical features of associated disease such as respiratory, cardiac or vascular disease?

INTERPRETATION OF SYMPTOMS IN RELATION TO HEMOGLOBIN LEVEL

Hb > 10g/dL Symptoms occur when the oxygen transport system is stressed by increased oxygen demand (e.g., exercise, fever) or by reduced oxygenation of the blood (e.g., impaired pulmonary gas exchange, high altitude, smoking, carbon monoxide exposure).

Hb 8 to 10g/dL Symptoms of increasing cardiac output at rest may be noted (e.g., palpitations) especially in elderly patients, but as a general rule the symptoms are not severe.

Hb < 8g/dL Increasing symptoms at rest, depending on cardiorespiratory reserve.
Anemia plus associated defect in oxygen transport (as a general rule the Hb is <10g/dL before these factors become significant):

- Patients with vascular disease associated with anemia may present with symptoms relating to the particular vascular bed in question, e.g., angina, intermittent claudication, transient cerebral ischemic attacks.
- Patients with impaired cardiac reserve and anemia may present in congestive cardiac failure.
- In patients with respiratory disease and impaired pulmonary gas exchange, a higher hemoglobin level is required to ensure the delivery of adequate oxygen for the reduced PaO_2 level. It should be remembered that approximately 5.0g/dL of Hb need be desaturated before central cyanosis is clinically apparent.
- In patients in whom there are red cell membrane or hemoglobin oxygen affinity defects, the peripheral blood Hb level may not correlate with the amount of oxygen which is actually available to the tissues. Such a situation may arise in hereditary spherocytosis, smoking, carbon monoxide exposure or massive blood transfusion.

COMMON TRAPS IN THE PRESENTATION OF ANEMIA

The Fluctuating Hemoglobin Level

- Excess intravenous fluids, especially colloids.
- Venous capacitance expansion will increase the size of the intravascular compartment and lead to transcapillary refill or the intravenous administration of fluids for the relative hypovolemia. Such a circumstance is most commonly seen in patients after surgery.
- Sudden alterations in cigarette smoking habits.

- Incorrect sample collection: wrong patient, collection from intravenous line, excessive tourniquet time.

Physiological "Anemia"

- Infancy, pregnancy.

Failure to See the Interaction of Anemia with Other Defects in Oxygen Transport

The hemoglobin level is only one component of the oxygen transport system and alterations in its level cannot be interpreted in isolation. The most important compensatory response for anemia is an increase in cardiac output but the clinical presentation of anemia may depend on the presence of other defects in the oxygen transport chain. Under normal circumstances there is no need for a person to increase cardiac output at rest until the hemoglobin level falls below 10g/dL and it will only be on exercise that symptoms of reduced aerobic capacity will be noticed. It is rarely necessary to transfuse a correctable anemia of >8.0g/dL unless blood loss or increased oxygen demands are imminent.

Treatment before a Definitive Diagnosis Has Been Established

The Sudden Onset of Anemia

The sudden onset of anemia nearly always implies there has been a loss of red cells as a result of bleeding or acute hemolysis. In most circumstances the cause is readily apparent, but a high index of suspicion is necessary in some cases. Where there is a combination of impaired red cell production, secondary to any cause, and acute red cell loss the onset of the anemia may be fulminant and life threatening.

The Coexistence of Anemia and Respiratory Failure

The combination of fulminant anemia and respiratory failure constitutes a medical emergency where astute clinical acumen is required. Central cyanosis does not occur in the presence of severe anemia, and the gravity of the defect in oxygen transport may not be immediately appreciated. The combination of respiratory failure and anemia may be seen under the following circumstances:

- Mycoplasma pneumonia with autoimmune hemolytic anemia.
- Pulmonary hemorrhage e.g., Goodpasture's syndrome, trauma.
- Lupus pneumonitis with pulmonary hemorrhage.
- Pulmonary infections in compromised hosts.
- Virus-associated hemophagocytic syndrome.
- Hemorrhagic shock and adult respiratory distress syndrome.

DIAGNOSIS OF THE CAUSE OF ANEMIA

A mechanistic approach to the etiology of anemia is usually advocated. Although this is valuable in understanding the pathophysiology and approaches to therapy it is of limited value in initially establishing the underlying cause. When the cause of anemia is multifactorial a combined problem-oriented and mechanistic approach may be necessary. Until the introduction of automated blood cell counters the diagnosis of anemia depended largely on the interpretation of the blood film in conjunction with the mean corpuscular hemoglobin concentration (MCHC) determination which was calculated from manually determined hemoglobin and hematocrit values. It was not possible to determine the mean corpuscular volume (MCV), mean corpuscular hemoglobin (MCH) nor red blood cell count (RBC) with any degree of accuracy. It should be emphasized that the MCV, MCH and MCHC are all mean figures for the population of red cells and if more than one population of cells is present (e.g., a dimorphic film) these indices are more difficult to interpret. With most of the newer cell counters it is possible to study the distribution of the cells on a histogram and determine whether there is more than one population of cells present. The red cell distribution width (RDW) is the crude measure of this cell characteristic. See Appendix 1 for a summary of the red cell indices and reference ranges.

If manual methods are used it is possible to identify the hypochromic anemias with a reasonable degree of confidence, but the separation of normocytic and macrocytic requires examination of the blood film by an experienced observer. However, most laboratories now provide an automated service and classification of the anemias into the broad categories of hypochromic-microcytic, normochromic-normocytic and normochromic-macrocytic can be done with accuracy. This separation is on the assumption that the anemia is unifactorial in origin; for the more complicated multifactorial anemias a more discriminating approach is required. There will always be a degree of overlap between the three major subdivisions and although mechanistically a particular anemia should be classified in one of the subgroups, its diagnosis may become apparent via more than one diagnostic route. This situation particularly applies to the anemia of chronic disease and sideroblastic anemias.

The importance of establishing a definitive diagnosis for the cause of an anemia, or at least collecting the appropriate samples, before therapy is initiated cannot be overstressed. It is most unusual for the cause of a significant degree of anemia to remain undiagnosed if a thorough investigation has been undertaken, if necessary in consultation with a hematologist.

Figure 3.1 outlines a diagnostic approach to anemia based on the initial MCV findings. It is important that a logical sequence of investigations be carried out, guided by constant reanalysis of the patient's clinical history and physical findings. A "shotgun" approach is not only uneconomical, but also runs the risk of failing to achieve a definitive diagnosis. The peripheral blood indices and film provide a high-yield, low-cost guide to the cause of most anemias. On the basis of these initial results more specifically directed and expensive investigations can be requested, in most cases to confirm the provisional diagnosis. If the immediate diagnostic course is not apparent, communication with the hematologist may be helpful. A two-way dialogue may quickly establish the diagnostic possiblities and probabilities.

COMMON PROBLEMS IN THE INVESTIGATION OF THE CAUSE OF ANEMIA

Multifactorial Anemia

The usual hematological features of specific anemias may not be found if there is more than one cause for anemia. Results may

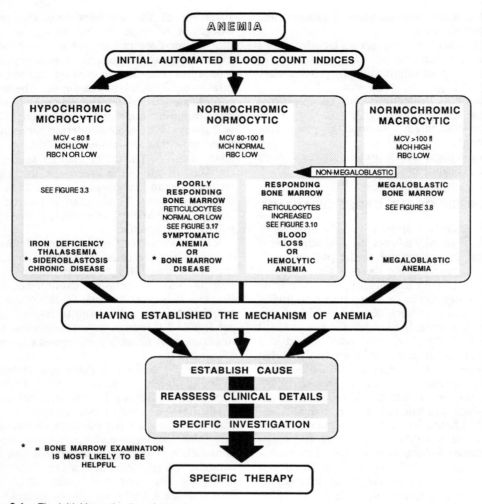

Figure 3.1. The initial investigation of anemia

sometimes be misleading and caution should be exercised when the initial clinical and laboratory features "don't compute"; multifactorial anemia may be responsible. Possible combinations include:

- Dimorphic anemia, a term loosely applied to anemias in which two populations of red cells are present and may be seen in a combined iron deficiency and megaloblastosis, responding iron deficiency, sideroblastic anemia and transfused iron deficiency.
- Hemolytic anemia without a reticulocyte response (discussed in the section headed Hemolytic anemia).
- A normal MCV in the presence of a combined microcytic and macrocyte anemia. The MCV is a mean value and if there are

two populations of cells or there are opposing influences on red cell size the nature of the anemia will not be revealed in the MCV. Examples of this situation would include combined iron deficiency and megaloblastosis; acquired sideroblastic anemia and megaloblastosis in thalassemia.

- Spurious blood cell indices may be misleading in the early investigation of anemia (see chapter 11).

GENERAL PRINCIPLES IN THE TREATMENT OF ANEMIA

After the obvious need to establish a correct diagnosis there are certain general principles in the management of anemia which are independent of the underlying cause. The urgency of therapy should be based on the clinical setting of the anemia and not physician or hospital related considerations (e.g., operation schedules). Inappropriate red cell transfusion is not only hazardous, but commonly delays response to definitive therapy by suppressing bone marrow response. The excuse that the patient has failed to respond to therapy and therefore needs transfusion is commonly a facile analysis of the clinical situation and important diagnostic and therapeutic principles have been ignored.

When to Transfuse the Patient with Anemia

- Prior to urgent surgery if Hb <10g/dL.
- Active or anticipated blood loss.
- No likelihood of specific therapy being effective.
- During bone marrow suppressive therapy (e.g., chemotherapy).
- When there are associated defects in oxygen transport (respiratory or cardiac decompensation).
- When there are increased oxygen requirements.

When Not to Transfuse the Patient with Anemia

- Mild anemia in young patients (especially females).
- When the anemia is reversible in the short term.
- As a preoperative "top-up" for elective surgery when there is definitive therapy available (e.g., iron deficiency).
- When the effects of hemodilution from the anemia may be beneficial (e.g., pregnancy, anemia of chronic disease, vascular disease).

Reasons Why Anemia May Not Respond to Therapy

- Incorrect diagnosis.
- Noncompliance to therapy.
- Incorrect or inappropriately administered therapy.
- Suppressive effects of blood transfusion.
- Multifactorial cause for anemia or the de-

velopment of another deficiency during response.
- Malabsorption.
- Blood loss.
- Low normal set point for hemoglobin (e.g., pregnancy or chronic disease).

Common Errors in the Management of Anemia

- Failure to establish a definitive diagnosis.
- Expecting the diagnosis to always be made on the initial blood count.
- Blindly ordering tests in a "poker machine" manner, in the hope that eventually the correct diagnosis will surface.
- Failure to interpret laboratory findings in the light of the clinical findings.
- Unnecessary red cell transfusion.
- Failure to analyze why a patient fails to respond to specific therapy for the anemia.
- Excessive concern about the hazardous effects of mild anemia.

THE HYPOCHROMIC-MICROCYTIC ANEMIAS

In this diagnostic category are included iron deficiency anemia, the thalassemic syndromes, sideroblastic anemias and some cases of the anemia of chronic disease. A red cell may become hypochromic as a result of problems in heme production, as in iron deficiency, reduced iron availability (as in the anemia of chronic disease) or disordered iron metabolism (as in sideroblastic anemia) (Fig. 3.2). On the other hand, heme synthesis may be normal, but there is a defect in globin chain synthesis, usually a congenital defect in alpha or beta chain synthesis (as seen in the thalassemic syndromes).

An unequivocally hypochromic-microcytic anemia usually turns out to be iron deficiency or a thalassemic syndrome. The racial origin may give a clue to the likelihood of a thalassemic syndrome, or a history of blood loss may point to iron deficiency, but these only assist in further diagnostic testing. The red cell indices may bias the assessment towards one or the other. In general the microcytosis in thalassemia trait is out of proportion to the degree of anemia and the MCHC is not significantly reduced, in contrast to iron deficiency where the red cell indices parallel the

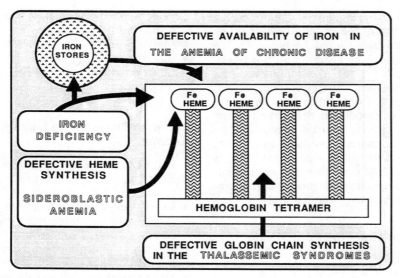

Figure 3.2. Mechanisms of hypochromic anemia

degree of anemia. As the subsequent investigation of a hypochromic-microcytic anemia is directly dependent on the cause, it is crucial to confirm that the patient is iron deficient before embarking upon a potentially long series of investigations.

LABORATORY INVESTIGATIONS IN THE DIAGNOSIS OF HYPOCHROMIC-MICROCYTIC ANEMIA

The Red Cell Indices

When there is a single cause for hypochromic-microcytic anemia (Fig. 3.3) the MCV and MCH are always low in iron deficiency, thalassemia and congenital sideroblastic anemia. However, in most patients with anemia of chronic disease the MCV will usually be normal or only slightly reduced. Paradoxically, the MCV in acquired sideroblastic anemia may be elevated and the hypochromic cells may only be present in small numbers on the blood film. As the cells are small in the microcytic anemias the red cell count is not as low in relation to the hemoglobin (or hematocrit) level as will be found in the normocytic and macrocytic anemias. The small cells do not pack as well and there is more plasma trapping when a manual hematocrit (packed cell volume) is performed. This is partly the explanation for the markedly re-

duced MCHC seen in iron deficiency when manual methods are used. Using automated cell counters, the MCHC has relatively narrow limits and small reductions are significant. Unless a patient has a significant hypochromic-microcytic anemia the hematocrit correlates well with the hemoglobin determination and can be used as a reasonably accurate measure of the oxygen-carrying capacity of blood. Microhematocrit centrifuges are economical, easy to use and provide a rapid and reliable bedside method for serial measurements of oxygen-carrying capacity in unstable clinical settings (e.g., hemorrhage, hemodilution).

Serum Iron and Total Iron Binding Capacity (TIBC)

Iron is carried in the circulation on transferrin in the ferrous state. Transferrin can be measured directly or indirectly as TIBC. Careful attention is needed in the interpretation of the serum iron and TIBC values. There is little justification for including a serum iron on a biochemical screen as it is liable to misinterpretation. Not only does the patient need to be fasting to avoid false normal levels, but the serum iron level is reduced in the two commonest causes of anemia (iron deficiency and the anemia of chronic disease) and is a poor test for diagnosing the cause of

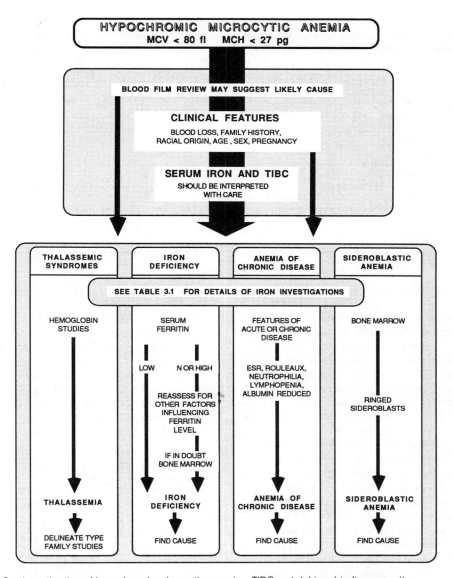

Figure 3.3. Investigation of hypochromic-microcytic anemia—TIBC = total iron binding capacity

an anemia. Serum iron falls as part of the acute and chronic phase reactions irrespective of the hemoglobin level and is thus a common finding on a biochemical profile where its reduction is part of the body's normal response to inflammatory or malignant disease. A TIBC should be performed in association with a serum iron measurement to assist in interpretation. In iron deficiency the TIBC is elevated and transferrin saturation reduced, in contrast to the anemia of chronic disease in which the TIBC is normal or reduced with only mild reductions in transferrin saturation. Table 3.1 summarizes the serum iron, TIBC, ferritin and bone marrow findings in various forms of hypochromic-microcytic anemia.

Ferritin Assay

Apoferritins are a series of iron binding proteins produced in many tissues which bind iron to form ferritin. The iron is stored in a hollow cavity in a molecule which protects the body from toxicity from elemental iron

Table 3.1
Laboratory Parameters in Hypochromic-Microcytic Anemia and Disorders of Iron Metabolism

	Serum Fe	TIBC	Saturation	Ferritin	Bone Marrow Stores	Sideroblasts
Iron deficiency	↓	↑	↓	↓↓	absent	↓
Chronic disease/infection/ inflammatory disorders or malignancy	↓	N or ↓	↓	N or ↑	N or ↑	↓
Sideroblastic anemia	N or ↑	N or ↓	N or ↑	↑	↑	↑ Ring sideroblasts
Thalassemia	N or ↑	N or ↓	N or ↑	↑	↑	↑
Pregnancy	N or ↓	↑	↓	N or ↓	N or ↓	N
Hemochromatosis	↑	N or ↓	↑	↑↑↑	↑↑↑	N or ↑

and the effects of "rusting." Iron stores are approximated by assuming that 1μg/L of ferritin represents 8 to 10mg of iron storage. Roles for this group of proteins other than the storage of iron in a safe form are still being elucidated. As ferritin accumulates the molecular structure alters, probably by a degree of denaturation, and hemosiderin is formed, which is stainable in the macrophage-monocytic system using Perl's stain. Serum ferritin measurement, usually by radioimmunoassay, is a helpful method for assessing iron stores. Although only the protein itself is being measured, under most circumstances there is a good correlation between the serum level of ferritin and the body's iron stores. This relationship does not always apply when there is a large amount of tissue breakdown (e.g., trauma, hepatitis) or in the presence of certain malignant diseases (especially lymphomas). The measurement of ferritin has allowed the elimination of bone marrow iron assessment in most patients with hypochromic-microcytic anemia.

Bone Marrow Examination

Except in the diagnosis of sideroblastic anemia bone marrow examination is rarely required in the investigation of hypochromic-microcytic anemia. However, in some complex anemias several different mechanisms may be operative and actual confirmation of the presence or absence of stainable marrow iron is helpful. Rheumatoid arthritis, systemic inflammatory or malignant disease with occult blood loss and when initial investigations give conflicting results, are situations in which marrow examination may be helpful. Under most circumstances bone marrow examination will be late in the investigations. In the hypochromic anemias, where there is impaired hemoglobinization of red cell precursors, the micronormoblastic changes in erythropoiesis with attenuation and vacuolation of the erythroblast cytoplasm may mask associated megaloblastosis.

PITFALLS IN THE DIAGNOSIS OF HYPOCHROMIC MICROCYTIC ANEMIA

The following are some of the common errors which may be made in the investigation of hypochromic-microcytic anemia.

- Misinterpretation of serum iron studies.
- Ferritin level not reflecting iron stores.
- MCV normal or high, but the underlying disorder is one of impaired heme or globin synthesis. This may occur in sideroblastic anemia, multifactorial anemia and in the anemia of chronic disease.
- Iron deficiency in a polycythemic patient may present with gross hypochromic-microcytic changes and abnormal hemoglobin level.

IRON DEFICIENCY ANEMIA

Worldwide, iron deficiency is the commonest cause of anemia and is one of the most eminently treatable. Its classification under the title of nutritional anemias has been unfortunate as this implies that nutrition is a major causal factor in most patients. This is far from the truth and although iron supplementation may reduce the incidence of iron deficiency anemia, nutrition should not be concluded as being the sole cause of iron deficiency until iron loss has been convincingly excluded. All patients with iron deficiency anemia are in negative iron balance, usually due to increased losses (usually blood loss) rather than a low dietary iron intake. In Third World countries the distribution of iron deficiency closely follows that of conditions such as hookworm infestation as well as borderline dietary iron intake. A sound knowledge of the basic facts of iron metabolism is essential if diagnosis and treatment of iron deficiency is to be logical and ultimately successful.

Iron Metabolism

Iron is an essential metal in metabolism and elaborate mechanisms have evolved to ensure its adequate supply. Despite this metal's vital importance it is enigmatic to contemplate the small size of the total amount of iron in the human body (4g) and the fine line existing between undersupply and oversupply. Figure 3.4 summarizes iron balance and metabolism. A normal male exchanges 0.5 to 1mg of elemental iron with his environment each day. Most of the body's iron is in hemoglobin (2250mg) with 1 ml of red cells containing 1mg of iron (500ml blood with a normal hematocrit contains approximately 250mg elemental iron). The normal unstressed bone marrow produces approximately 20ml red cells each day (20mg iron). The marrow does however have the potential to increase production by a factor of six, as long as adequate nutrients are available. Thus the normal bone marrow has a potential to utilize as much as 120mg iron per day, if such amounts can be supplied. In hemolysis the iron is rapidly recycled, but in blood loss iron is mobilized from normal hemosiderin/ferritin stores at the rate of 40mg/day. These fig-

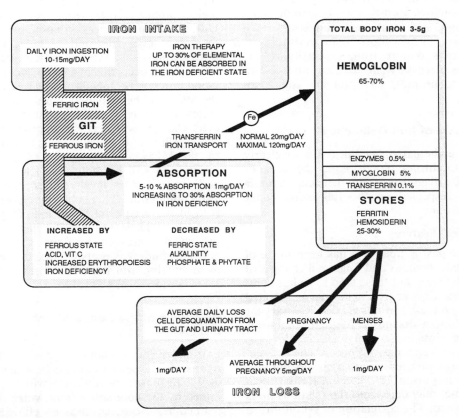

Figure 3.4. Iron metabolism and iron balance

ures explain how a population of iron deficient hypochromic red cells may be released from the bone marrow following an acute hemorrhage, despite adequate tissue iron reserves.

There is no effective excretory mechanism for iron in man and metabolic balance must be maintained by finely controlling absorption. The control of iron absorption is complex and not fully understood. Dietary iron in the heme form is better absorbed than in the elemental form (as ferric hydroxides and ferric protein complexes) and the gut has an absorptive mechanism for iron presented to it in either form. The absorptive mechanism is sensitive to increased requirements. The information concerning body iron requirements is generated somewhere in the body and transmitted as a message to the upper small intestine where absorption will increase. The average diet contains 15mg of iron of which 0.5 to 1mg (5% to 10%) is usually absorbed, but the gut has the capacity to increase absorption to 30% of ingested iron, a figure to remember in the oral treatment of iron deficiency anemia. Iron-rich foods include green vegetables, red meat, eggs and bread. Iron deficiency affects more than erythroblasts as all cells require iron, especially in the proteins necessary in aerobic metabolism (the cytochromes, flavoproteins and myoglobin).

Diagnosis of Iron Deficiency

Unless the patient's clinical history clearly points to chronic blood loss as the cause of anemia, a diagnosis of iron deficiency anemia is first suspected on the full blood count examination.

Clinical Features

In the past a great deal has been made of the mucocutaneous and fingernail changes of iron deficiency, but these tend to be less common these days as iron deficiency is detected earlier and these features are not necessary for establishing a diagnosis. Angular stomatitis, atrophic glossitis, koilonychia, brittle hair, pruritis and pica may all occur. The association of iron deficiency with a postcricoid web (Plummer-Vinson or Paterson-Kelly-Brown syndrome) may occur and the relationship is still debated. The correlation of symptoms to the hemoglobin level has been discussed above, but it is not uncommon to find that the symptoms are in excess of those expected for the hemoglobin level, probably due to a combination of the requirement for iron by the respiratory enzymes and defective hypochromic-microcytic red cells. The important clinical features in iron deficiency relate more to the finding of a cause rather than the diagnosis of iron deficiency, which is really a clinicopathological presentation of disease rather than a disease in its own right.

Laboratory Features

The initial parameters from a full blood count will usually point the clinician in the direction of iron deficiency. The low MCV, MCH and MCHC and hypochromic blood film are highly suggestive, particularly if the patient is known to have had a normal blood count in the past. The level of hemoglobin at which a patient develops the red cell indice changes and hypochromic blood film depends on the initial hemoglobin level, the rate of onset, and the presence of any other hematological abnormalities (e.g., polycythemia). During the initial stages of blood loss the hemoglobin level falls and reticulocytes rise until the body's iron stores are depleted. If the blood loss is occurring at a significant rate the blood film will be polychromatic initially and the MCV will be increased, but when the iron stores are depleted the hypochromic-microcytic changes will begin to appear with the MCV falling and RDW increasing, followed by the MCH and finally the MCHC. The serum iron will be reduced, TIBC elevated and serum ferritin level reduced. Occasionally a population of hypochromic cells may be seen in the peripheral blood following acute blood loss. These are iron-deficient cells although adequate iron stores may still be present. This finding is probably due to the delay in mobilizing iron from the stores following acute hemorrhage.

Diagnosis of the Cause of Iron Deficiency

Iron deficiency is not a diagnosis in its own right and a cause must always be sought. The likely diagnostic possibilities will be determined by the population from which the patient comes. However the astute clinician will

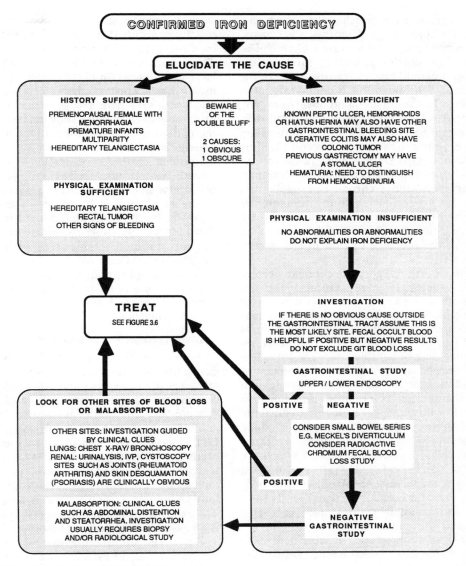

Figure 3.5. Management of iron deficiency

always be on the lookout for the "double bluff" where the obvious cause may distract attention from a second and possibly more sinister pathology. Possible causes for iron deficiency will vary in different populations and in different groups of patients, and these considerations will clearly determine approaches to diagnosis and management (see Fig. 3.5).

1. Infants (especially premature)—inadequate dietary intake.
2. Young children—negative iron balance during the growth spurts.
3. Menstruating women and pregnancy—negative iron balance.
4. Adult males and postmenopausal females—occult blood loss.
5. People in underdeveloped countries—decreased iron intake in conjunction with gut infestation with hookworm.

The first three do not usually require investigation for occult blood loss unless there are suggestive features in the history, and in patients from underdeveloped countries it may not be practical, nor necessary, to investigate all patients. It is the fourth group for which a tenacious approach to diagnosis is necessary. This is not to say that a cause will always be found, but sinister pathology must be excluded. A careful history relating to the bowel is necessary although this is commonly unrewarding. In contrast, blood loss from any other part of the body resulting in iron deficiency, is usually obvious (e.g., genitourinary tract, epistaxis, hemoptysis). Occult bleeding into solid organs is unlikely to result in iron deficiency as the iron is reabsorbed. Intrapulmonary hemorrhage, chronic hemoglobinuria (with hemosiderinuria) from intravascular hemolysis and disorders of transferrin are rare conditions in which iron deficiency may occur in the presence of iron in stores elsewhere in the body.

In the fourth category the clinician is committed to adequate investigation of the gastrointestinal system for an occult cause of chronic blood loss. Although it may seem paradoxical, if a patient's presenting symptom is blood loss from the gastrointestinal tract, respiratory tract or genitourinary tract it is less likely that he or she will be iron deficient at presentation as the pathology is brought to clinical attention before iron depletion can occur. For this reason it is unwise to attribute iron deficiency to such pathologies as peptic ulceration or esophageal varices, without firmly excluding other conditions which are likely to ooze blood slowly rather than bleed acutely. In contrast, to attribute iron deficiency to hiatus hernia, "gastritis" or diverticulitis may result in serious and remediable pathology being missed.

The important causes of iron deficiency which should be excluded include gastric carcinoma, colonic carcinoma, angiodysplasia and drug-induced GIT blood loss (especially nonsteroidal antiflammatory medications). Carcinomas of the stomach and cecum are two causes of iron deficiency which may present at a late stage and be associated with features of the anemia of chronic disease. These tumors may be bulky at the time of diagnosis because local GIT symptoms (e.g., bleeding or disturbed bowel function) may not occur.

Tests for Blood Loss

Tests for confirmation of gastrointestinal (GIT) blood loss have a limited role to play in the investigation of iron deficiency. Although

their use may seem logical, the clinician is usually committed to full GIT investigation in most patients irrespective of the result. Their main use is in the patient who may have two reasons for chronic blood loss (e.g., menorrhagia, epistaxis, hematuria) in association with GIT hemorrhage. If three consecutive stool examinations show no blood while the patient is on a meat-free diet and/or the patient is in category 1, 2 or 3 previously mentioned, further investigation is not warranted. Chromium-labelled red cell fecal blood loss studies rarely have a part to play, except as a research procedure. There may, however, be the occasional patient in whom there are two possible causes for iron deficiency, associated hemolysis, or where quantitation of blood loss may be helpful. The various angiographic and radionucleide investigations are useful for localizing acute hemorrhage, but have little place in the investigation of iron deficiency.

Investigations to Localize Pathology

Techniques for investigative access to the gastrointestinal tract have made spectacular advances in recent years and radiological procedures are having a lesser role to play. Endoscopic examination of the upper GIT and colon has revolutionized the investigation of GIT blood loss. Although the exact sequence of investigations is still debated it is becoming increasingly apparent that upper and lower endoscopy is necessary to exclude all important pathology. Angiodysplasia is a common cause of chronic blood loss, especially if there is an associated hemostatic disorder.

It is not uncommon that extensive GIT investigation fails to establish a cause for iron deficiency. Under these circumstances it may be worthwhile to perform investigations to firmly establish the GIT as the site of blood loss. A more careful search should be made, for the rare "trick" causes of iron deficiency, such as: chronic analgesic intake; rheumatoid arthritis; hematuria; hemosiderinuria; pulmonary hemosiderosis; exfoliative skin disease; dermatitis artefacta; surreptitious blood letting. Radiological investigation of the small bowel may be indicated in some patients. With the increasing popularity of exercise, unexplained iron deficiency may be found in joggers and long-distance runners. It appears that these people are in negative iron balance due to increased iron loss. There are various possibilities to consider, including sweating, urinary loss and March hemoglobinuria. However, GIT loss, the mechanisms of which remain to be elucidated, would appear to be a common finding in this population.

In an adult iron deficiency should never be attributed to poor dietary intake alone or malabsorption unless blood loss causes have been excluded or there is overwhelming evidence to support the diagnosis. In malabsorption there will usually be evidence of other deficiencies, such as folic acid, other vitamins and steatorrhea. Patients with polycythemia rubra vera are commonly iron deficient with the hypochromic microcytic red cell changes out of proportion to the degree of anemia. Such red cell findings should be a clue to such a diagnosis as the marrow is attempting to produce excessive red cells, but is limited by the availability of iron. This may be due to inadequate stores or GIT blood loss which is common in polycythemia rubra vera.

Treatment of Iron Deficiency

Correction of iron deficiency anemia can usually be considered independently of the basic pathology which requires definitive therapy. Despite iron deficiency being common and therapy readily available, its management still requires a sound understanding of iron metabolism and attention to detail. There have been many misleading and incorrect statements made in relation to iron therapy and bad therapeutic habits have resulted because application of the basic principles of diagnosis and management have been ignored. At the outset it should be pointed out that a large number of patients receiving iron therapy do not need it and the failure of presumed iron deficiency to respond to treatment is commonly due to an incorrect diagnosis.

Oral Iron Therapy

Effective treatment of iron deficiency requires the regular delivery of iron to the upper small bowel until the hemoglobin level is normal. Following this, a longer period of less intense iron therapy is necessary to replete the body's iron stores. The slightest intolerance of iron therapy is commonly interpreted as failure of therapy and if the physician does not stress the importance of compliance the patient will think it does not matter. Iron deficiency is no different from any other disorder which requires definitive therapy. Iron-deficient patients require iron in the same way as insulin-dependent diabetics require insulin and a subdural hematoma requires evacuation, and to achieve this is the physician's responsibility. If the physician is not interested, the patient is unlikely to think the therapy is important.

The majority of patients can be treated with oral iron therapy if certain important guidelines are followed. There are rare patients who are totally intolerant of oral iron or fail to absorb adequate iron. Under certain circumstances, when continuing blood loss cannot be controlled, it is difficult to deliver enough iron orally to prevent anemia and parenteral administration is necessary. Situations in which compliance to oral therapy is unlikely for reasons other than intolerance, such as other medical or psychiatric diseases, or in underdeveloped countries where follow-up may be inadequate may also necessitate parenteral administration. These considerations aside, every attempt should be made to administer iron therapy orally to avoid the potentially hazardous and cosmetic side effects of parenteral therapy.

A wide range of oral iron preparations is available. The introduction of **delayed-release iron** preparations has caused more problems than it has solved. As a general rule the side effects of iron therapy are related to the amount and availability of elemental iron in the preparation under consideration. Delayed-release iron preparations may be satisfactory for replenishing iron stores or treating mild iron deficiency. However, their use in the definitive management of severe iron deficiency is not only illogical, but sometimes ineffective. The concept of an oral iron preparation which delays the release of elemental iron beyond the optimal absorption sites and is advocated on a single daily dosage schedule flies in the face of scientific facts and is unlikely to result in optimal therapy. It is the author's view that the traditional forms of iron therapy should be used in the initial therapy of significant iron deficiency. Ferrous sulphate (225mg equivalent to 65mg elemental iron) is the cheapest, but unfortunately is not always readily available in standard formulation. Since the introduction of delayed-release preparations which contain ferrous sulphate there has been a tendency not to have the standard form available and if a physician writes a prescription for ferrous sulphate the pharmacist is likely to supply a delayed-release form. Ferrous gluconate (300mg equivalent to 35mg elemental iron) is thus usually the cheapest and most readily available preparation, but ferrous fumarate and succinate are also suitable.

Much has been written about the factors which may alter iron absorption by the gut, but their relevance in the practical management of iron deficiency is minimal. Compliant use of the appropriate iron preparation is of paramount importance. Despite the usual recommendations to the contrary, the author advocates the taking of oral iron with meals and in association with a high residue diet. It should be pointed out to the patient that there may be some upper gastrointestinal symptoms and alterations in bowel function with darkening of the stools. However, the initial intensive therapy of iron deficiency is short-term and if the patient understands the logic of the therapy and is being closely monitored, compliance is good and recovery is rapid. The rate of response will depend on the general considerations outlined above plus the following:

- Iron absorption, which is normally increased in the presence of iron deficiency.
- The ability to deliver iron to the upper GIT regularly throughout the day.
- The presence of continuing blood loss.
- The need to transfuse in the initial stages.

The ability of the marrow to utilize absorbed iron is related to the rate of erythropoiesis. The rate of erythropoiesis is intimately connected to the stimulus to red cell production (i.e., degree of deviation from the patient's normal hemoglobin set point) and the presence of other nutritional or suppressive factors which may impair the response. In the absence of other considerations the response to effective iron therapy relates to the amount of elemental iron delivered in conjunction with the fact that normal bone marrow has the potential to produce at six times the normal rate and thus to utilize as much as 120mg of iron a day. One ferrous gluconate tablet three times a day will make approximately 100mg of elemental iron available of which up to 25% (25mg) should be absorbed allowing the production of 25ml of red cells. Thus if the patient can tolerate a high iron intake, a maximal response of approximately 100ml of red cells each day results in a hemoglobin rise of 1 to 2g/week. However, as the hemoglobin rises the stimulus to erythropoiesis and iron absorption will decrease and the rate will slow down as the patient's hemoglobin approaches normal (see Fig. 3.6). In contrast to a megaloblastic anemia, where the bone marrow is hypercellular and ready for red cells to rapidly mature and produce a reticulocytosis, the marrow of a patient with severe iron deficiency is not hyperplastic (what is known as iron-limited or erythropoiesis) and needs time to "wind up" and produce new red cells. As reticulocytes are usually expressed as a percentage of the number of red cells, the total red cell count should be taken into consideration when assessing a patient's response to therapy. In microcytic anemia the red cell count in relation to the hemoglobin level is much higher than in a macrocytic anemia where the number of larger cells contributing to an equivalent hemoglobin level is considerably less. It is unusual to see a reticulocyte response much above 12% in a responding iron deficiency, in contrast to a severe megaloblastic anemia where responses as high as 60% may occasionally be observed.

Weekly blood counts should be performed initially to assess response to therapy. This not only encourages the patient to comply to therapy, but also allows early recognition of the patient who fails to show an expected hemoglobin rise, in which case appropriate measures can be taken to establish the reasons. Failure of, or delay in response to, therapy in iron deficiency should suggest the following possibilities:

- Noncompliance
- Incorrect diagnosis
- Multifactorial anemia
- Continuing blood loss
- Inappropriate iron therapy (e.g., single-dose, delayed-release preparations)
- GIT malabsorption
- Suppressive effects on marrow response and iron absorption by initial blood transfusion.

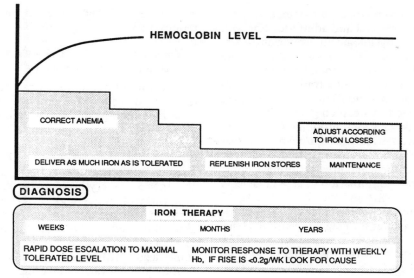

Figure 3.6. Treatment of iron deficiency

Parenteral Iron Therapy

The parenteral administration of iron should not be undertaken lightly and there should be good indications before resorting to this invasive mode of iron therapy. Staining of the skin and allergic reactions (arthralgias, fever, urticaria, bronchospasm and anaphylaxis) to intramuscular therapy may occur and severe anaphylactoid reactions are well documented with intravenously administered iron. Iron dextran is a stable complex of ferrous hydroxide and dextran and iron-sorbitol-citric acid complex is a rapidly absorbed intramuscular preparation. Intravenous iron therapy is even more hazardous and rarely indicated. Saccharated oxide of iron or iron dextran may be used.

Common Errors in the Diagnosis and Management of Iron-Deficiency Anemia

- Misdiagnosis of other hypochromic-microcytic anemias as iron deficiency.
- Regarding a low serum iron level as indicative of iron deficiency.
- Inappropriate iron therapy and a too-ready acceptance that oral therapy has failed.
- Failure to pursue a cause of blood loss in unexpected iron deficiency.
- Too-ready acceptance of the first-detected pathology as the cause of iron deficiency

(e.g., peptic ulceration, hiatus hernia, diverticular disease).

THE THALASSEMIC SYNDROMES

Failure to synthesize one of the globin chains (alpha or beta) of adult hemoglobin A will result in defective hemoglobin formation and inadequate hemoglobinization of the red cells and thus hypochromic-microcytic red cells. This group of the hemoglobinopathies has become increasingly heterogenous and complex. Although they are of great interest to the geneticist and molecular biologist their importance in clinical medicine is basically threefold. Firstly, the homozygous form of thalassemia results in severe clinical disease (thalassemia major) requiring constant medical attention. Secondly, the heterozygote states and the interaction of thalassemia genes with other hemoglobinopathies may produce a wide, and sometimes bizarre, spectrum of hematological abnormalities, and their correct diagnosis is essential if inappropriate therapy is to be avoided. Thirdly, with increasing understanding of these disorders accurate genetic counseling and intrauterine diagnosis are possible and it may not be in the too distant future that the rapid advances in genetic engineering may allow exciting therapeutic interventions.

Although several different hemoglobins are produced during fetal and adult life, HbF and HbA are the physiologically important ones. There is extreme clinical variability in the thalassemic syndromes ranging from hydrops fetalis to silent thalassemia trait where the patient has a normal blood film and the defect is only detected by detailed globin chain synthesis studies or DNA probing. The thalassemic syndromes can be simplistically classifed into major, intermedia, minor and trait, with these clinical pictures resulting from a heterogeneous combination of genetic defects involving the genes on chromosomes 16 (2 loci for alpha chain production) and chromosome 11 (genes for beta and gamma chain production). The defects may affect the globin chain production in varying degrees and have a variety of pathophysiological mechanisms, ranging from partial or complete deletion of globin genes, abnormalities of cleavage or splicing sites or point mutations in the original structural gene. In beta thalassemias no beta chains are produced whereas in the beta$^+$ some chains are produced. Figure 3.7 summarizes the pathophysiology of alpha and beta thalassemia.

Diagnosis

The thalassemias are commonly classified under the hereditary hemolytic anemias, but shortened red cell survival and acute hemolytic episodes are unusual clinical features. The failure of hemoglobin production fits them better into the hypochromic-microcytic anemias. The high frequency of the beta thalassemias in people of Mediterranean origin and alpha thalassemias in people of Asian extraction should increase the diagnostic threshold in these groups. However, these syndromes have been reported in all racial groups and have provided the anthropologically and genealogically oriented hematologists with a wealth of exciting information.

Clinical Presentation

Hydrops Fetalis (Bart's Hydrops)

Homozygous alpha thalassemia with total absence of alpha chain synthesis and gamma chains forming a poorly functioning tetramer (Hb Barts) results in hydrops fetalis and is in-

compatible with survival as alpha chains are required for all hemoglobins.

Thalassemia Major (Cooley's Anemia, Mediterranean Anemia)

A feature of homozygous beta thalassemia is failure of beta chain production and presents by 6 months of age. The babies are normal at birth as the major hemoglobin is HbF and it is not until the switch to HbA production that the disorder presents. Extramedullary hemopoiesis results in hepatosplenomegaly. Ineffective erythroid hyperplasia causes expansion of bones and increased iron absorption. Iron overload results from increased absorption and repeated transfusion. Dyserythropoiesis with ineffective *hemopoiesis* and some degree of hemolysis results in hyperbilirubinemia, elevated LDH and a grossly abnormal blood film.

Thalassemia Intermedia

These patients have milder disease presenting later than thalassemia major (usually by 5 years of age) with hypochromic-microcytic anemia and splenomegaly. It commonly presents as a result of decompensation during infections. Iron overload can be a problem later in life, as can pigment gall stones from the hyperbilirubinemia. The clinical picture can be produced by a variety of beta globin gene defects either in the heterozygous state or as homozygous forms of mild defects.

Thalassemia Minor

These patients are only mildly anemic and asymptomatic unless stressed (e.g., during pregnancy). The commonest problem is misdiagnosis as iron deficiency anemia and subsequent inappropriate iron therapy. It is usually due to heterozygous beta globin gene defects.

Hemoglobin H Disease

This is a variant of alpha thalassemia where three of the alpha gene loci are affected producing a clinical picture with similarities to thalassemia intermedia. The main difference is the shortened red cell survival and tendency to hemolytic episodes of the Heinz body type when exposed to oxidant stress. This form of thalassemia may develop iron deficiency due to hemosiderinuria, in contrast

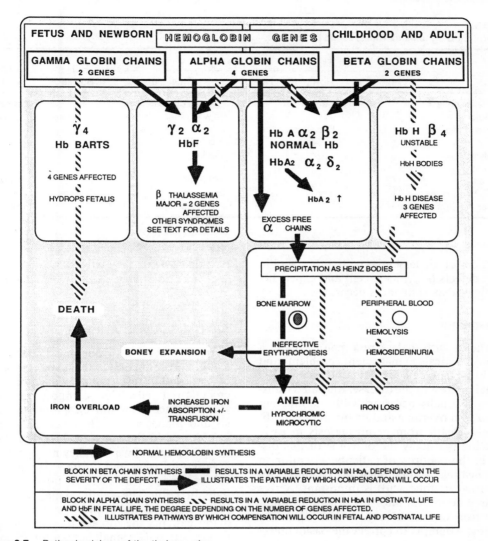

Figure 3.7. Pathophysiology of the thalassemias

to most thalassemias where iron excess tends to be the problem.

Thalassemia Trait

These patients are heterozygous for the mildest globin gene abnormalities and usually only have slight abnormalities in red cell indices. The peripheral blood may be normal in the case of alpha thalassemia if only one gene is affected.

Laboratory Diagnosis

Most patients with thalassemia come to clinical attention during the investigation of a hypochromic-microcytic anemia unless a family is being studied as a result of a propositus being identified.

Hemoglobin Electrophoresis

Table 3.2 summarizes the laboratory findings in the thalassemic syndromes. It is most important that the diagnosis be firmly established to avoid inappropriate therapy and the possibility of iron overload. Family studies should be done to identify further patients, not only for their own benefit, but also from the genetic counseling point of view. In some patients the genetic abnormality may be extremely complex, especially when there is in-

Table 3.2
Laboratory Diagnosis of Thalassemic Syndromes

		Hemoglobin Electrophoresis				HbH Bodies	Chain Synthesis
		HbF	HbA	HbA$_2$	Other Hb		
β	Thalassemia Major	↑↑	Absent or ↓↓	↑	Various combinations with other chain disorders Hb S, D, E, C	—	β absent or ↓↓↓
β	Intermedia	Variable	Depends on the severity			—	
	Minor Trait	↑	↑	↑	Hb Lepore	—	β ↓
α	Trait	N	N	N	Hb Barts at birth	+	α ↓
α	Hb H disease	N	N or ↓	N	HbH	+ + +	α ↓↓
α	Barts hydrops	—	—	—	Hb Barts	—	absent

teraction of thalassemia with other globin chain defects (e.g., sickle cell) and expert hematological assessment is necessary.

Management

Patients with thalassemia major present a serious clinical management problem and should be cared for by hematologists with a special interest in the disease. Repeated transfusion is usually necessary with the inherent risk of iron overload and its inherent complications. Death from hemosiderosis in early adult life is usually the outcome of this disease in the majority of patients. Attention to complicating factors, such as vitamin deficiencies (e.g., folic acid) is important. Active research continues into this disease to minimize iron overload, such as iron chelation therapy. Attempts to correct the basic molecular defect, such as bone marrow transplantation or gene manipulation therapy, may offer a better future to patients with thalassemia major.

The thalassemia intermedia, minor and trait syndromes are relatively simple syndromes to manage with the patients having an opportunity of a normal life expectancy. Correct diagnosis is the most important aspect of management in these patients, especially to prevent inappropriate iron therapy. During episodes of stress (e.g., pregnancy or infection) supplemental folate therapy is warranted. These patients may require advice regarding the likelihood of progeny being affected. If both parents are heterozygous for

beta thalassemia they will have a one in four chance of producing a child with thalassemia major.

SIDEROBLASTIC ANEMIA

In the sideroblastic anemias there is a defect in the production of the heme component of hemoglobin resulting in hypochromic-microcytic red cells. They compose a complex group of anemias requiring specialist diagnosis and management. However, they are of importance to the nonspecialist from the diagnostic point of view as they may present in a variety of ways and create enigmatic difficulties if the patient is not "channelled" in the right direction. The condition may be congenital or acquired and primary or secondary. In many patients the disease may be clonal in nature with only a small population of abnormal hypochromic-microcytic cells in the peripheral blood, but erythropoiesis may be grossly ineffective causing severe anemia. Under these circumstances the anemia may present as normocytic or macrocytic.

Diagnosis

Clinical Features

As can be seen from the long list of causes of sideroblastosis it should be thought of in several clinical settings after the more common causes of anemia have been excluded. The commonest causes seen in clinical practice are either secondary to alcoholism, hematological malignancy, or acquired idiopathic disease.

Laboratory Features

The definitive diagnois of sideroblastic anemia is made in the laboratory on the basis of the typical sideroblastic changes in the bone marrow seen in the iron stain. However, to the experienced hematologist it is rarely an unexpected finding as other clinical and pathological features point to the probability and marrow examination serves as the final confirmation.

- Decreased red cell indices and microcytic hypochromic red cells are found in congenital sideroblastic anemia. In acquired anemia the indices commonly reveal a macrocytosis due to the dyserythropoiesis or megaloblastosis in the marrow and the blood film needs to be examined carefully for the presence of hypochromic-microcytic cells.
- Leukocyte abnormalities or thrombocytopenia may be a feature when sideroblastosis is secondary to a hematological malignancy.
- Bone marrow examination shows increased stainable iron, heavy granulation of the red cell precursors and the diagnostic ring sideroblasts in which iron granules are seen accumulated around the nucleus. It is also common to find dyserythropoietic or megaloblastic changes in erythropoiesis. An underlying hematological malignancy or preleukemic syndrome may also be apparent.
- Associated hematological and biochemical changes of alcoholism may be present, especially macrocytosis.
- Ferritin is usually elevated indicating iron overload.
- Serum iron may be elevated with a normal transferrin (TIBC).

Causes of Sideroblastic Anemia

As specific therapy such as pyridoxine is only occasionally effective, it is important to identify any possible underlying cause which may be reversible. In other circumstances the identification of a cause may help in prognostication. The causes of sideroblastic anemia are:

- Acquired sideroblastic anemia
  Primary idiopathic
    Onset late in life, usually associated with marked iron overload and evidence of hemosiderosis. May be pyridoxine responsive.
  Secondary
    Associated with hematological or other malignancy or as a preleukemia syndrome.
    Toxic—lead poisoning, alcohol.
    Drugs—antituberculous drugs, chloramphenicol, some cytotoxic agents.
    Nutritional—malnutrition, alcoholism.

Management

Any identifiable cause should be removed, a trial of pyridoxine therapy in increasing dosage up to 100 to 200mg four times a day and folate supplements. Regular blood transfusion is necessary in some patients with idiopathic and preleukemic sideroblastic anemia. Androgen therapy is occasionally helpful.

Macrocytic-Normochromic Anemia

Anemia with the MCV > 100 fl directs the clinician along the macrocytic anemia investigative line, however direct consideration and investigation for the classical textbook causes of macrocytic anemia should not be immediately undertaken (Fig. 3.8). There are certain key questions which have to be asked and several anemias, in which patients may present with elevated MCV's, need to be identified and "redirected" via more appropriate investigative channels outlined under normocytic-normochromic anemia.

What Is the Degree of Macrocytosis?

If the MCV is >110 fL it is highly likely that the cause will be megaloblastosis or a dyserythropoietic anemia and investigations should proceed along these lines.

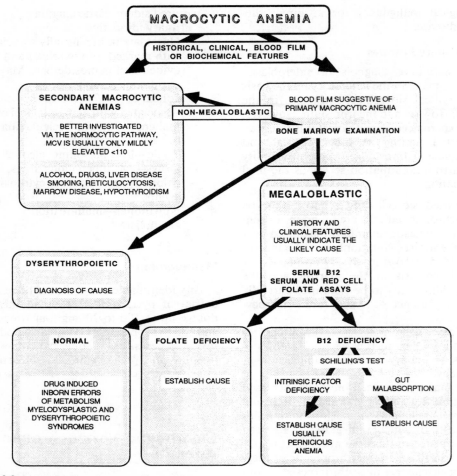

Figure 3.8. Investigation of macrocytic anemia

What Does the Blood Film Show?

Oval macrocytes, marked anisocytosis and poikilocytosis are pointers towards megaloblastosis. Round, thin macrocytes, target cells, mild anisocytosis and poikilocytosis suggest liver disease with or without alcoholism (especially if stomatocytes are present). Polychromasia, suggesting an elevated reticulocyte count, will increase the MCV and red cell features of hemolysis may also be present. Severe pancytopenia or circulating leukemic cells indicate underlying bone marrow disease and dyserythropoiesis is likely to result in peripheral blood macrocytosis. Occasional hypochromic microcytic cells should arouse the suspicion of acquired sideroblastosis.

Are There Any Clinical Findings Which May Assist?

Alcohol, smoking, jaundice, liver disease, hypothyroidism, dietary history, malabsorption, past bowel surgery, neurological findings suggestive of B12 deficiency, drug history (especially cytotoxic agents), glossitis or atrophy and a sallow complexion, may all be helpful.

Is Bone Marrow Examination Indicated?

When it is likely that the macrocytic anemia is due to megaloblastosis it is desirable, but not essential, to perform a bone marrow biopsy to confirm the diagnosis. As the commonest cause of mild macrocytosis is the variable combination of alcohol, liver disease and smoking, bone marrow biopsy should be avoided in this group as it is usually unhelpful. Although a mild degree of folate deficiency is common in the alcoholic and cirrhotic patient it is more appropriate to perform a folate assay.

What Other Investigations Need to Be Performed?

The need for other investigations will be directed by the answers to the above questions. Folate and B12 analyses are readily available and relatively economical and their performance on the basis of suggestive clinical information or to exclude associated megaloblastosis is reasonable. More detailed investigations for the cause of a megaloblastic anemia which is not apparent from the clinical findings should only be pursued after megaloblastosis has been confirmed on bone marrow examination. Iron deficiency can mask a megaloblastosis in the bone marrow and under some circumstances it may be necessary to establish folate or B12 deficiency in the absence of a megaloblastic marrow.

NONMEGALOBLASTIC MACROCYTIC ANEMIAS

There are several conditions which may present with a macrocytic anemia in the absence of megaloblastic erythropoiesis. These conditions, like early B12 or folate deficiency, may be macrocytic in the absence of significant anemia. Although this may seem a rather intimidating list of causes, in the majority of patients the cause is obvious from the clinical findings or the initial investigations. Unexplained macrocytic anemia is usually readily diagnosed following hematological consultation. If megaloblastosis has been excluded investigation is best pursued via the normocytic-normochromic pathway and most of the ultimate causes of such a macrocytic presentation will be elucidated. As a bone marrow biopsy is usually performed to confirm megaloblastosis any unexpected marrow disease will be detected and appropriate action taken. The causes of macrocytosis (with or without anemia) without any evidence of frank megaloblastosis are:

Reticulocytosis—hemolysis, blood loss or neonates
Toxins—alcohol, arsenic
Hypothyroidism and hypopituitarism
Aplastic anemia, red cell aplasia
Dyserythropoietic anemia
Some acquired sideroblastic anemias
Preleukemic syndromes
Malignant infiltration of the marrow
Some hematological malignancies with marked dyserythropoiesis
Scurvy
Protein malnutrition
Postsplenectomy
Pregnancy
Chronic obstructive lung disease.

MEGALOBLASTIC-MACROCYTIC ANEMIA

Vitamin B12 and folic acid are both required for normal deoxyribonucleic acid (DNA) synthesis. Deficiency of one or other of these substances will result in defective nuclear maturation of the cells, with continuously replicating cells (bone marrow, gut mucosa and skin) being most affected. The exact pathophysiological mechanisms are still hotly debated, but the clinical effects, techniques for investigation and therapy are all well understood. Figure 3.9 summarizes the essentials of B12 and folate metabolism.

The definitive investigation to confirm the presence of megaloblastic erythropoiesis is bone marrow examination and the identification of the cause is by assessing vitamin B12 and folate status by specific assays. Most clinicians would agree that it is not necessary to perform marrow examination in milder degrees of folate or vitamin B12 deficiency unless there is some other specific indication. However, in severe macrocytic anemia in which the cause is not immediately apparent examination of the bone marrow becomes an important investigation.

Diagnostic Approach to Megaloblastic-Macrocytic Anemia

Clinical Features

The clinical features of megaloblastic anemia are determined by:

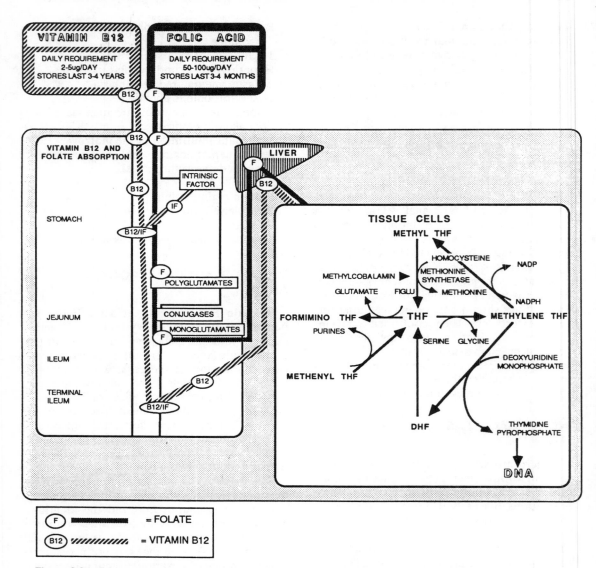

Figure 3.9. Folate and vitamin B12 metabolism—DHFA = dihydrofolic acid; THFA = tetrahydrofolic acid

1. Rate of onset—vitamin B12 deficiency is usually of slow, insidious onset as stores last up to two years and the vitamin B12 is not consumed in metabolism. Folate deficiency can have a variable onset, but in some cases where demands are high and intake low the limited stores are rapidly consumed and acute megaloblastosis results. Drug-induced megaloblastosis is usually of rapid onset, unless due to antiepileptic agents (e.g., phenytoin sodium).

2. Nonhematological effects of vitamin B12 deficiency include parasthesia, ataxia, visual deterioration, dementia, anorexia and glossitis. These features may occasionally be seen with folate deficiency.

3. Complicating factors—other causes of anemia such as hemolysis, blood loss, and malnutrition or increased demands for folate may all complicate the presentation of folate deficiency.

The cause of a megaloblastic anemia can usually be determined from the clinical history with the specific investigations serving as confirmation.

Vitamin B12 Deficiency

- Except in vegans B12 deficiency is caused by malabsorption either due to intrinsic factor deficiency or small bowel disease. Supportive evidence for the various possibilities is usually forthcoming in the history.
- Associated neurological abnormalities—subacute combined degeneration of the cord.
- Family history of pernicious anemia or other autoimmune diseases (especially thyroid, adrenal, allergies, malabsorption syndrome) may be found.

Folate Deficiency

- Except in the malabsorption syndromes folate deficiency is most commonly due to inadequate dietary intake (especially the elderly, alcoholics and diseases causing anorexia) or increased requirements (pyrexia, sepsis, malignancy, pregnancy). Folate deficiency is more commonly associated with iron deficiency than is vitamin B12 deficiency, as seen in the malabsorption syndromes, pregnancy and GIT malignancy with occult bleeding.

Drug-induced Megaloblastosis

- A drug history will usually elicit the therapeutic agents which are likely to be responsible for megaloblastosis (see below).

Laboratory Investigation

Confirmation of Megaloblastic Macrocytic Anemia

Blood Examination—if there is a moderate degree of anemia present MCV is usually >110fL, with elevated MCH, reduced RBC and reticulocytopenia. Variable degrees of thrombocytopenia and neutropenia or pancytopenia may be found.

Blood film—anisocytosis, poikilocytosis, oval macrocytes, hypersegmented neutrophils, but as the anemia becomes more severe teardrop cells, fragmented cells, Howell-Jolly bodies and stippled cells may be present.

Biochemistry—unconjugated hyperbilirubinemia and elevated LDH may be present due to ineffective erythropoiesis, occasionally a positive Schumm's test result is found and haptoglobins may be reduced.

Bone marrow:

- Hypercellular due to the arrest in maturation of all cell lines.
- Megaloblastic hematopoiesis—all cell lines are larger than normal with excess immature forms present.
- Erythropoiesis shows increased nucleocytoplasmic ratio with advanced cytoplasmic hemoglobinization in relation to nuclear development.
- Granulopoiesis is left shifted, giant metamyelocytes and giant band forms are present with twisted and deformed forms present.
- Megakaryocytopoiesis shows giant hyperlobulated forms.
- Iron stores and siderotic granulation are usually increased.
- The bone marrow biopsy should be interpreted with caution as megaloblastic cells may appear "worryingly" primitive on an hematoxylin and eosin preparation.

Establishing the Cause of Megaloblastosis

Unless the patient has received antifolate drugs such as methotrexate or other megaloblastosis-inducing drugs (e.g., cytosine arabinoside) megaloblastosis occurring de novo is due to vitamin B12 or folate deficiency in 90% of the cases. As already mentioned, the specific investigations for the cause of megaloblastosis are usually to confirm a strong clinical suspicion. Initially the presence of vitamin B12 or folate deficiency must be confirmed and subsequently the underlying disease responsible.

Vitamin B12 Deficiency

Vitamin B12 is synthesized by microorganisms and humans obtain it by eating products from ruminating animals; it is not present in vegetables or fruits. Vitamin B12 is made up of a group of compounds called cobalamins which contain cobalt in the centre of a corrin ring. Methylcobalamin and deoxyadenosyl cobalamin are the two principle forms in the diet (7 to 30µg/day), and they are not affected by cooking. Ingested cobalamin binds to a glycoprotein intrinsic factor, which is produced by the gastric parietal cells. This complex then attaches to ileal receptors permitting B12 absorption to occur. Following absorption the B12 is transported by transcobalamin II. Vitamin B12 is stored primarily in the liver, but significant amounts are also bound by transcobalamin I in the blood and in granulocytes. On a B12 deficient diet stores will last for up to two years or more.

The Investigation of Vitamin B12 Deficiency

Vitamin B12 Assay

This test is usually done by an immunoassay technique which is not affected by antibiotics, in contrast to the microbiological assays.

Schilling's Test

In this test the absorption of vitamin B12 labelled with two radioactive isotopes of cobalt is compared with and without intrinsic factor. It is measured by collecting the urine and also comparing the ratio of the two isotopes in the peripheral blood and urine. From this test the ability of the gut to absorb vitamin B12 can be determined, and if abnormal, whether the defect is a deficiency of intrinsic factor or due to small bowel malabsorption. If the test suggests a small bowel cause it should be repeated after a course of antibiotic therapy (tetracycline) especially if there is any suspicion of a blind loop syndrome or upper gastrointestinal diverticula. A Schilling's test is still valid in a patient under treatment with B12. A B12 injection is given as part of the test, to which the patient may make an immediate symptomatic and hematological response.

Tests for Autoimmunity

Parietal cell antiboidies, intrinsic factor antibodies and thyroid antibodies all may support a diagnosis of pernicious anemia.

Tests for Gastric Mucosal Atrophy and Achlorhydria

These are rarely indicated in diagnosis.

Other Tests for Underlying Pathology

The result of the Schilling's test in conjunction with other clinical and laboratory information will direct the clinician to the performance of more detailed investigations if necessary. If pernicious anemia has been excluded, small bowel investigations, such as a small bowel radiological series and biopsy may be necessary.

Causes of Vitamin B$_{12}$ Deficiency

Inadequate Intake

Vegans.

Intrinsic Factor Deficiency

- Addisonian pernicious anemia is an autoimmune disease usually occurring in the elderly where gastric atrophy occurs in association with parietal cell antibodies. There is failure of intrinsic factor production. It may be associated with other autoimmune diseases and classically occurs in northern European people with pale skin, blue eyes and premature greying. Antibodies to intrinsic factor are present in 60% of patients, parietal cell antibodies in over 90% and thyroid antibodies in 50%.
- Congenital intrinsic factor deficiency.
- Childhood pernicious anemia.
- Gastrectomy.

Dissociation of B$_{12}$/Intrinsic Factor Complex

Bacterial overgrowth in blind loop syndrome, diverticula, scleroderma, Whipple's disease.

Small Bowel Disease

- Celiac disease: folate deficiency is more common as the proximal small bowel is more severely affected.
- Tropical sprue: the terminal ileum is commonly affected.
- Crohn's disease: the terminal ileum is the classical site of disease.
- Distal ileal resection of greater than 60 cm.
- Specific selective ileal malabsorption of B12 (Immerslund's syndrome).
- Fish tapeworm (Diphyllobothrium latum) which occurs around major lake areas, especially in Scandinavia.
- Other rare causes: severe pancreatic deficiency; hypothyroidism; drugs (prolonged nitrous oxide); giardiasis.

Treatment of Vitamin B12 Deficiency

If the underlying cause cannot be corrected in the short or long term, the patient is committed to life-long vitamin B12 therapy on a 1 to 3 monthly basis. Blood transfusion should be avoided, particularly in a severe megaloblastic anemia which has developed over a long period of time. The deficiency state affects all the body's tissues, including the heart and there is a risk of precipitating pulmonary edema and death. In rare circumstances when the patient is already in congestive cardiac failure an exchange transfusion with fresh blood may be necessary.

In the United States, if B12 is given orally, it is usually given as a 1000 μg/day dosage. For parenteral administration, in the United States, generally a minimum of six intramuscular injections of 1000 μg of cyanocobalamin given at two- or three-day intervals is required for initial saturation. In situations where the underlying disease process is irreversible, as in pernicious anemia, lifelong maintenance therapy is administered following the replenishment of the body stores of vitamin B12, usually 250 μg monthly.

Maintenance therapy varies in concentration given and intervals administered from one institution to another, depending on the severity of the deficiency and preference of the clinician.

Principles of therapy include:

- Treat the cause.
- Parenteral vitamin B12 therapy is available in two forms, cyanocobalamin is the most widely used, but is less well retained in the body than hydroxy cobalamin. Initially the patient is given several loading injections of 1000 μg twice a week of either preparation until the response to therapy is well established. As a megaloblastic bone marrow is hypercellular with cells arrested in development the reticulocyte response is rapid (3 days) as soon as the B12 is made available, peaking at 1 week. As well as the hazards of blood transfusion, hypokalemia (especially if diuretics are used) and reactive thrombocytosis (with the possibility of vascular occlusive events) may occur.
- Folate alone should not be administered to a patient with megaloblastic anemia unless B12 deficiency has been excluded. Although B12 deficiency may initially respond to folate the neurological features may become more severe. If there is doubt about the cause of megaloblastosis it is advisable to give B12 and folate therapy until assay results are available. It can sometimes be difficult to differentiate even after the results are available as severe folate deficiency may reduce the B12 level, in contrast to B12 deficiency where the folate level is high unless there is a combined deficiency.

Folate Deficiency

The terms folic acid and folate refer to a group of compounds containing pteridine, para-aminobenzoic acid and a variable number of glutamic acid moieties. The tetrahydrofolates are the active folates in various enzyme reactions. Humans are unable to synthesize folate and thus require it performed as a vitamin in the diet (average daily intake 700μg, requirement 50 to 100μg). Folates are present in most foods with high concentrations in liver, vegetables and yeast, but in contrast to B12, they may be destroyed by excessive cooking. The polyglutamates in the diet are broken down to monoglutamate by folate hydrolases prior to absorption by the duodenum and jejunum. Folates are transported in the blood as monoglutamate-5-methyl-tetrahydrofolate bound to proteins. Polyglutamates are the main intracellular and storage form of folate. Folates are required in several biochemical reactions involving single carbon transfer, including synthesis of purines pyrimidines and DNA. The one-carbon fragments may be bound to different sites on the pteridine moiety of tetrahydrofolic acid.

Investigations for Folate Deficiency

Folate Assays

The serum folate and red cell folate are both reduced in folate deficiency. The serum folate reflects current dietary intake whereas the red cell folate is a measure of folate status at the time the cells were formed and is thus a better indication of the body's folate status. The assays are usually done by an immunoassay method although microbiological assays are occasionally used.

Specific Absorption Tests

These are not a routine investigation in folate deficiency and when deficiency has been demonstrated by the assays above attention is directed towards finding the cause.

Causes of Folate Deficiency

Inadequate Intake

Dietary deficiency, anorexia, inability to eat satisfactorily and alcoholism.

Increased Utilization or Loss in Excess of Dietary Availability

Under most circumstances there is adequate folate in the diet to satisfy demands, but sometimes folate stores are low secondary to factors listed above and any increase in demands or urinary loss results in the onset of megaloblastosis. These increased demands include:

- Pregnancy and lactation.
- Prematurity.
- Childhood growth spurts.
- Febrile illnesses.
- Malignancy.
- Acutely ill patients, especially with trauma and/or sepsis.
- Hemolytic anemia and myeloproliferative disease.
- Severe inflammatory disease (especially dermatological).
- Dialysis.
- Homocysteinuria.
- Urinary loss in active liver disease and congestive heart failure.

Malabsorption

In contrast to vitamin B12 deficiency, disorders affecting the upper small bowel are more likely to result in folate deficiency. Again, in contrast to B12 deficiency it is easy to overcome folate malabsorption by swamping the gut with pharmacological doses, whereas this is difficult to do in B12 deficiency due to the transport mechanism involving intrinsic factor and the specific absorption mechanisms in the ileum.

Small bowel disease (especially that affecting the jejunum) may be responsible for folate deficiencies in the following conditions: celiac disease; tropical sprue; bowel resection; Crohn's disease and anticonvulsant therapy (especially phenytoin). Unless the history indicates the cause of malabsorption small bowel investigation is usually indicated.

Treatment of Folate Deficiency

Megaloblastosis due to folate deficiency is a simple condition to treat. In many of the conditions outlined above which may cause folate deficiency prophylactic therapy is warranted. This particularly applies to conditions where there is increased utilization (e.g. pregnancy, malignancies, hemolysis). Whatever the cause of the folate deficiency it will usually respond to pharmacological doses of folic acid (1mg/day), but the underlying cause must be established and if possible corrected. Once the folate stores are replenished a single daily dose is all that is necessary if the underlying cause is not correctable. The parenteral sodium salt of folate may be used in severely ill patients unable to take therapy orally (15 mg/ml).

Megaloblastosis in the Presence of Normal Vitamin B12 and Folate Assays

There are several circumstances in which a patient may have varying degrees of acute or chronic megaloblastosis which is not due to the direct effects of folic acid or vitamin B12 deficiency. Except for antifolate medications which interfere with folate metabolic pathways this is a rare finding and requires specialist investigation. In some circumstances the appearance of erythropoiesis in the bone marrow may be bizarre and not classically megaloblastic and the term megaloblastoid may be used.

Direct Blockade of Folate Metabolism

Methotrexate and aminopterin are powerful inhibitors of the enzyme dihydrofolate reductase.

Pyrimethamine and trimethoprim occasionally produce a mild megaloblastosis, especially in patients with preexisting folate deficiency.

Antimetabolic Drugs

These drugs interfere with DNA synthesis with the effects not being reversible with folic acid: inhibitors of purine synthesis (thioguanine, 6-mercaptopurine and azathioprine), inhibitors of deoxyribonucleotide synthesis (cytosine arabinoside, hydroxyurea).

Interference with Vitamin B12 Metabolism

Prolonged nitrous oxide anesthesia.

Inborn Errors of Metabolism

Hereditary orotic aciduria; rare defects in folate metabolism.

"Unexplained Megaloblastosis"

Megaloblastosis may be found in several circumstances, usually in association with evolving preleukemic or leukemic syndromes: sideroblastic anemias; refractory anemia with dysplastic marrow; erythroleukemia.

Pitfalls in the Diagnosis of Megaloblastic Anemias

Associated Hypochromic-Microcytic Anemia

Any condition impairing the hemoglobinization of red cell precursors may mask to a variable degree the presence of megaloblastosis. These opposing influences on the red cell size may produce confusing red cell indices, requiring careful interpretation. The MCV may be in the normal range despite severe anemia due to a hypochromic microcytic influence being balanced by megaloblastosis. Under these circumstances the MCHC is usually markedly reduced. Hypersegmented neutrophils may be a clue to underlying megaloblastosis.

Sudden Onset

With the normal life span of the red cell being 120 days it will take some weeks for a macrocytic influence to manifest from the point of time that the patient becomes megaloblastic. In contrast the shorter life span of the neutrophil and platelet means acute megaloblastosis may present with neutropenia and thrombocytopenia before a macrocytic anemia has time to evolve.

Confusion with Hemolysis

The ineffective erythropoiesis found in some of the megaloblastic syndromes may be misinterpreted as hemolysis by the unwary. The intramedullary destruction of red cell precursors may give many of the laboratory features of hemolysis.

Low B12 in Severe Folate Deficiency

Relying on Serum Folate Levels for Diagnosis

A red cell folate assay is necessary for definitive diagnosis of megaloblastosis secondary to folate deficiency.

The Nonmegaloblastic Macrocytic Anemias

The myelodysplastic syndromes (see chapter 9) and acquired sideroblastic anemias are commonly misdiagnosed as megaloblastic anemias. An initial partial response to therapy may further confuse the picture.

For technical reasons a low normal B12 level may still be consistent with B12 deficient megaloblastosis.

THE NORMOCYTIC NORMOCHROMIC ANEMIAS

This is the group of anemias where the red cell size and hemoglobinization are not affected, thus the patient presents with anemia, a reduced red cell count, normal MCV, MCH and MCHC. It is this group of anemias which results in the greatest confusion and difficulty in diagnosis. If certain basic questions are addressed in the early stages of investigation a diagnosis is relatively simple to achieve. There are some anemias which usually present as normocytic normochromic, but may in some patients present with mild microcytosis (e.g., the anemia of chronic disease) or macrocytosis (reticulocytosis, aplastic and dyserythropoietic anemias, hypothyroidism, liver disease, alcoholism). Under these circumstances when the clinician is happy that the patient does not have a megaloblastic anemia, on the basis of the clinical setting, other hematological features or the results of bone marrow examination, the further investigations are best approached in line with the normocytic normochromic anemias.

The following questions should be addressed early in the diagnostic process (Fig. 3.10).

Is the Bone Marrow Responding Appropriately to the Anemia?

If there is a reticulocytosis, which will be noted as polychromasia on the blood film, it

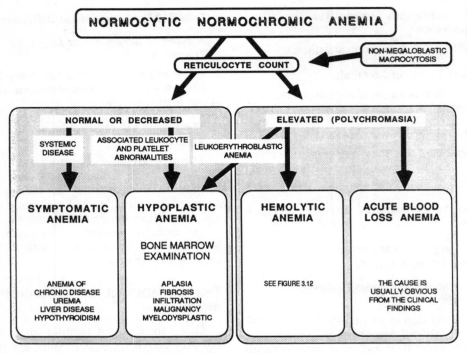

Figure 3.10. Investigation of normocytic normochromic anemia

means there is unlikely to be any abnormality of the bone marrow and microscopic examination is unlikely to be helpful in diagnosis. The only exception is leukoerythroblastic anemia where red and white cell precursors are prematurely released into the peripheral blood. In some cases of sudden blood loss or hemolysis there may not have been time for a reticulocytosis to develop, however, the diagnosis is usually obvious from other clinical or pathological features.

If the Reticulocyte Count Is Normal or Reduced in the Presence of Anemia, Is There Evidence of a Nonhematological Disease Which May Be Responsible for a Symptomatic (Secondary) Anemia?

In all the symptomatic anemias the marrow is suppressed and microscopic examination of a marrow sample is unlikely to give any helpful information. The causes of symptomatic anemia are discussed below.

Are There Associated Alterations in the Leukocytes, Platelets, or Plasma?

If there are quantitative or qualitative abnormalities in the non-red cell elements of the

blood important clues or diagnoses may become apparent, especially in the identification of hematological malignancy or bone marrow dysfunction.

Are There Any Morphological Abnormalities in the Red Cells?

Alterations in red cell shape are especially important in the diagnosis of hemolytic anemia, but may also assist in directing diagnosis towards a dysplastic, fibrotic or infiltrative disorder of the bone marrow.

Are There Any Clinical Features from the History or Physical Findings of the Patient to Suggest Hematological Disease and from What Nonhematological Diseases Does the Patient Suffer?

Abnormal findings in the hemopoietic system may clearly point the clinician towards a primary hematological diagnosis and assist in expediting the appropriate investigations. Clinical features to support the diagnosis of a symptomatic anemia may be present.

Normocytic-Normochromic Anemia with Increased Reticulocyte Count

Where there is evidence that the bone marrow is appropriately responding to the presence of anemia it is most likely that red cells are being lost from the circulation or red cell life span is shortened. If bleeding is occurring into the soft tissues or solid organs the extravasated hemoglobin will be resorbed and handled in the usual manner to produce bilirubin. In such circumstances care must be taken to delineate the anemia from hemolysis.

Blood Loss Anemia

Blood loss occurring at such a rate as to produce a reticulocytosis, while iron stores are still sufficient to support erythropoiesis, will result in a normocytic normochromic anemia. Clearly, there is a limit to such blood loss before iron depletion and the onset of a hypochromic microcytic anemia supervenes. Unless the patient has a psychiatric disturbance, blood loss occurring at such a rate is either clinically obvious to the patient (or his attendants) or produces severe pain. There are the inevitable exceptions which will test even the most astute clinician. Massive occult GIT hemorrhage may not produce an episode of hypotension or it may be missed and the melena may not appear for a day or more. Occasionally, retroperitoneal hemorrhages may be silent in the initial stages and only produce the classical flank hematoma some days later. Probably the commonest "trap" is the trauma patient who may have undiagnosed occult hemorrhage with continuing oozing. With multiple soft tissue injuries patients may not localize pain adequately or there may be a head injury suppressing the level of consciousness.

Hemolytic Anemia

The investigation of hemolytic anemia can be challenging and interesting. Many clinicians see it as "all too complicated" and prefer to refer the patient with the question: Has this patient got a hemolytic anemia? As hemolysis is an important diagnosis to establish and may present in a plethora of clinical settings and in many deceptive ways it does behoove most clinicians to have a basic prob-lem solving approach to the initial assessment. If hemolysis is suspected the following questions need to be addressed.

Are There Any Clinical Features Suggestive of Hemolysis?

- Family history.
- Past history e.g., jaundice, gall stones, leg ulcers.
- Recent history e.g., jaundice, dark urine, pains, Raynaud's phenomenon, shivers and sweats, pyrexia, blood transfusion, drug administration, toxin exposure, envenomation, burns.

Are There Any Laboratory Features of Hemolysis?

Figure 3.11 summarizes the pathways of hemoglobin degradation and the biochemical abnormalities found in hemolysis.

Naked Eye Examination of the Urine and Urine Analysis

Urobilinogen in the urine indicates increase bilirubin turnover. Bilirubinuria indicates conjugated hyperbilirubinemia. Positive testing for "blood" should be further examined. Frank bright red hematuria or "smoky" urine indicates the presence of red cells. Dark "muddy" urine suggests the presence of oxidized hemoglobin or myoglobin. In both circumstances it is desirable to further examine the urine microscopically and biochemically to clarify the situation. The separation of hemoglobinuria from myoglobinuria does need expert knowledge and careful interpretation. Immunoassays are now available for the measurement of minute amounts of myoglobin and hemoglobin in plasma and urine, but these are not readily available.

Naked Eye Inspection of the Plasma

Red or brown plasma in the presence of dark urine is highly suggestive of hemolysis. Clear plasma in the presence of dark urine suggests myoglobinuria. Yellow plasma due to unconjugated hyperbilirubinemia with clear urine suggests hemolysis, whereas yellow plasma with dark urine (frothy shaking) suggests conjugated hyperbilirubinemia.

Blood Film Examinaton

The first suggestion of hemolysis is frequently made on the basis of routine blood

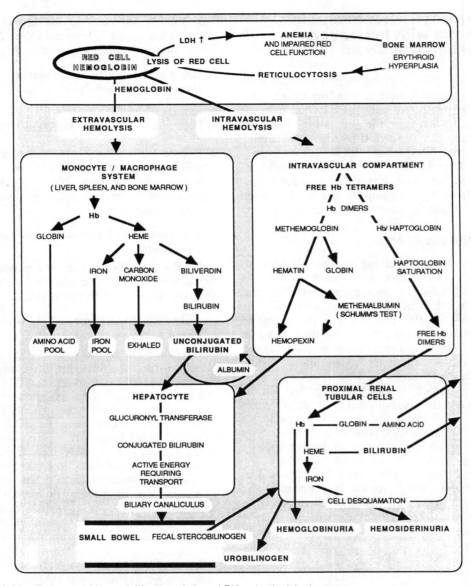

Figure 3.11. Pathways of hemoglobin degradation—LDH = lactic dehydrogenase

film examination. The presence of anemia with polychromasia raises the possibility and any specific red cell changes may be highly suggestive or diagnostic of hemolysis. If there is a question of hemolysis it is always worthwhile asking the hematologist to review the blood film.

Hyperbilirubinemia

If liver and biliary function are normal an unconjugated hyperbilirubinemia occurs in hemolysis and the only real differential diag-

nosis is that of Gilbert's syndrome which is usually a diagnosis of exclusion. The standard teaching that a conjugated hyperbilirubine-mia excludes hemolysis is incorrect. Firstly, the techniques used for measuring conjugated bilirubin are indirect and not truly accurate. A normal person should not have any detect-able conjugated bilirubin present, but up to one third of the bilirubin may appear conju-gated by the methods used in most laboratories.

There are several clinical situations in

which there may be a combination of hemolysis in conjunction with impaired hepatobiliary handling of conjugated bilirubin. The system may thus be stressed by hemolysis with hepatic conjugation proceeding normally, but a buildup occurring at the excretory level. Excluding the obvious biliary obstruction from gall stones (possibly pigment stones in a chronic hemolytic anemia) the commonest defect seen in seriously ill patients (who are high-risk candidates for hemolysis secondary to blood transfusion, drugs, infections etc.) is at the energy-requiring level of the active transport of conjugated bilirubin from the hepatocyte into the biliary canaliculus. Many patients with acute hemolysis are also likely to have impaired bilirubin transport due to the effects of shock or sepsis. Under these circumstances bilirubin from hemolysis will be rapidly conjugated but will have delayed excretion and manifest as a conjugated hyperbilirubinemia.

Reticulocytosis

Reticulocytes are usually expressed as a percentage of the red cells. The count should be corrected to an absolute reticulocyte count by using the red cell count (normal range 20,000–100,000 per mm^3). In acute hemolysis there may not have been time for the bone marrow to respond, as some days are usually necessary for erythropoiesis to increase to a point where the reticulocytosis is manifest in the peripheral blood.

As long as the hematocrit and level of erythropoietin stimulation are normal, the observed reticulocyte percentage may also be considered an index of production (normal reticulocyte production index = 1). With a lower than normal hematocrit level, however, the retic count must first be corrected to a hematocrit of 45 before calculating the reticulocyte production index (RPI). A further correction is required when erythropoietin stimulation results in premature delivery of marrow reticulocytes to circulation ("shift reticulocytes"), since these younger cells require 2 to 3 days to lose their reticulum. With increasing anemia, there is a progressive lengthening of the reticulocyte maturation. The reticulocyte production index may be calculated as follows:

$$\frac{\text{Retic count (\%)} \times \dfrac{\text{Patient's Hematocrit (Hct)}}{45 \text{ (Normal Hct)}}}{\text{Retic Maturation Time}}$$

Example: A patient has a reticulocyte count of 9%, a hematocrit of 25%, and easily visible "shift" red cells (polychromasia) on the peripheral smear.

$$RPI = \frac{9\% \times \dfrac{25}{45}}{2.0} = 2.5\%$$

Elevated Lactic Dehydrogenase (LDH), or Isoenzyme Hydroxybutyric Dehydrogenase (HBDH)

Lactic dehydrogenase is a cytoplasmic enzyme and can be helpful in determining the presence of hemolysis. An isolated marked elevation of LDH with other "profile" enzymes remaining normal (AST, ALT, CPK, ALP) is highly suggestive of red cell destruction (hemolysis or ineffective erythropoiesis). Red cells do not contain mitochondria so the level of other "standard" enzymes for tissue damage (e.g., ALT and AST) which are mitochondrial in origin are normal or only marginally elevated. LDH has five isoenzymes with LD1 being present in red cells. This isoenzyme is also active against hydroxybutyrate and can be measured as HBDH, further helping to identify the origin of the LDH. Muscle (cardiac or skeletal) damage or acute rhabdomyolysis will markedly elevate all enzymes especially the CPK (creatine kinase), thus helping in the differentiation of hemolysis from rhabdomyolysis.

Haptoglobins

This family of hemoglobin binding plasma proteins will be reduced if significant hemolysis is occurring. However, their measurement is not always as helpful as one would like. Haptoglobins are acute phase reactants and may be elevated in infection and inflammation. In contrast they may be rapidly reduced by blood transfusion as a result of nonsurviving stored red cells. If they are present or increased significant hemolysis can be reasonably excluded, but their reduction or absence must be interpreted with caution.

Plasma Hemoglobin

This obvious test would appear to be of logical assistance in diagnosing hemolysis, but it too is susceptible to several measurement and interpretative difficulties. Blood may be hemolyzed during collection and small elevations are probably not of clinical significance.

Schumm's Test

When severe intravascular hemolysis occurs, free hemoglobin is released into the circulation. It initially binds to haptoglobins which are rapidly cleared from the circulation by the liver. This mechanism for clearing hemoglobin is limited and probably not of major functional significance. Haptoglobin probably has a much more important role as a bacteriostat in hematomas. In its tetrameric form free hemoglobin is not filtered by the kidney and accumulates in the blood, splitting into dimers which can be filtered as hemoglobinuria. The hemoglobin molecule in the circulation becomes further oxidized to methemoglobin and the globin chains are separated from the heme molecule. This metheme binds to a protein, hemopexin, which is responsible for its clearance from the circulation and conservation of the iron. When this hemopexin is overloaded the metheme (hematin) binds to albumin to form methemalbumin. The methemalbumin remains in the circulation until hemopexin can complete the clearance.

The Schumm's test is a method for detecting the presence of methemalbumin. In most patients, if other clinical and laboratory data has been carefully analyzed, a positive result should not be a surprise finding. In most patients with a positive Schumm's test the plasma is discolored with a brown appearance. A positive result is sometimes found in severe pernicious anemia and severe hemorrhagic pancreatitis.

Hemosiderinuria

A week after an episode of intravascular hemolysis, or in patients with chronic intravascular hemolysis, examination of the urine with a Prussian Blue stain for iron may confirm the presence of hemosiderinuria. After the dimers of hemoglobin are filtered by the kidney they are resorbed by the proximal tubules and metabolized. The resultant iron can be found in the tubular cells shed into the urine.

Red Cell Survival Studies

The use of radioactive chromium-labelled red cells to demonstrate shortening of red cell life span is rarely needed to establish the diagnosis of hemolysis. In some patients it may be valuable in localizing the site of red cell destruction.

Having Confirmed That Hemolysis Is Present, What Steps Should Be Taken to Establish the Cause?

There are over 50 causes of hemolysis so it is not surprising that the nonexpert (or indeed the expert) may find the investigation of a patient with hemolysis rather daunting. The mechanistic classifications of hemolytic anemia into intracorpuscular, membrane and extracorpuscular have served well in extending our understanding of the causes, but are sometimes a hindrance to clinicians trying to wend their way through the diagnostic maze of complex investigations. The division into intravascular and extravascular may assist to a certain degree, but the overlap may be so great that confusion rather than clarity is produced.

As a result of these mechanistic approaches the clinician has been forced to order investigations in a "poker machine pathology" fashion, in the hope that he will hit the jackpot. To make matters worse he is commonly trying to make a retrospective diagnosis of hemolysis and what could have been the possible causes. The clinician is thus justified in viewing the field of hemolytic anemia as a veritable "mine field" for the unwary.

The author has found that the problem-oriented approach put forward here is workable and results in reduction in the ordering of unnecessary investigations. The system is centered around expert examination of the blood film. This requires close liasion with an experienced medical technologist who understands the diagnostic decision process, or a consultant hematologist who is regularly examining blood smears. If this vital link in the diagnostic chain can be achieved the investigation of hemolytic anemia takes on new dimensions. A certain liberty is taken in broadening the use of the term spherocyte to include all abnormal cells which appear to have lost membrane and are dense hyperchromatic cells. This lost membrane may result in completely spherical spherocytes or irregular fragmented "spherocytes," sometimes referred to as "shistocytes."

What Does the Blood Film Show?

Figure 3.12 summarizes the decision tree in the investigation of hemolytic anemia. Al-

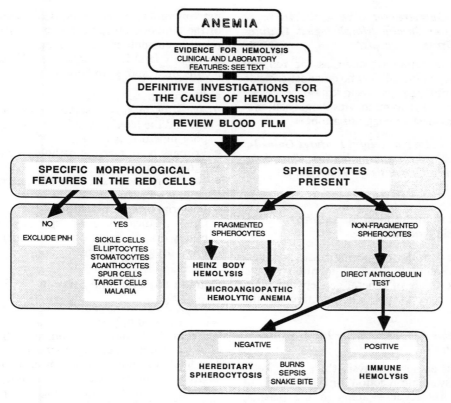

Figure 3.12. Investigation of hemolytic anemia—PNH = paroxysmal nocturnal hemoglobinuria

though the patients don't always have "text-book" findings this general approach will result in the diagnosis of the majority of patients with hemolytic anemia. However, the astute clinician will always weigh up the "diagnostic odds" and pursue alternative approaches when indicated.

Are There Spherocytes Present?

Whatever the cause of hemolysis, the end result is rupture and destruction of the red cell. This rupture involves membrane damage which need not be complete from the outset (except in fulminant intravascular hemolytic reactions) so degrees of development of red cell damage may be observed in the circulating red cells.

If So, Are the Spherocytes Regular or Irregular?

If membrane is lost evenly from the red cell, as seen in hereditary spherocytosis and autoimmune hemolysis, smooth regular hy-perchromic spherocytes will be seen in the blood film.

If the Spherocytes Are Irregular Fragmented Cells, What Are the Specific Morphological Changes?

Red cells have the ability to reseal following rupture resulting in varying shapes of cells (poikilocytosis). If a single intracytoplasmic particle has been removed (usually by the spleen) a cell with a "bite" out of it will result. These are known by several names (Heinz body cells, "moth-eaten" spherocytes, bite cells, drug cells), but essentially the mechanism is the same in most patients (i.e., Heinz body hemolysis) except when the cells are produced as a result of removing malarial parasites. If the fragmented cells result from random red cell damage a heterogeneous collection of irregularly fragmented cells may result. The term microangiopathic hemolytic anemia (MAHA) is used in these circumstances.

If the Cells Are Not Spherocytic, Are There Any Specific Morphological Features to Assist in Diagnosis?

In some hemolytic anemias the red cell morphology in itself may be diagnostic: sickle cells; elliptocytes; pyruvate kinase deficiency "satellite" cells; stomatocytes; target cell; malarial parasites; autoagglutination.

If There Are No Helpful Features Gained From Blood Film Examination, Should the Presumed Diagnosis of Hemolysis Be Reconsidered?

General Management Measures for Hemolytic Anemias

Before considering specific causes and therapy for hemolytic anemia mention should briefly be made of general concepts of management which apply, irrespective of the cause.

Problems Related to Acute Intravascular Hemolysis

During acute hemolysis there may be a marked systemic reaction with activation of several proteolytic systems in the plasma, such as the kinin-kininogen, complement and coagulation systems. A state of shock may occur with the development of prerenal or renal failure. Acute apprehension and pain in the abdomen, chest or back may be severe and lead to the suspicion of other diagnoses. Attention to circulatory perfusion and urinary output is essential and an alkaline diuresis should be established. Disseminated intravascular coagulation should be suspected if hemostatic failure is manifest.

Problems from Increased Bilirubin Load

Pigment gall stones and biliary sludge may result in biliary obstruction.

Factors Affecting the Bone Marrow Response to Shortened Red Cell Survival

Hemolysis places acute or chronic demands on the marrow to produce more red cells. In young and healthy patients this presents no difficulties as long as they are well nourished. There are several factors which may alter the ability of a patient to tolerate acute or chronic hemolysis. The development of acute hemolysis in the context of impaired marrow function or sudden decompensation of the marrow in established hemolysis may result in an acute medical emergency and can be rapidly fatal if not recognized. Factors affecting the response to hemolysis include:

- Rate of onset.
- Age—the marrow reserve diminishes with age and the likelihood of other diseases and poor nutrition is higher.
- Primary bone marrow pathology, e.g., malignant infiltration.
- Nutritional factors, a good diet and supplemental folic acid.
- Bacterial or viral infections.
- Other medical diseases, especially hepatobiliary disease, renal disease, endocrinopathies, drug-induced myelosuppression.

Causes of Hemolytic Anemia

Table 3.3 lists the causes of red cell hemolysis on a pathophysiological basis, but the best route to diagnosis is by pursuing the morphological abnormalities in the blood film. The final common pathway of all hemolytic anemias is the premature disruption of the red cell membrane with hemoglobin release. The outlined classification is centered on the red cell membrane and the mechanism of damage.

The Spherocytic Hemolytic Anemias

Hereditary Spherocytosis (HS)

This is a dominantly transmitted hereditary hemolytic anemia with variable expression of the gene. It is usually suspected after examination of the blood film in the appropriate clinical setting. There is a red cell membrane defect with progressive loss of membrane during the life span of the cell. The nature of the membrane defect remains *sub judice,* but involves the membrane cytoskeleton (spectrin in particular) and it is likely that there will be heterogeneity in relation to the specific molecular causes. The spleen is the main site for this "eating away" at the membrane until the cells are no longer able to survive.

Clinical Features

Patients with HS are commonly asymptomatic and are detected incidentally on a

Table 3.3
A Mechanistic Classification of Hemolysis

Primary disorders of the red cell membrane
  Congenital: Hereditary spherocytosis
              Hereditary stomatocytosis
              Hereditary elliptocytosis
              Blood group deletion syndromes
              Abnormal cation transport syndromes
              Muscular dystrophies
  Acquired: Paroxysmal nocturnal hemoglobinuria
Secondary disorders of the red cell membrane
  Intracytoplasmic defects
  Enzymopathies: Disorders of the pentose phosphate pathway
              e.g., G6PD deficiency, uremia, iron deficiency
              Disorders of the glycolytic pathway
              e.g., PK deficiency, hypophosphatemia
  Globin disorders: Defects of globin structure
              e.g., unstable hemoglobinopathies
              Defects in globin synthesis
              e.g., thalassemias
  Heme disorders: Porphyrias
  Nuclear maturation defects: e.g., megaloblastic anemia
  Extracellular disorders
  Lipid abnormalities: Hereditary acanthocytosis
              Lecithin/cholesterol acyl transferase deficiency
              Liver disease
              Clostridial infection
              Anorexia nervosa
              Vitamin E deficiency
  Immunological destruction: Autoimmune hemolytic anemia
              Transfusion reaction
              Drug induced hemolysis
  Fragmentation syndromes: Cardiac induced hemolysis
              Microangiopathic hemolysis
  Miscellaneous disorders: Infectious agents
              Physical agents
              Drugs, chemicals and venoms

blood count. Common clinical presentations include: neonatal jaundice; episodes of jaundice with infections; leg ulcers; poor exercise tolerance; biliary colic or investigation as a part of a family study. Splenomegaly is a common finding.

Laboratory Features

Blood Count. The red cells are normocytic spherocytes, but hyperchromic with an elevation of the MCHC. Due to the rigidity of the spherocytic red cells and a low 2,3-diphosphoglycerate (DPG), the patient's symptoms of impaired exercise tolerance tend to be greater than the level of hemoglobin would suggest. Such a patient can be significantly hemolyzing with a hemoglobin of 14 gm/dL.

This has resulted in the misapprehension that HS is a well-compensated hemolytic anemia.

Osmotic Fragility and Autohemolysis Studies. These are tests which examine the ability of the red cell to withstand osmotic and metabolic stress. They are not definitive diagnostic tests for hereditary spherocytosis as they may be positive in any spherocytic hemolytic anemia. After 24-hour incubation of red cells a degree of hemolysis occurs which is increased in HS, but correctable with the addition of glucose to the incubation medium.

Family Studies. As there is no definitive test for HS one must rely on demonstrating the defects outlined above in other members of the patient's family. However, if no other family members can be shown to be affected the clinician has to rely on the exclusion of other causes before "labelling" a patient with HS. It may not be long before definitive identification of the molecular membrane defect in the disease is readily available.

Management

Although splenectomy provides a definitive form of therapy, returning the red cell life span towards normal, it should not be performed without due consideration. Chronic anemia, repeated hemolytic episodes, pigment gall stones and leg ulcers would be accepted as indications for splenectomy in any patient over the age of 7 years. Constant lethargy and poor exercise tolerance may also be accepted and the beneficial effects reported through the family by members who have had their spleen removed may encourage others to do likewise. With increasing understanding of splenic function and the risk of the post-splenectomy state a more conservative approach is being taken.

Immune Hemolysis

In the immune hemolytic anemias there is a specific antibody-mediated attack on the red cell membrane. The antibodies involved are usually IgG or IgM and may or may not involve the complement system in mediating their damaging effects. The antibodies may be directed against autoantigens in the red cells (as in autoimmune hemolytic anemia), be alloantibodies directed against transfused red cells or transferred from a mother across the placenta to attack the fetal red cells. They may also be stimulated by exogenous agents (especially medications). The red cells are usually destroyed by the macrophage-monocyte system, in either the liver or the spleen. In rare cases there may be complete activation of the complement system through all its nine components, with direct lysis of the cells in the circulation, without the involvement of the monocyte-macrophage system (see Fig. 3.13).

General Clinical Features

As well as a history suggestive of hemolysis there may be clues to an underlying medical disorder, such as autoimmune or connective tissue disease, hematological malignancy, medications, recent blood transfusion or re-cent infections. Splenomegaly may be found in patients with chronic hemolysis, so there may be physical signs consistent with underlying disease.

Laboratory Features

The laboratory has an important role to play in the investigation, diagnosis and management of immune hemolysis. The correct collection of samples and performance of appropriate tests is critical for a logical analysis of the problem.

Direct Antiglobulin Test (DAT) or Coombs' Test. In this pivotal test for the diagnosis of an immune hemolysis, the patient's red cells are tested for evidence of antibodies or complement on the cell surface. If either can be detected using a Coombs' antiglobulin reagent on washed cells a diagnosis can be made. However, this test does not define the nature or specificity of the immune reaction, which must be interpreted in the light of other clinical and laboratory findings. It is difficult to make a diagnosis of immune red cell damage in the absence of a positive DAT unless there is strong supportive evidence from the clinicopathological findings.

Antibody Screen of the Patient's Serum. The patient's serum should be examined for the presence of antibodies. The nature of the investigations will depend on the suspected diagnostic possibilities. A standard test is the screening of the serum against a panel of group O red cells and reacting the serum with the patient's own cells at various temperatures. This will usually establish if there are any red cell antibodies present. Further tests will be necessary to identify their alloimmune or autoimmune nature and their specificity. The presence of cold agglutinins will raise the possibility of cold autoimmune hemolysis.

Immunological Investigations. Complement levels, plasma protein electrophoresis, immuno-electrophoresis and antinuclear antibodies may all help in the investigation for any underlying cause.

Autoimmune Hemolytic Anemia (AIHA)

The autoimmune hemolytic anemias have provided a prototype of autoimmune disease, which has led the way in our understanding of the pathophysiology of this group of disorders. Many insights gained in these readily

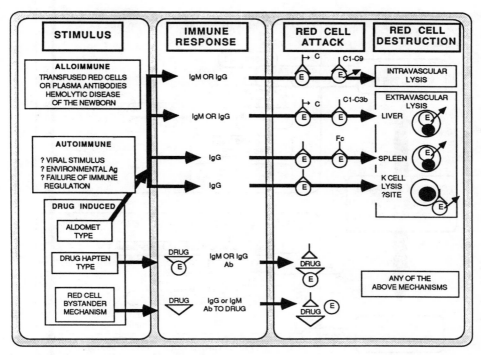

Figure 3.13. Mechanisms of immune red cell destruction—E = erythrocyte; C = complement, Ab = antibody, Fc = Fc end of the immunoglobulin molecule

studied diseases have had far-reaching implications for our understanding of other autoimmune disorders. The autoimmune hemolytic anemias are broadly divided into the warm and cold reacting antibody types, primary or secondary in etiology and acute or chronic in their clinical presentation. Figure 3.14 outlines a classification of autoimmune hemolytic anemia.

Clinical Features

As a general rule the clinical features of autoimmune hemolytic anemia correlate with the in-vitro behavior of the autoantibody. The severity and time course of the hemolysis depends on the lytic ability of the antibody and the rate of appearance, peak level and disappearance from the blood. Unless there is an underlying disease associated with the antibody, cases of autoimmune hemolysis, especially in children, are usually self-limiting and only supportive therapy, including corticosteroid medication, is usually all that is necessary.

History. Possible underlying malignant, autoimmune or infectious disease, especially a recent history of "viral" infection, is common. Recent or concurrent chest infection may be relevant in mycoplasma-induced cold AIHA.

Examination. Features of hemolysis as above, splenomegaly, evidence of associated infectious, autoimmune or malignant disease.

Management

Acute Supportive Therapy. Some patients with AIHA may have a fulminant clinical presentation and intensive supportive therapy may be needed. Adequate hydration, warmth and attention to renal function are important. Blood transfusion may be necessary and present serological difficulties for the blood transfusion laboratory. It is usually safe to transfuse with the most compatible blood available. Blood should not be withheld from a profoundly anemic patient on the basis of crossmatch incompatibility. As long as ABO compatible blood is administered the transfusion may be life saving. Occasionally plasma exchange therapy may be indicated. Under some circumstances the management of patients with AIHA can be extremely com-

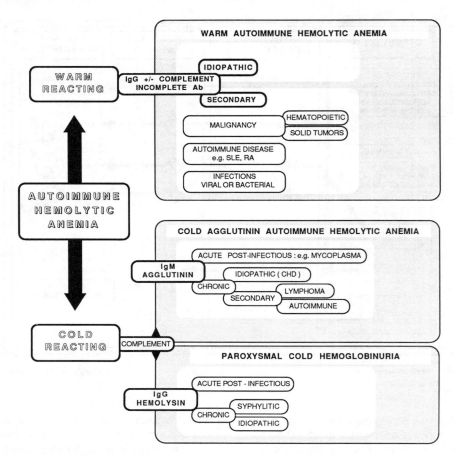

Figure 3.14. Classification of autoimmune hemolytic anemia—Ab = antibody

plex and referral to a specialized unit is essential.

Corticosteroids. Corticosteroids are the mainstay of therapy for AIHA of the warm antibody type. They act by suppressing phagocytosis and by their immunosuppressive effect. In general they only need to be used in the short-term, especially if the disease is self-limiting. If the disease is chronic, attempts should be made to use the lowest doses possible, using cytotoxic immunosuppressive therapy if necessary or resorting to splenectomy. Corticosteroids are not effective in the cold AIHA syndromes unless there is an underlying lymphoproliferative disease.

Other Immunosuppressive Therapy. If the hemolysis cannot be controlled with corticosteroids alone drugs such as alkylating agents (cyclophosphamide, chlorambucil) or azathioprine may be used.

Splenectomy. It is uncommon to require splenectomy for the control of AIHA. It should only be done after a good trial of therapy as outlined above. The presence of massive splenomegaly in association with a lymphoproliferative disease can be considered an exception warranting early splenectomy.

Monitoring. Regular monitoring for control of hemolysis and the possibility of an underlying disease manifesting itself is important.

Specific AIHA Syndromes

Paroxysmal Cold Hemoglobinuria. This is a rare form of AIHA generally occurring in children and used to be due to congenital syphilis in many patients. The antibody (Donath-Landsteiner) is unusual in that it is an IgG biphasic hemolysin which reacts at low temperatures and firmly fixes complement. On warming, there is a violent intravascular hemolysis. This syndrome remains rare, but these days is more commonly related to childhood viral infections.

Chronic Cold Hemagglutinin Disease. This is a syndrome of the older age group in which there is a cold-reacting IgM red cell agglutinin which causes acral cyanosis and Raynaud's phenomenon when the patient is exposed to the cold. In a small percentage of patients it is associated with an underlying lymphoma. Unless there is a lymphoma, the condition can be difficult to treat and avoidance of exposure to cold is the most important advice one can give. Alkylating cytotoxic agents are usually worth a trial.

Evan's Syndrome. This is the association of warm autoimmune hemolytic anemia and immune thrombocytopenia.

Alloimmune Hemolysis

Alloimmune hemolysis occurs whenever patients receive red cells against which there is an antibody in their plasma. It may also occur if an antibody is infused in plasma or crosses the placenta. The former is most commonly observed with an incompatible blood transfusion reaction and the latter in hemolytic disease of the newborn. The laboratory investigations are similar to those outlined for autoimmune hemolysis except that the interpretation is different in the light of the clinical and laboratory features.

Hemolytic Transfusion Reactions

There are several mechanisms by which blood may be hemolyzed in relation to a blood transfusion. Most of them are obvious and can be avoided if the appropriate precautions are taken. The most important, from the immune point of view, are the immediate or delayed incompatible red cell transfusions where the patient's plasma contains a preexisting antibody (immediate transfusion reaction) or develops one after the transfusion (delayed transfusion reaction).

There are several mechanisms by which blood may be hemolyzed before or after transfusion including:

Immune Destruction
Donor red cell serological incompatibility:
(a) Acute incompatible blood transfusion

(b) Delayed transfusion reaction
High titer hemolysin in donor plasma
Interdonor incompatibility
Destruction of donor cells without detectable antibodies.

Nonimmune Destruction
Transfusion of incorrectly stored or outdated blood
Inadvertently frozen blood
Overheated blood
Infected blood
Mechanical destruction, e.g., infusion under pressure.

Acute Hemolytic Transfusion Reaction

In most immediate immune-mediated transfusion reactions serological incompatibility can be demonstrated if the pretransfusion tests are reassessed and most errors that occur are of a clerical nature. The most dreaded incompatibility is that involving the ABO system as they may cause massive, life-threatening, intravascular hemolysis and disseminated intravascular coagulation. As the anti-A and anti-B are naturally occurring antibodies in the plasma of group O (anti-A and anti-B), group A (anti-B) and group B (anti-A) individuals, ABO compatibility must always be adhered to if these reactions are to be avoided. Strict attention to detail at each point in the blood supply chain is essential. Group-specific blood should be used wherever possible for transfusions with the saline agglutination test remaining the best test for confirming ABO compatibility before transfusion. Most other antibodies responsible for acute transfusion reaction are stimulated by previous transfusions or pregnancy and are usually detected on the antibody screening of the patient's pretransfusion serum specimen.

Delayed Hemolytic Transfusion Reaction

A delayed hemolytic transfusion reaction is defined as one occurring some hours or days after homologous blood transfusion where the blood was serologically compatible on cross-matching at the time of transfusion. An alloantibody has manifest itself after the transfusion. Unless it is realized that a transfusion has been given in the recent past the clinical and laboratory findings may be interpreted as indicating the presence of an autoimune hemolytic anemia.

Drug-induced Immune Hemolysis

There are several mechanisms by which medications may be responsible for immune-mediated hemolysis. The diagnosis of drug-induced immune hemolysis should be entertained in any patient in whom immune hemolysis is diagnosed. It is only by careful assessment of the drug history of all patients that this potentially remediable form of hemolysis will be appropriately diagnosed. There are mechanisms for immune-mediated, drug-induced hemolysis.

The Drug Adsorption (Hapten) Mechanism

(penicillin, cephalosporins, insulin)
The drug is adsorbed onto the red cell membrane surface and the antibody is directed against the drug on the cell.

The Immune Complex (Innocent Bystander) Mechanism

(stibophen, quinidine, ibuprofen, sulfonamides, some antituberculous drugs, chlorpromazine, tetracycline)
The drug and antibody form an immune complex which adsorbs onto the red cell surface. As a result of the adsorption and associated complement fixation the cell is lysed.

Membrane Modification (Nonimmunologic Protein Adsorption) Mechanism

(cephalosporins)
The drug modifies the red cell membrane so that normal plasma proteins are adsorbed nonimmunologically. While this mechanism will give a positive DAT, it has not been associated with hemolysis.

The Alpha-Methyldopa Mechanism

(alpha methyldopa, mefenamic acid, L-dopa, chlordiazepoxide)
The drug stimulates the production of autoantibodies to red cell antigens, especially the rhesus system. This probably occurs as a result of the drug affecting immunoregulation.

Heinz Body Hemolytic Anemias

This is a group of hemolytic anemias in which the hemoglobin molecule is oxidized and "falls apart" in the red cell. A final product of this oxidation process is the precipitation of insoluble aggregates of degraded hemoglobin (Heinz bodies), leading to lysis of the red cell. These refractile particles attach to and rigidify the red cell membrane. On subsequent passage through the spleen these alterations in the red cell are detected by the splenic macrophages as the cells pass from the cords into the splenic sinuses and the Heinz bodies are removed. This results in the production of the "bite" spherocytes. The resultant cells have a limited life span, the older cells dying first. The hemoglobin molecule and cell membrane may become oxidized by 3 mechanisms (Fig. 3.15).

Enzyme Defects in Aerobic Glycolysis

Faulty reductive capacity of the red cell due to enzyme deficiency in the hexose monophosphate shunt (HMS) or the glutathione pathways impair the red cell's ability to handle normal and abnormal oxidant stresses. The red cell is constantly exposed to stresses which oxidize hemoglobin and certain vital sulfydryl groups in the membrane. The HMS provides the major reductive capacity of the normal red cell. Defects in this system will expose the red cell and the hemoglobin molecule to intolerable oxidative influences. The red cell has several mechanisms for dealing with oxidizing species such as, superoxides and hydrogen peroxide, which have the potential to lyse the red cell. Superoxide dismutase is the main defense against superoxide (O^-_2). The H_2O_2 produced can be eliminated by catalase, but the main mechanism is the glutathione antioxidant system. Reduced glutathione (GSH) is oxidized to the disulfide form (GSSG) in the process of converting H_2O_2 to water. NADPH is necessary for the reduction of GSSG back to GSH for the process to continue. Glucose-6-phosphate dehydrogenase (G6PD) catalyzes the first step in the HMP shunt resulting in the reduction of NADP to NADPH to produce the only NADPH in the red cell. Deficiency of this enzyme is the most frequent cause of Heinz body hemolysis and is also the commonest known enzyme deficiency.

G6PD Deficiency. This is a heterogenous group of disorders with as many as 250 variants known. There are two forms of G6PD which are regarded as normal, the commonest—the B form—is found in the majority of

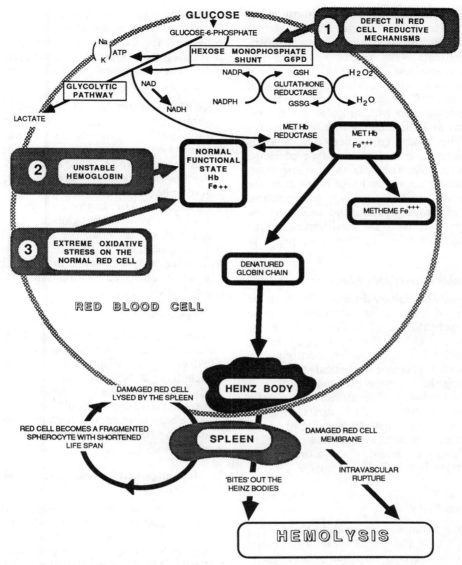

Figure 3.15. Mechanisms of Heinz body hemolysis—G6PD = glucose-6-phosphate dehydrogenase; GSH = glutathione; GSSG = oxidized glutathione; ATP = adenosine triphosphate; NAD = nicotinamide adenine dinucleotide; NADP = nicotinamide adenine dinucleotide phosphate

people and the A form in some Africans. The clinical severity is usually classified on the basis of enzyme activity.

- Class I $<10\%$ enzyme activity—life-long hemolysis
- Class II $<10\%$ enzyme activity—acute episodes of hemolysis
- Class III 10% to 60% enzyme activity—episodic hemolysis on exposure to oxidant agents
- Class IV Normal—interest to geneticists

The variable expression of the G6PD variants leads to a wide spectrum of hemolytic syndromes that range from mild hemolysis to severe life-threatening neonatal jaundice. Any of the variants are susceptible to varying degrees of acute intravascular hemolysis in association with oxidant chemicals or drugs (see Appendix 2), infectious episodes or acidosis. Most patients with G6PD deficiency are asymptomatic until stressed. The classical Mediterranean variant, which is the cause of favism in children exposed to fava beans, may be associated with more severe clinical problems and the enzyme levels are usually lower. The African type, referred to as A⁻, is more likely to give a chronic type of Heinz body hemolysis. The African type also characteristically has normal G6PD levels in the reticulocytes and the episode of hemolysis will be self-limiting even if the insult persists. This is in contrast to the Mediterranean type in which cells of all ages are susceptible to lysis.

Unstable Hemoglobin Molecule

There are hereditary disorders in which the hemoglobin tetramer is inherently unstable due to substitution of amino acids in the alpha or beta chains, introducing hydrophilic amino acids into the interior, modifying the heme pocket, affecting the helical structure or modifying the interface between the alpha-1 and beta-1 subunits. The molecule thus has a constant tendency to "fall apart" spontaneously or on the slightest exposure to an oxidant stress. The same unstable state occurs in HbH disease, a variant of alpha thalassemia in which the beta-4 HbH is unstable.

Drug or Toxin Oxidation of an Otherwise Normal Red Cell

There is a limit to the oxidant stress a red cell can handle and a total breakdown is seen in such conditions as moth ball poisoning and in relation to certain drugs. The sulfonamides have a particularly bad name in this respect, especially sulfasalazine and dapsone. The reason for this probably relates to the slow metabolic acetylator status of some patients.

Laboratory Investigations for Heinz Body Hemolysis

Blood Film. The typical fragmented "bite cell" spherocytes are found on the blood film during and after hemolytic episodes.

Heinz Body Test. Supravital staining of Heinz bodies using a wet preparation confirms the pathogenic mechanism of hemoly-sis, but does not determine the basic red cell defect. As most of the Heinz bodies are removed by the spleen they may be difficult to find unless the sample is collected early in hemolysis or when splenic function is saturated.

Specific Tests for the Cause.
- G6PD screening test and a specific assay should be performed when the patient is not hemolyzing, as reticulocytes may have normal or adequate enzyme levels for normal function and it is the older cells which are low in enzyme that are the most sensitive to hemolysis.
- Heat stability or isopropanol precipitation tests for unstable hemoglobin.
- Methemoglobinemia.
- Hemoglobin electrophoresis.
- Test for acetylator status may be helpful if a cause cannot be identified and a drug is implicated.

Management

Identify precipitants and avoid them in the future; this especially applies to drugs (see Appendix 2). In patients commencing drugs which have a high association with Heinz body hemolysis, such as sulfasalazine or dapsone, the blood count should be checked one week after commencing therapy. Infections should be rapidly identified and treated expeditiously.

Microangiopathic Hemolytic Anemia (MAHA)

Red cells may be irregularly fragmented under several circumstances and the finding of these microangiopathic changes on the peripheral blood film is of considerable diagnostic value. MAHA was originally described in relation to defective prosthetic cardiac valves causing red cell trauma. However, this is a relatively uncommon cause and most patients with MAHA have evidence of a disease in which the basic pathophysiology is occurring in the microvasculature, due to alteration in the endothelium or the deposition of fibrin.

Clinical Features

As this group of disorders may affect a variety of microvascular beds alone or in combination, a wide spectrum of clinical pictures may result, with severity ranging from mild chronic disease to life-threatening fulminant syndromes. Hemolytic anemia is a variable feature depending on the degree and rate of red cell fragmentation.

Laboratory Features

The peripheral blood may demonstrate the following features:

- Fragmentation of the red cells with schistocytes and "helmet" cells, polychromasia and, in some cases, thrombocytopenia.
- Evidence of hemolysis.
- There may be laboratory features of disseminated intravascular coagulation.

Clinical Syndromes Associated with MAHA

Disorders which may be associated with microangiopathic hemolytic anemia are:

Hemolytic uremic syndrome (HUS)
Thrombotic thrombocytopenic purpura (TTP)
Malignant hypertension and toxemia of pregnancy
Vascular malformations
Autoimmune disorders—arteritis and vasculitis, Wegener's granulomatosis
Hemorrhagic fevers
Malignancy
Disseminated intravascular coagulation
Cardiac and large vessel diseases—prosthetic valves, patches and occasionally valvular lesions and congenital heart defects.

As MAHA is not a disease in its own right the diagnosis of the underlying cause is a major aspect in management. The cause may or may not be reversible or self-limiting in the short or long term and supportive therapy, plus therapy directed at some of the possible pathophysiological mechanisms outlined in relation to TTP may be warranted.

Thrombotic Thrombocytopenic Purpura (TTP)

This is a rare disorder of uncertain etiology, but probably has a range of different causes and pathophysiological mechanisms. The essential features are a microangiopathy affecting primarily the cerebral circulation and gut, with variable involvement of the kidney, lung and liver. Hemolysis and thrombocytopenia with severe hemostatic failure oc-

curs. The prognosis has improved in recent years, but it remains unclear as to which modalities of therapy are most important. In fulminant cases a combination of multiple therapies including corticosteroids, antiplatelet therapy, heparin, fresh frozen plasma, fresh blood, plasma exchange, dextran, prostacyclin and splenectomy may be used. A chronic relapsing form also exists.

Hemolytic Uremic Syndrome (HUS)

This syndrome has many similarities to TTP but renal involvement is the hallmark in association with MAHA and thrombocytopenia. It usually occurs in children, but may rarely be seen in adults. The prognosis and approach to management are similar to TTP.

Other Red Cell Fragmentation Anemias

Red cell fragmentation may also be seen in march hemoglobinuria, karate hemolysis and burns. In each of these the history provides the relevant information.

Nonspherocytic Hemolytic Anemias

If there is no suggestion of spherocytosis on the blood film any specific morphological changes in the red cells should be examined for and appropriate investigations requested.

There are several hemolytic anemias due to hereditary defects in the red cell membrane, the hemoglobin molecule or enzyme deficiencies which may be diagnosed by specific morphological alterations in the red cells on the blood film. In some instances there are specific tests to confirm the diagnosis, in others the diagnosis depends on the morphological features, sometimes in conjunction with a family history.

Sickle Cell Disease and Trait

Sickle cell disease results from the homozygous inheritance of an abnormal hemoglobin in which a glutamic acid in the beta-chain is replaced by valine. This was one of the first molecular diseases to be recognized. The solubility of hemoglobin is defective with precipitation occurring when the cell is exposed to a hypoxic or acid environment. The aggregates form in fibrils which distort the cells into the typical sickle shape. Initially this sickling is reversible on reoxygenation, but eventually becomes irreversible with the cells being hemolyzed (Fig. 3.16).

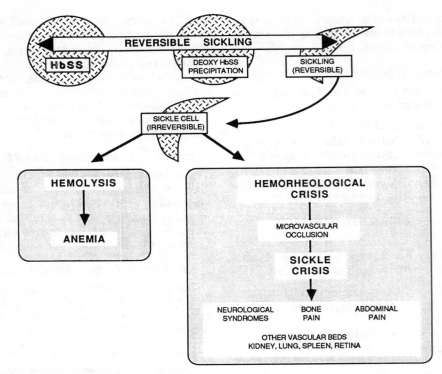

Figure 3.16. Pathophysiology of sickle cell disease

Clinical Features. Symptoms appear after 6 months when hemoglobin S is in full production. The presence of HbF tends to protect the patient against sickle cell crises.

- Anemia: hemolytic crisis, aplastic crisis, splenic sequestration, nutritional deficiency (especially folate).
- Microvascular occlusive crises: splenic, bone marrow, gut, retinal, leg ulcers, renal papillary necrosis, pulmonary.
- Bone and joints: aseptic necrosis of femoral head, dactylitis, osteomyelitis.
- Gall stones.

Laboratory Findings

- Normocytic normochromic anemia, anisocytosis, poikilocytosis, polychromasia, target cells and the diagnostic sickle cells. In older children and adults the features of splenic atrophy may be found. Sickle cell trait usually has a normal blood film and can only be diagnosed by performing the screening test.
- Sickle cell screening test gives positive results.
- Hemoglobin electrophoresis: HbS and var-

iable amounts of HbF in homozygous disease; in sickle cell trait HbS band of 35% to 50% and a normal HbA band.
- Various combinations of HbS with other hemoglobinopathies or thalassemia may give clinical syndromes of variable clinical severity. These include: HbS + hereditary persistence of HbF, various HbS-thalassemia interactions, HbS/C disease. Most of these need expert investigation to clarify their true nature. Knowledge of the genotype is important in genetic counselling. High HbF levels tend to protect the red cells from sickling.
- Prenatal diagnosis is possible using DNA probes to detect HbSS.

Management. Prophylaxis against sickle cell crisis:

- Hypovolemia, hypoxia, dehydration, acidosis and exposure to cold should be avoided.
- Early diagnosis and treatment of infection.
- Preoperative hypertransfusion or red cell exchange prior to elective surgery or during pregnancy. Hyperoxygenation or hyper-

baric oxygen may help in surgical emergencies.

- Screening for the heterozygous state in high-risk racial groups.
- Prophylactic folic acid therapy.

Therapy of sickle cell crisis:

Close attention to adequate cardiopulmonary function and peripheral perfusion. This is best achieved with good hydration, warming, oxygen therapy, correction of acidosis, blood transfusion or exchange transfusion if indicated. Infection should be sought and treated and nutritional support and vitamin supplements should be given (especially folic acid). Various drugs have been advocated, including urea and potassium cyanate, but without convincing evidence of their efficacy. Aplastic crises may occur which have recently been identified as being associated with parvovirus infection in a high proportion of patients.

Other Abnormal Hemoglobinopathies

Numerous target cells may suggest Hb C or E disease which is confirmed by hemoglobin electrophoresis.

Hereditary Elliptocytosis. Mild autosomal dominant disease.

Hereditary Stomatocytosis. Heterogeneous group of disorders which may be associated with mild thrombocytopenia.

Hereditary Acanthocytosis. Autosomal recessive disorder with malabsorption, retinitis pigmentosa and peripheral neuropathy due to a-betalipoproteinemia.

Spur Cell Anemia in Severe Liver Disease. See symptomatic anemias.

Malaria. Malaria is diagnosed and typed by peripheral blood examination. It may be noted or diagnosed on the normal blood smear, but thick preparations appropriately stained are more accurate.

If there are no features on the blood film indicating a definite or possible diagnosis for the cause of a hemolytic anemia expert consultation is advisable as numerous rare and complex disorders may need to be considered.

Enzyme Defects in Anaeorobic Glycolysis: Embden Myerhoff Pathway Pyruvate Kinase (PK) Deficiency

Pyruvate kinase deficiency is the commonest red cell enzyme defect after G6PD deficiency, but deficiency of hexokinase, triose phosphate isomerase (TPI) and phosphoglycerate kinase (PGK) may rarely occur. PK deficiency is an autosomal recessive disorder which may be due to a heterogeneous variety of defects in qualitative or quantitative enzyme function. The deficiency causes a non-spherocytic hemolytic anemia but occasional "spikey" spherocytic red cells may be seen on the blood film ("satellite cells"). The 2,3-DPG level is elevated secondary to the metabolic block, resulting in a right shift in the oxygen dissociation curve and the patient has less symptoms of anemia than would normally be expected for the degree of anemia. The hemolysis shows considerable variation in severity. Unless the typical cells are seen in the peripheral blood there are no diagnostic clinical or laboratory features. The patients usually have a chronic compensated hemolysis. The autohemolysis test yields abnormal results, with no correction with added glucose, but correction with ATP. Screening tests are available as are quantitative enzyme assays.

Rare Hereditary Red Cell Enzyme Defects

Hypersplenism. Discussed in chapter 8.

Paroxysmal Nocturnal Hemoglobinuria (PNH)

PNH is a rare disorder which stimulates an inordinate amount of interest from hematologists and some would argue that it provides the wealth of clinical features and system involvement that diabetes does for the endocrinologist, syphilis for the infectious disease physician and systemic lupus erythematosus for the immunologist. The basic pathophysiology of this acquired disorder remains an enigma, but there appears to be a clonal red cell membrane defect in which the cells are excessively sensitive to complement lysis, especially at low pH.

Clinical Features. A variety of clinical features may be seen with PNH overlapping with other hematological syndromes.

- Episodes of hemolysis with hemoglobinuria, usually worse at night. Hemolysis may be precipitated by infections, vaccinations, blood transfusions or iron injections.
- Venous thrombosis, including atypical sites such as mesenteric, cerebral and hepatic veins.

- Pain syndromes of unknown etiology: abdomen and back.

  Laboratory Features

- Blood film does not show any specific features.
- Evidence of intermittent hemolysis.
- Hemosiderinuria, which may lead to iron deficiency.
- Pancytopenia in some patients or isolated cytopenias.
- Bone marrow may be hypoplastic, sideroblastic, dysplastic or show evidence of evolving leukemia.
- Positive result on Ham's test or sucrose lysis test.

  Management

- Transfusion as necessary. Reactions may be a problem and specially prepared, leukocyte-poor blood may be necessary.
- Treat iron deficiency.
- Treatment for aplastic anemia may be indicated, including bone marrow transplantation in selected patients.
- Treatment of venous thrombosis as necessary.

Pitfalls in the Diagnosis of Hemolytic Anemia

There are many traps in the diagnosis of hemolytic anemia for both the inexperienced and experienced alike.

The Association with Hepatobiliary Disease

As already mentioned, the presence of a cholestatic hyperbilirubinemia does not exclude the diagnosis of hemolysis but may in some cases be the clue to diagnosis.

Hyperbilirubinemia Secondary to Nonhemolytic Causes

Ineffective erythropoiesis due to intramedullary death of red cell precursors may give many of the peripheral blood features of hemolysis, except the reticulocytes are reduced. Pernicious anemia, dyserythropoietic anemias, thalassemias and sideroblastosis may cause this picture. Resorption of hematoma, especially if the hemorrhage has been occult (e.g., retroperitoneal, fractures and other trauma) may also masquerade as hemolysis.

Hemolytic Anemia without Reticulocytosis

Hemolysis may be of sudden onset before the marrow has had time to respond. Bone marrow failure due to associated or unrelated cause (e.g., aplastic crisis, malignant infiltration, folate deficiency) will prevent reticulocytosis.

Hemolysis Where Reticulocytes Are Also Affected

In most hemolytic anemias the reticulocytes are relatively protected from hemolysis, but occasionally they suffer the same rapid fate as older red cells, sometimes seen in autoimmune hemolytic anemia.

Failure of the Definitive Test to Confirm the Diagnosis

Clinicians are sometimes surprised how difficult it may be to firmly establish the cause of a hemolytic anemia when there are so many sophisticated tests available. In some hemolytic diseases it is essential that the tests be performed at the time of hemolysis. In other cases the tests will only be diagnostic when hemolysis is not occurring. The effects of transfusion should never be forgotten. Consultative help is necessary if the tests "don't make sense."

Retrospective Diagnosis of Hemolysis

It may sometimes be necessary to pursue a retrospective diagnosis of a hemolytic episode. This may be extremely difficult, but there are some laboratory investigations that may help.

- Alterations in retrospective biochemical profiles performed for other reasons—bilirubin, LDH.
- Reduced haptoglobins.
- Hemosiderinuria.
- Hemoglobin casts in the urine or on renal biopsy.
- Hemolytic red cell changes in the blood film (spherocytes or fragmented cells).
- The appearance of an alloantibody after a blood transfusion.

Normocytic Normochromic Anemias with Normal or Reduced Reticulocyte Counts

When a patient has an established normocytic normochromic anemia in which there is

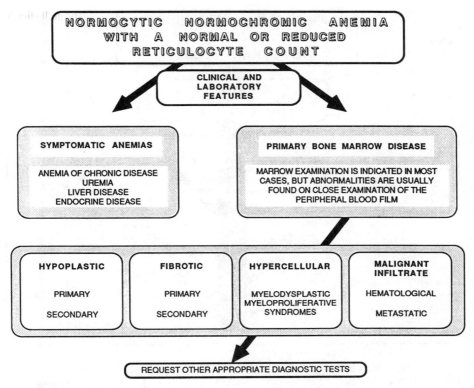

Figure 3.17. Investigation of normocytic-normochromic anemia with normal or reduced reticulocytes

inadequate or no marrow response to the anemia it can be concluded that the marrow is suppressed by either external factors, as seen in the symptomatic anemias, or there is primary marrow failure. Leukoerythroblastic anemia is an exception to this principle in that the blood film is polychromatic and the reticulocyte count increased due to premature marrow release of red cells, despite the fact that the marrow is failing or has decreased reserve. In this group of anemias a bone marrow examination is usually indicated after the symptomatic (secondary) anemias have been identified (Fig. 3.17).

Symptomatic Anemias

Sometimes known as secondary anemias there are several normocytic normochromic anemias included in this category. A bone marrow examination is not usually necessary, and indeed is unhelpful for their identification as there are clinical and laboratory features present which should alert the clinician to the diagnosis. A degree of overlap may occur with the microcytic anemias in the case of the anemia of chronic disease and the macrocytic anemias in the case of hypothyroidism and liver disease.

The Anemia of Chronic Disease

The anemia of chronic disease would be the second commonest anemia seen on a worldwide basis, but probably the commonest in a general medical and surgical hospital population of patients. The anemia of chronic disease is not a primary diagnosis in its own right, but normal secondary response to disease elsewhere in the body. The anemia of chronic disease is a component of the acute/chronic phase response and is discussed in chapter 10. There are numerous reactive changes which occur in the blood in response to infectious, inflammatory or malignant disease which are all part of the host defense and healing mechanisms of the human body. Mild anemia is part of this reaction and should be regarded as normal for the clinical setting and not to be "corrected." There is some evidence that the development of anemia in this setting

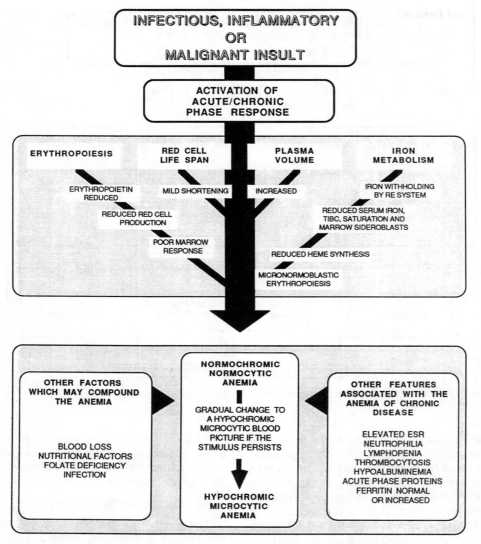

Figure 3.18. Pathophysiology of the anemia of chronic disease—TIBC = total iron binding capacity

is a compensatory mechanism to ensure fluidity of the blood is maintained during a time when numerous cellular and humoral changes in the acute phase response may work to the contrary. The importance of the anemia of chronic disease is threefold:

- Correct recognition to avoid inappropriate diagnosis and treatment, especially an incorrect diagnosis of iron deficiency.
- As a hematological clue to occult infectious, inflammatory or malignant disease somewhere in the body.

- As it is commonly associated with other causes of anemia it is important to recognize the multifactorial nature of the problem.

The pathophysiological mechanisms include a combination of the following (Fig. 3.18):

- Reduced erythropoiesis, reduced erythropoietin.
- RES iron withholding.
- Mildly shortened red cell life span.
- Mild plasma volume expansion.

Clinical Features

The anemia of chronic disease occurs in association with any condition in which there is a systemic reaction to an infection, inflammation or malignancy. The patient may have pointers in the history to the likely location or nature of the problem, but on the other hand the detection of the anemia and associated hematological changes may be the first finding to alert the clinician to the presence of organic disease of this nature. Having established a diagnosis of the anemia of chronic disease the clinician should extend investigations to establish the cause, primarily with the aim of excluding serious and treatable conditions. It is not uncommon for the search for a cause to be unsuccessful and a self-limiting disease resolves.

Laboratory Investigation

Hematology. In most patients the blood examination reveals a normocytic normochromic anemia, but if the underlying disease has been developing for several weeks or months a microcytic hypochromic element may be found and differentiation from iron deficiency is essential, and may be difficult in the first instant.

- Elevated ESR due to hyperfibrinogenemia or polyclonal hypergammaglobulinemia.
- Ferritin is normal or commonly increased due to tissue damage or malignancy.
- Neutrophilia, lymphopenia, thrombocytosis.
- Bone marrow examination usually shows reactive nondiagnostic changes with normal or increased iron stores and reduced or absent sideroblasts. Occasionally a specific cause may be found (e.g., metastatic malignant cells, granulomas), but in general the bone marrow examination is unhelpful and should only be performed when specifically indicated. It is common to recommend culture of the marrow, but this in the author's experience is unlikely to yield additional information.

Biochemistry

- Reduced serum iron with normal or reduced transferrin (TIBC).
- Mild reductions in albumin.
- Slight hyponatremia.

- LDH may be elevated if there is significant tissue damage.
- Plasma protein electrophoresis may show changes consistent with acute/chronic phase reaction, i.e., albumin reduced, elevation of alpha-2 and beta globulins and sometimes polyclonal hypergammaglobulinemia.

The Search for a Cause

If the patient's history and clinical findings do not alert the clinician to the underlying diagnosis (e.g., rheumatoid arthritis, bacterial infections, carcinoma) a detective approach is commonly necessary, but should be performed in a systematic fashion. Review of the history and physical examination should be done before detailed costly and invasive investigations are requested. Careful checking for fever, review of the chest X-ray, and urine examination are simple investigations which will establish the cause in a high proportion of patients. Investigation of the acute and chronic phase response, fever of unknown origin and elevation of the ESR may follow similar lines (see chapters 10 and 11). The conditions likely to present with the anemia of chronic disease with minimal or subtle clinical findings include:

Infectious Diseases

- TB, brucellosis, mycoplasma, endocarditis, urinary tract infection, abscesses (e.g., lung, renal, liver).

Inflammatory Diseases

- Autoimmune disease—SLE, Sjogren's syndrome, systemic vasculitis, temporal arteritis, polymyalgia rheumatica, polyarteritis nodosa.

Allergic Diseases

- Extrinsic allergic alveolitis, drug reactions.

Diseases of Unknown Cause

- Hereditary Mediterranean fever, sarcoidosis.

Malignant Disorders

- Hematological—especially Hodgkin's disease and macrophage-monocytic system malignancy.
- Solid Tumors—especially intra-abdominal (such as stomach, cecum, pancreas, liver,

cholangiocarcinoma, hypernephroma) lung, cardiac atrial myxomas.

Management

There is no effective specific therapy for the anemia of chronic disease and, for the reasons outlined above, therapy may be counterproductive. Diagnosis and treatment of the cause will lead to resolution of the anemia. There are several factors which may lead to accentuation of the anemia to the point that treatment may be necessary. Associated nutritional deficiency may be present in relation to the underlying disease (especially folic acid). Excessive blood sampling or occult bleeding should always be borne in mind, especially if there is associated iron deficiency present. As the bone marrow is suppressed it is unable to respond to any additional insults and blood transfusion is likely to be required if sudden hemorrhage occurs, surgery is undertaken or complicating infection is a problem.

Uremia

Patients with chronic renal failure usually develop anemia when their creatinine is above 3.4mg/dL or when the GFR is less than 25% of normal. There is generally a good correlation between the degree of uremia and the hemoglobin level. A combination of factors is responsible, including bone marrow suppression from uremic toxins, deficiency of erythropoietin from reduced renal mass, shortened red cell survival and in some patients plasma volume expansion. Other factors may contribute to the anemia which are either specific for the disease state (e.g., hemolytic uremic syndrome), related to nutrition (e.g., folic acid), related to associated disease (e.g., blood loss), related to therapy (e.g., immunosuppression) or dialysis (e.g., aluminium). In the case of the specific anemia of uremia, dialysis is the only effective therapy and otherwise transfusion may be warranted.

Liver Disease

The anemia in liver disease is usually macrocytic MCV (100 to 110fl). The red cells are normochromic and "thin" round macrocytes are seen on the blood film. Target cells are prominent and if there is severe liver failure spur cells may be seen. Other causes of macrocytosis may be seen in conjunction with liver disease, such as alcohol, or folate deficiency. Patients with liver impairment are usually in a precarious balance and are easily "tipped over" into a decompensated state from which they may have great difficulty regaining the status quo when demands are being made on the synthetic functions of the liver and bone marrow.

Endocrine Diseases

Hypothyroidism

Erythropoiesis is dependent on thyroid hormones for normal function. Patients with hypothyroidism commonly have a mild anemia with a tendency towards macrocytosis. The blood film sometimes shows marked poikilocytosis with numerous irregularly crenated cells. The carotenemia or myxedema in conjunction with the anemia may give the patient a pale, sallow complexion. Iron deficiency may complicate the picture due to a combination of increased loss from menorrhagia and decreased iron intake and absorption. There is also an increased incidence of pernicious anemia. The patient's total blood volume is contracted so the reduction in red cell mass may be greater than suggested by the hemoglobin level. This is probably due to the vasoconstriction reducing cutaneous blood flow to conserve heat. These facts are to be taken into account when treating severe myxedema or myxedema coma where therapy should be gradual and closely monitored.

Hypopituitarism

Deficiency of thyroid hormones is probably the major factor in the anemia of hypopituitarism, but testosterone and corticosteroids probably also play a role. Due to the reduced pigmentation, the pallor is usually in excess of that to be expected from the hemoglobin level.

Hypoadrenalism

Patients with Addison's disease may have a mild normocytic-normochromic anemia with mild eosinophilia.

Normocytic-Normochromic Anemias Due to Primary Hypofunction of the Bone Marrow

If there are no clinical or laboratory features to indicate a normocytic-normochromic anemia which is secondary in orgin, diagnostic efforts move towards primary bone marrow dysfunction.

Most of these causes are of a primary hematological nature and require bone marrow examination and expert hematological diagnosis and management. In the majority of patients there are clinical features or associated abnormalities in the blood film pointing toward likely diagnoses. The experienced hematologist will rarely perform a bone marrow examination in the hope of making a chance diagnosis. The marrow examination in general confirms or refutes a strong impression that the patient has a certain diagnosis. Disorders which may be responsible for primary bone marrow hypofunction are:

Hypoplastic or aplastic anemia
Red cell aplasia
Myelofibrosis
Hematological malignancy
Metastatic marrow infiltration
Primary infection of the bone marrow

Questions to be addressed in the investigation of primary bone marrow dysfunction:

1. **Is there a history of hemopoietic or immune failure?**
- Anemia, infections, bleeding or bruising.
2. **Are there any physical findings?**
- In the hemopoietic system—hepatosplenomegaly, lymphadenopathy, hemostatic failure, infections.
- In other systems—masses or infiltrates, skin rash, jaundice.
3. **Are there any associated abnormalities in the blood count?**
- Quantitative or qualitative alteration in other cellular components—leukocytes, platelets.
- Red cell morphological alterations—anisocytosis, poikiocytosis, macrocytes, teardrop cells, stippled cells, nucleated red cells.
4. **Are there any abnormalities in the biochemical profile or plasma protein electrophoresis?**
- Total protein, calcium, LDH, bilirubin, alkaline phosphatase, uric acid, abnormal monoclonal protein on EPG.
5. **How will a bone marrow aspirate and/or biopsy help in diagnosis? Should any special investigations be done at the time of marrow examination (e.g., chromosomal analysis, cytochemistry, electron microscopy, cell markers, culture)?**
6. **Should any other biopsies or diagnostic examinations be performed (e.g., lymph node, liver, aspiration cytology)?**

INVESTIGATION OF PANCYTOPENIA

The majority of patients with pancytopenia are suffering from primary marrow disease due to decreased production of all *hemopoietic* cell elements. It is thus appropriate to consider the investigation of pancytopenia at this juncture. The approach to the diagnosis of pancytopenia is similar to the investigation of primary marrow failure and the above questions are appropriate. If it turns out that the pancytopenia is due to peripheral destruction or utilization of cells, this will become apparent when a bone marrow biopsy is performed. Table 3.4 lists the conditions which may be associated with pancytopenia.

APLASTIC ANEMIA

In aplastic anemia the bone marrow is hypocellular with a reduced or absent production of all *hemopoietic* cell lines resulting in pancytopenia.

Table 3.4
Conditions Which May Be Associated with Pancytopenia

Primary marrow failure
  Aplastic anemia
  Marrow infiltration
    Hematological malignancy
    Metastatic malignancy
    Myelofibrosis
    Granulomatous diseases
  Myelodysplastic and preleukemic syndromes
  Direct marrow toxins
    Cytotoxic drug therapy
    Heavy metals
    Alcohol
  Infections
    Tuberculosis
  Bone marrow necrosis
Severe megaloblastosis
Systemic lupus erythematosus
Acute peripheral consumption
  Disseminated intravascular coagulation
  Overwhelming sepsis
Hypersplenism
Paroxysmal nocturnal hemoglobinuria

Pathophysiology

Aplastic anemia may occur as a primary disease in which the basic cause is unclear or secondary to a marrow insult. In the secondary aplastic anemias the pathophysiology may be quite variable, ranging from an autoimmune mechanism to a direct toxic effect of chemicals or drugs. *Hemopoiesis* is a continuously replicating process and as such is susceptible to numerous insults (e.g., radiation, cytotoxic therapy and toxic agents), causing immediate and direct effects on the dividing progenitor cells in the bone marrow in a dose-related manner. The net effect on the numbers of end cells in the peripheral blood will be determined by the life span of each cell, which may in turn be affected by the rate of consumption (e.g., infection or hemorrhage). The depressive effect on the marrow is usually reversible when the insult is removed.

Direct bone marrow toxins include:

- Ionizing radiation: medical, industrial, experimental.
- Cytotoxic therapy.
- Other drugs: chloramphenicol, gold.

In the more classical aplastic anemias where the cause is more difficult, or impossible, to identify, the underlying pathophysiology is not as well understood and several different mechanisms may be operative, alone or in combination. Postulated and proven pathophysiological mechanisms include:

- Bone marrow stem cell defects.
- Cellular or humoral immunological suppression or damage to stem cell or committed stem cells.
- Defects or deficiency in growth and/or differentiation factors.
- Disorders of marrow microenvironment.

With all these, genetic and/or acquired mechanisms may be operative. In some patients acquired environmental factors may be identified including:

- Genetic (congenital)—Fanconi's anemia.
- Chemicals: benzene, insecticides, hair dyes, toluene.
- Infectious agents—hepatitis, parvovirus.
- Drugs—anticonvulsants, antimicrobials (chloramphenicol), antithyroid, antiinflammatory (phenylbutazone, indomethacin).

- Miscellaneous—pregnancy associated, paroxysmal nocturnal hemoglobinuria, preleukemic syndromes.

There is accumulating experimental, clinical and therapeutic evidence that autoimmune mechanisms are operative in a high proportion of patients with aplastic anemia.

Clinical Features

The onset is usually insidious with anemia, bleeding or infection. As with bone marrow failure from any cause, the onset may seem to be sudden due to a serious bleeding or infection. However, the disease probably evolves over some period of time and it is not until a complication occurs spontaneously in a situation where the host defenses cannot respond due to total depletion and failure of production that a crisis is created. Except for signs relating to marrow failure there is usually nothing else to find on physical examination.

Laboratory Features

Blood Count

Pancytopenia, reticulocytopenia, normochromic-normocytic red cells occasionally macrocytic.

Bone Marrow

The marrow is hypocellular with almost total absence of hemopoietic cell development; occasionally there are hypercellular nests of hemopoiesis. Lymphocytes and plasma cells are present and sometimes increased.

Other Investigations

Serum iron and ferritin may be elevated, erythropoietin is increased, hemoglobin F may be increased on Hb EPG, especially in the recovery phase.

Management

Attention to complications and an "expectant" approach to the outcome has been the traditional approach to this frustrating and devastating disease. With better understanding of the disease, therapy is being more scientifically based and there are some glimmers of hope appearing for unfortunate patients with this disease.

Supportive Therapy

- Blood component therapy: this should be kept to a minimum to delay the onset of immunization and thus resistance to transfusion (especially platelet concentrates). In general, therapy should be for symptomatic deficiency rather than prophylactic therapy.
- Prevention and early therapy of infection and bleeding episodes. This may on occasions involve isolation and prophylactic antibiotics.
- Avoid invasive procedures such as intramuscular injections and traumatic shaving.
- Correct any vitamin deficiencies, attend to areas of potential infection or hemorrhage with close attention to bowel habits, menstrual bleeding, oral hygiene and shaving.

Specific Therapy

- All identifiable possible causative agents should be removed.
- Marrow stimulating therapy: several approaches may be taken in an attempt to stimulate the marrow, but the results are usually disappointing and commonly associated with unwanted side effects. Approaches used include corticosteroids, androgens, lithium, splenectomy, etiocholanolone and others. The wide range of agents used confirms the usual lack of efficacy in many patients.
- Immunosuppressive therapy (high dose corticosteroids, cytotoxic drugs and antilymphocyte or antithymocyte globulin): on the basis that some cases of idiopathic aplastic anemia may be caused by immune mechanisms, immunosuppressive therapy is well founded. Unfortunately the results are unpredictable and associated with complications.
- Bone marrow transplantation: this is a good option for patients with severe aplastic anemia who are fortunate enough to have an HLA compatible donor. The procedure is most successful if performed early and pretransplant blood transfusions have been kept to a minimum and totally avoided from related donors. Rejection and graft versus host disease remain signif-

icant hurdles to overcome despite HLA compatibility. Bone marrow transplantation with the use of concomitant immunosuppression may be used when the aplastic anemia is caused by active suppression of stem cell function.

Prognosis

The outcome of aplastic anemia depends on the cause and severity and it is difficult to predict the prognosis for many patients. In the untreated classical severe idiopathic disease the prognosis is poor with up to a 75% mortality in adults and 50% in children. Of those who survive, only a small number achieve a complete remission of the disease, the remainder either receive continuing therapy or have persisting cytopenias. If a causative agent can be identified the patients may do slightly better.

PURE RED CELL APLASIA (PRCA)

In the pure red cell aplasia syndromes there is acute or chronic failure of erythroid development in the bone marrow. As with classical aplastic anemia there are several mechanisms by which erythropoiesis is suppressed.

Acute Pure Red Cell Aplasia

This condition may be seen in children in association with chronic hemolytic anemia or as an isolated condition. It is a self-limiting disease probably virally related (especially parvovirus), but in some cases drugs such as diphenylhydantoin and chloramphenicol have been implicated.

Chronic Pure Red Cell Aplasia

The Diamond-Blackfan syndrome is a congenital form of PRCA which may be associated with other congenital abnormalities. Regular transfusion is usually necessary with its inevitable problems of iron overload in the majority of patients.

Acquired pure red cell aplasia usually affects adults and appears in the majority of patients to be immune mediated by cellular or humoral mechanisms. It has been reported in association with SLE, thymoma, myasthenia gravis, lymphoproliferative disease, paraproteinemia and hypogammaglobulinemia. Initial therapy is with blood transfusion, but some patients repond to immunosuppressive therapy in the form of corticosteroids, cytotoxic drugs or plasma exchange.

DYSERYTHROPOIETIC ANEMIA

In this group of disorders erythropoiesis is defective resulting in ineffective and abnormal red cell production. Dyserythropoiesis may occur in conjunction with clearly identifiable disease states such as iron deficiency, sideroblastosis, infection, thalassemia, megaloblastosis, hypoplastic anemias and hematological malignancy. On the other hand they may occur as a rare primary congenital disorder of erythropoiesis. The patients have isolated anemia (commonly macrocytic) with marked morphological changes in bone marrow erythropoiesis and circulating red cells. Hyperbilirubinemia is common secondary to the intramedullary destruction of red cell precursors. Three congenital types are recognized. Primary acquired dyserythropoiesis is usually associated with sideroblastic anemia and/or the myelodysplastic syndromes.

Further Reading

Chanarin, I: *The megaloblastic anaemias.* Oxford, Blackwell Scientific Publications, 1979.

Schrier, SL (ed): *Clinics in haematology: the red blood cell membrane.* Feb. 1985. Vol. 14 No. 1. Philadelphia, W.B. Saunders.

Weatherall, DJ and Clegg JB: *The thalassaemic syndromes* 3rd ed. Oxford: Blackwell Scientific Publications, 1981.

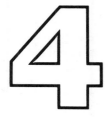

Polycythemia and Other Hemorheological Disorders

A man is as old as his arteries

Thomas Sydenham (1624–1689)

The physics of a man's circulation are the physics of the waterworks of the town in which he lives, but once out of gear, you cannot apply the same rules for the repair of the one as of the other.

Sir William Osler (1849–1919)

General Concepts of Hyperviscosity

Blood hyperviscosity is considered to play an important role in the clinical manifestations of a number of disease states. The hyperviscosity may be secondary to abnormalities in the cellular or plasma components of the blood and polycythemia has always been the classical hyperviscosity disease for which venesection has been the mainstay of therapy.

Tissue perfusion is proportional to perfusion pressure, radius of the vessel and the viscosity of blood (including deformability of the individual cellular components). Figures 4.1 and 4.2 summarize the hemorheological components of blood flow. Microcirculatory failure may thus result from inadequate perfusion pressure, vessel narrowing or reduced blood fluidity. Figure 4.3 summarizes the causes of microvascular failure. The central concepts of Virchow's triad are discussed in chapter 5. The hematologist has a particular interest in the blood viscosity factors as they affect microcirculatory flow, but these factors must be taken in combination with the vessel diameter and perfusion pressure which are of greater interest to the cardiologist and vascular clinician. The term hyperviscosity may be used in a general sense, implying reduction in blood fluidity, which may or may not be measured in the laboratory as increased whole blood or plasma viscosity. These measurable abnormalities are usually due to a quantita-

tive increase in one or more of the blood components. However, significant hyperviscosity may be present in the blood due to interactions of cellular and plasma components, increased rigidity of individual cells or particular physicochemical characteristics of an abnormal plasma protein (e.g., cryoglobulin) which will not usually be detectable by standard in-vitro blood viscosity measurements. Whatever the cause, microcirculatory failure or insufficiency is the end result of blood hyperviscosity.

CLINICAL FEATURES

Whatever the pathophysiology, the net effect of reduction or cessation of tissue perfusion is ischemia or infarction. However, the clinical presentation may be a strong pointer to the basic pathology. The oxygen transport system is a complex multi-linkage chain starting with the inspiration of oxygen and ultimate delivery to mitochondria in the tissues (see chapter 1) and it is only as strong as its weakest link. On this basis the hyperviscosity syndromes may present in several different ways.

The "Classical" Hyperviscosity Syndrome

This syndrome is typically seen in association with Waldenstrom's macroglobulinemia and polycythemia rubra vera where there is a

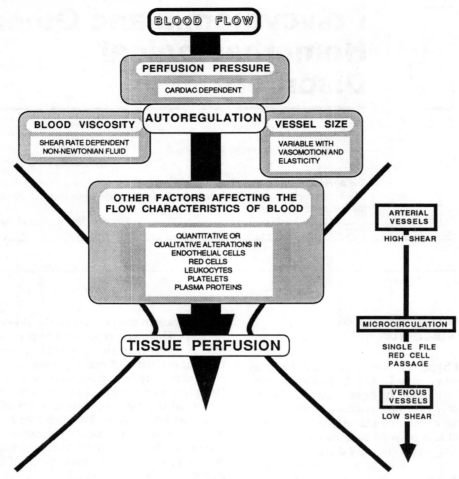

Figure 4.1   Basic concepts of blood flow

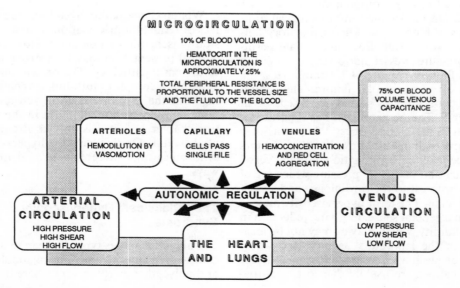

Figure 4.2.   Determinants of microcirculatory blood flow

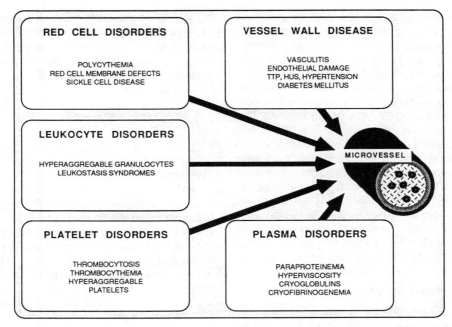

Figure 4.3. Pathophysiology of microcirculatory failure—TTP = thrombotic thrombocytopenic purpura; HUS = hemolytic uremic syndrome

combination of hyperviscosity and hypervolemia. The following clinical features may be seen in the syndrome: visual or auditory disturbances; headache; neurological dysfunction and hypervolemia. There may also be clinical findings suggestive of congestive cardiac failure. The chest x-ray may show pulmonary congestion with a normal cardiac shadow, jugular venous pressure may be elevated, the patient looks and feels congested in the head (plethoric in the case of polycythemia), hemostatic failure, such as epistaxis, bruising and purpura, due to a combination of hypervolemia and platelet dysfunction. Examination of the retinal fundus reveals marked venous engorgement with "cattle trucking" of the veins, hemorrhages and, in severe cases, papilledema. In this setting the patient has precarious microcirculation and anything which may aggravate the hyperviscosity such as dehydration, diuretics, hypotension and blood transfusion should be avoided.

Primary Microcirculatory Failure Syndromes

In some disorders there is primary microcirculatory obstruction with end organ failure in the presence of normal large vessels. This may manifest as digital ischemia with normal peripheral pulses or multisystem organ failure in the presence of normal blood pressure and macrocirculation. Such a presentation is typically seen in vasculitis, disseminated intravascular coagulation and thrombotic thrombocytopenic purpura.

Hypertension

Hypertension, especially when the diastolic pressure is disproportionately elevated, may be indicative of hyperviscosity. As flow depends on the viscosity, radius and the perfusion pressure, flow will only be effectively maintained in the presence of hyperviscosity if the perfusion pressure rises.

A corollary to this is reduction of perfusion pressure in the presence of hyperviscosity may precipitate a perfusion crisis, a fact which must be carefully considered before reducing the blood pressure in a patient with vascular disease of any nature.

Combination of Large Vessel and Small Vessel Hypoperfusion or Occlusion

As with anemia, hyperviscosity may present with what appears, at first sight, to be solely large vessel disease, such as coronary artery disease, cerebrovascular disease or peripheral vascular disease. Atheroma is common in the age group at risk from the hyperviscosity syndromes. Large vessel occlusion and hyperviscosity are a bad combination. In these circumstances lesser degrees of hyperviscosity are likely to produce symptoms. The normal hemodilution mechanism of the microcirculation, controlled by vasomotion, is inactivated beyond a large vessel block and this occurs in the presence of a low perfusion pressure, leading to inevitable sludging of the blood and loss of fluidity in the microcirculation. A presentation such as this (especially when the heart or brain is affected) constitutes a medical emergency requiring careful analysis of the pathophysiology involved (Fig. 4.3).

Cold-Related Syndromes

Many microcirculatory syndromes are precipitated by exposure to cold, such as seen in Raynaud's syndrome, cryoglobulins and cold agglutinins.

An Unexpected Laboratory Finding

Full blood counts and biochemical profiles are the commonest blood tests performed and incidental findings are common (see chapter 11).

Polycythemia
Leukocytosis
Thrombocytosis
Elevated ESR
High total protein
Red cell changes: spherocytes and fragmented spherocytes
Sickle cells
Cryoglobulins, cold agglutinins, cryofibrinogen

LABORATORY FEATURES

There would be few other disorders in which in-vitro or in-vivo laboratory study could be potentially more complex, yet so much valuable information be available from two of the cheapest and most frequently performed investigations (i.e., the full blood count and the biochemical profile). Although specific measurements of blood fluidity may be helpful in the diagnosis and management of hyperviscosity and microcirculatory disease most information can be gained from simple investigations and the clinical effects inferred when interpreted in the light of the clinical findings.

Full Blood Examination

Simple examination of the peripheral blood will detect most cellular causes of hyperviscosity and at the same time indicate the underlying diagnosis (e.g., leukemias, sickle cells, microangiopathic red cell changes). Elevation in plasma proteins and cold agglutinins will be reflected in the erythrocyte sedimentation rate or background staining on the blood film. The only exception where the ESR may be misleading is in extreme plasma hyperviscosity or in the presence of a cryoglobulin, where the plasma may be too thick for the red cells to settle.

Biochemical Profile

A multiparameter biochemical screen will usually raise the suspicion of the presence of an abnormal monoclonal protein if it is present in large enough amounts to be responsible for a hyperviscosity syndrome.

Immunological and Other Protein Investigations

Serum electrophoresis, cryoglobulins, cold agglutinins and examination for cryofibrinogen will usually exclude most causes of plasma hyperviscosity. Antinuclear antibodies, rheumatoid factor and complement levels may all help in identifying autoimmune diseases which may be complicated by small vessel vasculitis.

Test of Blood Fluidity

Whole Blood and Plasma Viscosity

Plasma viscosity relative to water is a simple investigation, but its interpretation is difficult as it does not take into account any of the cellular components of the blood. Whole blood viscosity is a truer measurement of what is likely to be occurring *in vivo*. High and low shear rates are used in the viscometer to simulate the flow in larger arterial vessels versus the flow characteristics of the microcirculation and venous systems. Unfortunately the normal range is wide and highly hematocrit dependent.

Tests of Red Cell Deformability

These may find an important place in clinical medicine when suitable methods become available. To date the methodology has been plagued with interpretive problems.

Tests for Microvascular End-Organ Dysfunction

Microvascular disease classically causes diffuse fluctuating end-organ involvement. Sophisticated methods are now available for the study of most organs of the body. The following investigations may be of assistance in specific circumstances: nail fold capillary microscopy; retinal fundus examination; EEG; renal blood flow scan; urine examination for evidence of glomerular disease; pulmonary, mesenteric and renal angiography and more recently cerebral flood flow studies.

General Principles of Management of Impaired Blood Fluidity

Avoidance of Aggravating Factors

- Dehydration
- Diuretics
- Hypotension
- Radiological contrast media
- Infection
- Blood transfusion
- Cold exposure and other vasoconstrictive influences
- Hypoxia
- Stasis
- Hypoglycemia

Correct Other Weak Links in Oxygen Transport

- Hypoxemia.
- Cardiac failure.
- Salt, water and intravascular volume depletion.
- Factors increasing hemoglobin affinity: alkalosis, carbon monoxide, hypothermia.

Initial Therapy Aimed at Improving Blood Fluidity

Although long-term management of a hyperviscosity syndrome requires definitive therapy directed at the basic cause, immediate temporizing therapy may reduce mortality and morbidity. Most definitive therapy requires days to weeks to become effective. The initial therapy will depend on the specific alteration in the blood leading to reduced blood fluidity. Table 4.1 summarizes the causes and general approaches to initial therapy and figure 4.4 outlines the agents which may be used in the treatment of various forms of vascular obstruction.

An Overview of Antithrombotic Therapy

There are a variety of therapeutic agents which act on the hemostatic mechanism and/or affect the rheological characteristics of blood which may be used in disorders in which fluidity of the blood is threatened.

HEPARIN

Heparin is a heterogeneous substance composed of negatively charged sulfurated mucopolysaccharides with a molecular weight ranging from 6,000 to 25,000. It was discovered in 1916, introduced into clinical medicine in 1931 and established its place in the definitive management of pulmonary embolism in 1960.

Mode of Action and Pharmacology

Heparin binds to and potentiates the action of antithrombin III, the principal control protein of the coagulation cascade. When used prophylactically in low doses heparin's action with AT III is predominantly directed against activated factor X before the common pathway is activated. Small doses are therefore necessary as thrombin has not been generated. When heparin is used therapeutically the aim is to neutralize circulating thrombin, in which case high doses may be required. Heparin has several other effects, but the ones of significance in relation to its hematological effects include enhancement of plasminogen

Table 4.1
Hematological Causes of Vascular Obstruction and General Principles of Therapy

Pathophysiology	Initial Therapy
Erythrocytes	
Polycythemia	Phlebotomy and hemodilution
Defects in red cell fluidity	Hemodilution
Leukocyte disorders	
Leukostasis syndrome	Leukapheresis
Neutrophil aggregation syndromes	Corticosteroids
Platelet disorders	
Thrombocytosis	Antiplatelet therapy
Thrombocythemia	Antiplatelet therapy +/− thrombopheresis
Platelet aggregation syndromes	Antiplatelet therapy
Plasma disorders	
Paraproteinemia IgM > IgA > IgG	Plasma exchange
Cryoglobulinemia	Plasma exchange
Hyperfibrinogenemia	Defibrination therapy +/−
Cryofibrinogenemia	Plasma exchange
Cold agglutinins	Warming +/− plasma exchange
DIC	See chapter 6
Vessel wall	
Vasculitis	Corticosteroids +/− plasma exchange
Microangiopathies	Controversial (see Chapter 3)
Arterial obstruction	Correct hemorheological factors as above, direct attack on vessel blockage
Venous thrombosis	Anticoagulants, mobilization correction of any hemorheological factors as above

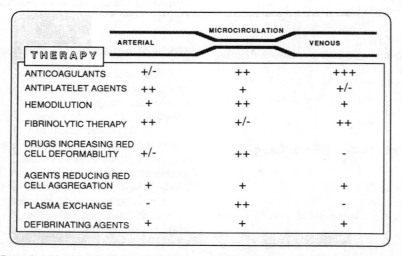

Figure 4.4. Role of antithrombotic, fibrinolytic, and hemorheological therapy in various forms of vascular disease

activator release and thus potentiation of fibrinolysis; an aggregating effect on platelets and reversal of some of the vasoactivity in the initial phases of a pulmonary embolus. Heparin must be given systemically, has a biological half-life of slightly more than one hour and is predominantly inactivated by the liver with small amounts being excreted by the kidney. Hepatic and renal impairment will delay clearance. Heparin is available as sodium and calcium salts which have slightly different pharmacological characteristics which are not of practical clinical significance.

Dosage and Mode of Administration

There is considerable patient variation in response to a standard dose of heparin and it is difficult to advocate a standard approach to initial therapy. A bolus loading dose of 5,000 to 10,000 units is usually recommended followed by a continuous infusion of 30,000 to 40,000 units over 24 hours depending on the clinical effects and the results of monitoring tests. As a general rule, in the initial instance, it is reasonable to give higher doses to patients with major pulmonary embolism in order to ensure effective control of the thrombotic process. It is better to "err" on the side of excess dosage in the initial 48 hours of therapy until control of thrombosis is gained. Dosage needs close observation and may require reduction as thrombin generation is brought under control.

Constant infusion, using an infusion pump, is the most accurate and safest method for the administration of therapeutic heparin. However, under certain circumstances a therapeutic dose can be given subcutaneously or as an intermittent bolus dose (generally not more than 2 hourly). In patients with difficult venous access or in whom multiple venous lines are already in use this approach is warranted. With prolonged therapy with heparin there may be a fall in antithrombin III levels by up to 15%. This is usually not of great clinical significance, unless the patient has preexisting low levels or the heparin is suddenly ceased without alternative anticoagulant therapy.

Monitoring of Therapy

Laboratory monitoring of heparin therapy remains a controversial issue and has been overstated by many authors. It matters little how heparin therapy is monitored as long as it is done carefully with the correct aims in mind. If the patient's clinical condition is improving obsessive monitoring is less important. There are two main reasons why heparin therapy is monitored. First, to ensure adequate heparin effect and secondly to reduce the likelihood of bleeding. If a patient does not appear to be responding to therapy it is important to demonstrate heparin effect in the laboratory tests. In most laboratories the activated partial thromboplastin time (APTT) is the most appropriate and simplest test to monitor heparin. The thrombin time can be used, but varies in its sensitivity to heparin. Some laboratories use a sensitive thrombin time test which will also detect the lesser amounts of heparin used for prophylactic therapy. In most laboratories an APTT of approximately twice normal is considered adequate heparinization. In the initial phases of a severe pulmonary embolus it is reasonable to perform tests every 12 hours, but after the patient has been stabilized daily monitoring is adequate.

Resistance to Heparin

When heparin resistance is encountered the following should be considered:

- Major stimulus to thrombus, e.g., malignancy.
- Inadequate dosage on a body-weight basis.
- Antithrombin III deficiency.
- Heparin-induced thrombosis-thrombocytopenia syndrome.
- Rapid clearance in some individuals.

Reversal of Action

Protamine sulfate 1mg IV is the recommended reversal dose for each 100 units of heparin. As a rough guide 50% of the neutralizing dose is given one hour after heparin and 25% two hours after heparin. Reversal should be assessed using the APTT or thrombin time (TT). A further dose may need to be administered some time later. This has been attributed to heparin rebound, but is more likely due to protamine sulfate having a shorter half-life than heparin.

Complications

Heparin is a potentially dangerous drug and is high on the list of iatrogenic causes of death.

Bleeding

Bleeding is the commonest and most serious hazard of heparin therapy. It rarely occurs under 48 hours unless there is an associated defect in the hemostatic system. The following are factors to consider as contributory towards increasing the risk of bleeding:

- Overdose and/or increased sensitivity to heparin.
- Pre-existing defects in the hemostatic system.
- Other agents affecting the hemostatic system such as antiplatelet therapy or oral anticoagulants.
- Local lesions, invasive procedures, trauma (particular care with physiotherapy), surgery, age (especially elderly females).

Heparin Induced Thrombosis-Thrombocytopenia Syndrome (HITTS)

This is an important complication of heparin therapy which warrants greater attention than it currently receives. In this complication an immune reaction occurs to heparin after 7 to 10 days of therapy at which time the patient's platelets aggregate and thrombocytopenia develops. In contrast to other causes of drug-induced thrombocytopenia there may be arterial, microvascular or venous thrombosis associated with the platelet aggregation. This paradoxical thrombosis induced by heparin will present the clinician with a diagnostic dilemma. The overall incidence of this complication of heparin is unknown, but may be on the increase with the wider prophylactic use of subcutaneous heparin. The best way to avoid this potentially devastating complication is to keep heparin therapy as brief as possible and always be alert to the diagnostic possibility of HITTS in any patient who develops thrombocytopenia or any arterial or venous thrombotic episode while receiving therapy.

Allergic Reactions, Osteoporosis, Alopecia and Abnormalities in Liver Enzymes May Rarely Occur

VITAMIN K ANTAGONISTS

The oral anticoagulants are vitamin K antagonists derived from coumarin or indandione.

Mode of Action and Pharmacology

Warfarin, a coumadin derivative, is the most widely used oral anticoagulant and interferes with the reduction of vitamin K resulting in accumulation of phylloquinine epoxide. This prevents the carboxylation of the glutamic acid residues of prothrombin, factors VII, IX and X and coagulation inhibitor proteins C and S. These coagulation factors circulate but are unable to bind calcium or phospholipid, an essential property for their action in the coagulation cascade. The therapeutic effect of oral anticoagulants is delayed until the circulating clotting factors have decayed at a rate dependent on their respective half-lives. The first affected are factor VII (extrinsic system) and protein C with a half-life of approximately 5 hours, followed by IX (25 hours), X (40 hours) and II (60 hours). As factor VII is unique to the extrinsic system full anticoagulation is not achieved until the APTT is prolonged. The early fall in protein C may possibly in fact initially predispose the patient to thrombosis.

As the rate of onset of action of oral anticoagulants is determined by the half-life of the coagulation factors there is no point in administering a large loading dose. This practice is potentially hazardous as it is likely to expose the patient to the risk of bleeding even though intrinsic anticoagulation has not been affected. For the same reasons repeated frequent dosage adjustment is inappropriate and makes it difficult to stabilize a patient's therapy, a practice colloquially known as "Himalayan therapeutics" due to the wild, unpredictable fluctuations in the prothrombin time and subsequent dosage adjustments.

Factors Affecting Oral Anticoagulant Action

Hepatic Function

Patients with impairment of hepatic function will be exquisitely sensitive to vitamin K antagonists and significant dose reductions are necessary. This also applies to patients with hepatic congestion from cardiac impairment. Some drugs may inhibit the metabolism of warfarin (cimetidine, sulphinpyrazone, amiodarone, phenylbutazone, metronidazole, cotrimoxizole, ketoconazole) and potentiate its action. Some drugs (e.g., barbiturates, glutethamide, phenytoin, carbamazepine, rifampicin) will induce the cytochrome P450 enzyme system and enhance warfarin metabolism. In contrast cessation of the drugs in a stabilized patient will do the reverse. Chronic alcohol ingestion acts in this way to some extent but the action has been overstated. Patients with normal liver function receiving oral anticoagulant therapy are able to take alcohol in moderation.

Age

The elderly appear to be more sensitive to oral anticoagulants.

Vitamin K Availability

The activity of oral anticoagulants depends on vitamin K availability. Action may be potentiated by antibiotics which may reduce bacterial synthesis in the colon and by cholestyramine binding vitamin K and reducing its absorption.

Protein Binding

Warfarin may be displaced from protein binding when other protein-binding drugs are introduced, but this only has a transient effect on anticoagulant action until the new steady state is reached. This type of drug interaction has been an overstated problem.

Drugs Which Do Not Interact with Oral Anticoagulants

The following drugs have been investigated in association with warfarin and do not affect its anticoagulant action. However, some of these drugs may have antiplatelet action (e.g., nonsteroidal antiinflammatory drugs) which may compound the hemostatic defect.

- Analgesics: indomethacin, ibuprofen, naproxen, paracetamol.
- Antiarrythmics: atropine, lignocaine.
- Antibacterials: aminoglycosides, cephalosporins, penicillin.
- Anticonvulsants: ethosuximide, sodium valproate.
- Antihypertensives: hydralazine, methyldopa, prazosin.
- Beta-blockers are probably safe.
- Bronchodilators: aminophylline, salbutamol, terbutaline.
- Hypnotics: benzodiazepines.
- Hypoglycemics: sulphonylureas, biguanides.
- Oral contraceptive: progestogen-only pills.

Initiation of Therapy

For the reasons outlined above it takes up to one week for vitamin K antagonists to achieve their full anticoagulant effect. The rate at which this is achieved is not significantly affected by increasing the drug dosage and large loading doses are not recommended. After consideration of all the factors which may affect the action of oral anticoagulant, an appropriate starting dose is given (usually between 5mg and 7.5mg of warfarin) and the prothrombin time (PT) measured at 48 hours. At this point the PT is only representing a reduction in factor VII and the intrinsic system is unaffected. It is not until the APTT is prolonged that effective anticoagulation is achieved.

In patients with major or recurrent venous thromboembolic disease it is important that during the induction phase of oral anticoagulant therapy there is sufficient overlap of heparin therapy to ensure adequate anticoagulation. Two days with full-dose heparin and two with half dose is usually adequate unless there is a marked hypercoagulable state, in which circumstance overlap time is dictated by the results of PT. The reduction of antithrombin III levels during heparin therapy may be important in this respect. There may also be grounds for concern in the first few days of vitamin K antagonists due to reduction in the coagulation inhibitor protein C, before II, IX and X are reduced.

Monitoring of Therapy

The monitoring of oral anticoagulants using the PT has been plagued with problems of standardization, reporting methods and therapeutic ranges. These problems have been difficult for the clinician to understand and thus their clinical significance was not appreciated. The tissue factor (thromboplastin reagent) used in the PT test is the critical component in determining the sensitivity of the test. Of the different types of thromboplastin available, human brain thromboplastin is the most widely available reagent which is sensitive to the effects of oral anticoagulants. Unfortunately, the arrival of the human immunodeficiency virus (HIV) has cast a shadow over the use of human brains for the manufacture of thromboplastin.

With an insensitive rabbit brain reagent the leeway between anticoagulation and bleeding complications is small and many patients tend to receive too much anticoagulant with a high risk of bleeding. When a sensitive human brain reagent is used the PT is a better guide to the degree of anticoagulation and spontaneous bleeding is uncommon when the PT is within the accepted therapeutic range. When a human brain reagent has been standardized against a reference reagent, such as the British reference thromboplastin, the therapeutic ratio is between 2 and 4, in contrast to the rabbit brain preparations where the ratio is 1.5 to 2.5 (with an increased risk of bleeding). As rabbit brain is still widely used (especially in North America) there has been a recent trend towards the use of "low-dose warfarin." This is really an acknowledgement of the fact that insensitive reagents are not capable of accurately measuring the anticoagulant effect in many patients until the coagulation factors are dangerously low.

It is thus important to know the type of reagent used in the laboratory and if a patient travels detailed information should be carried. A real problem exists under these circumstances where a patient's drug dosage is constantly altered due to varying results in different laboratories when in fact the degree of anticoagulation has not altered.

The PT may be expressed as a ratio (patient's time/control time) or an index (control time divided by patient's time expressed as a percentage). More recently the International Normalized Ratio (INR) has been recommended for the reporting of PT in an attempt to correct for the differences in thromboplastin sensitivities. A commonly used test is the thrombotest in which the result is expressed as a percentage coagulation activity. As this is a standardized commercial test the information provided by the manufacturer should be followed.

Pregnancy and Anticoagulants

Heparin does not cross the placenta and is a relatively safe reagent to use during pregnancy. Warfarin crosses the placenta and may have teratogenic effects in the first three months of pregnancy. Patients receiving long-term warfarin therapy should carefully plan any pregnancies and either discontinue warfarin therapy or use alternative forms of antithrombotic therapy from conception through the first trimester. In the third trimester and during delivery there is a risk to the fetus from hemorrhage and again alternative therapy should be used. Warfarin does not pose a risk to breast-fed babies and no precautions need be taken.

Antiplatelet Therapy

There are numerous pharmacological agents which may inhibit platelet function and impair hemostasis, however, only a few are used specifically for this purpose in antithrombotic therapy. Antiplatelet therapy is generally used in clinical conditions where the primary phase of hemostasis may have a pathophysiological role in vascular obstruction. These include atheromatous disease, arterial emboli and microangiopathy. Numerous clinical trials have been carried out to establish efficacy of such therapy, but controversy still holds sway in most disorders in which antiplatelet therapy would seem logical. Most antiplatelet agents interfere with prostaglandin metabolism.

Aspirin

Aspirin irreversibly acetylates cyclooxygenase in the platelet and megakaryocyte and thus prevents thromboxane A_2 synthesis. There is continuing debate as to the appropriate dose and frequency of aspirin administration. Small doses (80mg/day) substantially inactivate the platelet prostaglandin pathways with lesser, but reversible, effects on prostacyclin production by the endothelial cell. As platelets are unable to resynthesize the acetylated cyclooxygenase the antiplatelet action of aspirin persists for the life of the platelet. It is thus 7 to 10 days until the function of all circulating platelets returns to normal. The ideal dose of aspirin for maximal antiplatelet action and minimal inhibitory effects on prostacyclin production by the endothelial cell remains *sub judice*. Small frequent doses (50 to 100mg) would seem logical, but trials using widely differing dosages have failed to demonstrate any difference in efficacy.

Sulphinpyrazone

Sulphinpyrazone is a uricosuric agent, but has a similar structure to some of the nonsteroidal antiinflammatory agents. As with most nonsteroidal antiinflammatory drugs sulphinpyrazone is a competitive inhibitor of cyclooxygenase. This means the drug must be given on a regular basis (200mg qid) and the effects are reversible.

Dipyridamole

This coronary vasodilator is an inhibitor of platelet phosphodiesterase, the enzyme which converts cyclic AMP to AMP. The net effect of this inhibition is to potentiate the action of prostacyclin on the platelet as prostacyclin inhibits platelet function by elevating cyclic AMP. Dipyridamole is usually administered in a dosage of 75 to 100mg qid before food, but lower starting doses may be necessary, if vasodilatation is a problem.

Newer Agents

Thomboxane synthetase inhibitors and thromboxane receptor antagonists have been developed and are currently undergoing clinical evaluation. Ticlopidine is a compound which appears to act on the fibrinogen/von Willebrand interactions with membrane glycoproteins.

Reevaluated Older Agents

There are an increasing number of well established medicinal and other compounds which, similar to aspirin and sulphinpyrazone, are being found to have antiplatelet action. Among these are:

- Clofibrate—reduces platelet adhesion.
- Nitroglycerine and bendrofluazide—stimulate prostacyclin production.

- Alcohol—impairs platelet factor 3 release.
- Adrenergic-receptor blockers.
- Nutritional factors—see chapter 6.

Dextran

The dextrans were developed as plasma volume expanders, but subsequently much interest has been shown in their flow-promoting and antithrombotic properties. Dextran is produced by the action of the bacterium *Leuconostoc mesenteroides* on sucrose. Dextran consists of a long string of glucose units linked together by alpha 1-6 bonds. At intervals of about 20 glucose units short side-chains of one or two further glucose residues are linked by alpha 1-3 linkage. Dextran 70 with a molecular weight of 70,000 is commonly used for plasma volume expansion. Dextran 40 with a molecular weight of 40,000 is predominantly used for its flow-promoting properties. The products are available in electrolyte or dextrose solution.

The dextrans are ideal agents for short-term hemodilution to improve microcirculatory flow. As discussed above, this is an area of increasing importance as greater understanding of the rheological properties of blood in various disease states is gained. The properties of intravascular persistence, red cell deaggregation and antithrombosis make dextrans ideal for hemodilution. In patients with hyperviscosity, this hemodilution is usually performed in association with venesection. The dextrans are also recommended as a form of prophylaxis against venous thromboembolism. Dextran has effects on all components of Virchow's triad of factors involved in the pathophysiology of vascular occlusion. The antithrombotic effect has aroused great interest, as the hemostatic defect produced has similarities to von Willebrand's disease. The regular use of dextran as thrombosis prophylaxis has been tempered by conflicting trial results, occasional allergic reactions and impairment of hemostasis.

FIBRINOLYTIC THERAPY

Thrombolytic drugs have been available for clinical use for over 30 years and there is no doubt regarding their fibrinolytic action in dissolving fibrin clots. However, their lack of wide acceptance into regular clinical use has been due to a number of factors. Skepticism regarding their clinical efficacy, potential for inducing hemostatic failure and high cost have all played their part. Streptokinase and urokinase; plasminogen activators, have been used both systemically and locally for the dissolution of both arterial and venous thrombi or thromboemboli. More recently the development of tissue plasminogen activators has introduced the promise of more specific and localized therapy, overcoming the disadvantage of systemic fibrinolytic activation which accompanies the systemic use of streptokinase and urokinase and sometimes also their local use. The reader is referred to the specialized literature for information regarding the indications and protocols for administration of acute fibrinolytic therapy. In general, it is only advocated for use by clinicians with knowledge and experience in this type of therapy.

Long-term fibrinolytic therapy may be used in disorders where reduced fibrinolytic activity is thought to play a pathophysiological role (e.g., recurrent venous thrombosis) or when hyperfibrinogenemia is implicated in rheological or thrombotic disorders (e.g., retinal vein occlusion, some cases of arterial disease). In the latter it is the fibrinogenolytic action in normalizing the circulating fibrinogen level that is the aim of therapy. Phenformin, metformin, arabolin and stanazol are all agents which will stimulate the fibrinolytic system. Therapy can be monitored using the euglobulin lysis time and the fibrinogen level.

Polycythemia

The term polycythemia has been given several different meanings. Strictly, the term should be used in its broadest sense to mean excess red cells per unit volume of blood, irrespective of the underlying cause. Some clinicians have restricted the term polycythemia to conditions where there is a demonstrable increase in the red cell mass and used the term relative polycythemia for all disorders where plasma volume contraction is responsible. As a result of this approach some clinicians have been guilty of neglecting the hyperviscosity implications of polycythemia secondary to plasma volume contraction. Many hematologists lose interest in the further investigation of polycythemia as soon as contraction of plasma volume is identified as the cause. This is a most restrictive approach and may be detrimental to the patient because it ignores significant blood fluidity problems.

BASIC PHYSIOLOGY AND PATHOPHYSIOLOGY OF BLOOD VOLUME, RED CELL VOLUME, PLASMA VOLUME AND HEMATOCRIT CONTROL

The factors determining an individual's "set point" for hematocrit are not well understood and any patient whose hematocrit is in the middle or lower part of the normal range may have marked plasma volume contraction before the hematocrit rises above two standard deviations from the mean. This is in contrast to a patient whose hematocrit is at the upper limit of normal in whom the slightest reduction in plasma volume will result in polycythemia in relation to the normal reference range. Patients may thus have significant elevation in hematocrit in relation to their own particular "set point" which will only arouse attention if sequential blood counts have been performed.

The subject of blood volume, plasma volume and red cell mass control remains complex and confusing (Fig. 4.5). The literature contains controversy and contradictions, many of which reflect our lack of basic understanding in the field. The total blood volume, red cell mass and plasma volume have closely interrelated control mechanisms. There appears to be a specific "set point" for each of these parameters at which level the body's circulation functions most efficiently, while, at the same time allowing reserve for the stress of increased oxygen requirements or acute blood loss. Blood volume control sensors are located centrally to ensure adequate filling of the heart, but each specific microvascular bed also has its own autoregulation determined by local needs. The detailed mechanisms by which the body is able to accurately sustain total blood volume, osmolality, pH, temperature, oxygen-carrying capacity and viscosity, around predetermined "null points" is receiving increasing attention, particularly when there are large volumes of blood contained in inactive capacitance depots.

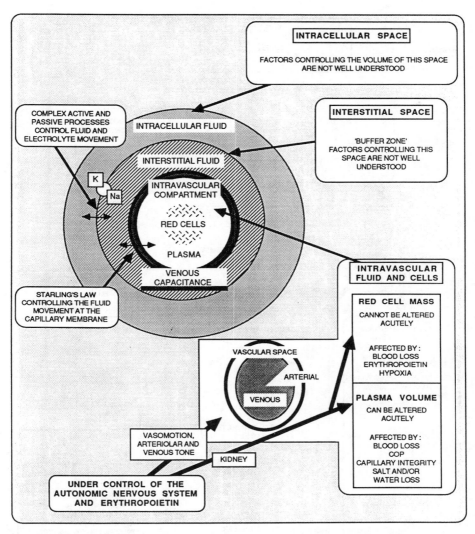

Figure 4.5. The body fluid compartments and their control—COP = colloid osmotic pressure

In order to maintain a correct balance of blood volume distribution between the central and peripheral circulations, acute changes in either plasma volume or capacitance vessel volume will be initiated. As it is not possible to acutely alter the total red cell mass and assuming the total intravascular space remains constant, blood volume can only be controlled by changes in plasma volume, via interstitial fluid shifts or alterations in urine volume. By the same reasoning any sudden alterations in the capacitance volume (venous tone) will have significant effects on the central blood volume and thus the cardiac filling pressures which can only be compensated for by altering the plasma volume.

It is interesting to contemplate the teleological reasons for the kidney being the site of red cell mass control via erythropoietin production. The renal cortex has the highest blood flow in relation to oxygen requirements of any tissue in the body and basically operates on minimal oxygen extraction, with efferent hemoglobin remaining well saturated. It thus does appear logical that this organ should be given the responsibility of sensing small reductions in hemoglobin saturation and stimulating erythropoiesis via erythropoietin pro-

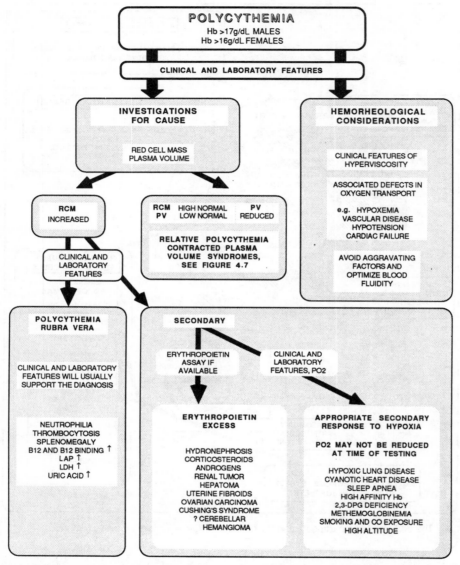

Figure 4.6. The investigation of polycythemia—RCM = red cell mass; PV = plasma volume; LAP = leukocyte alkaline phosphatase; LDH = lactate dehydrogenase; DPG = diphosphoglycerate

duction. It also seems logical that the organ responsible for plasma volume control also has some responsibility in red cell mass control.

APPROACH TO THE INVESTIGATION OF POLYCYTHEMIA

In the initial assessment of polycythemia there are certain key questions which need to be addressed from the outset (Fig. 4.6).

1. At what level of hemoglobin should a patient be investigated? There is continuing debate in relation to the reference range for the hemoglobin level and there is increasing agreement that a hemoglobin above 17.0g/dL in a male and 16.0g/dL in a female requires explanation and should be considered as a significant risk factor for vascular disease.
2. Is the patient suffering from acute hyperviscosity and at risk of a vascular event?

If there is already evidence of vascular compromise or there is a significant risk present, initial therapy may take precedence over diagnosis.

3. Is the cause obvious from the clinical history?

    If it is, the investigations can be more specifically directed or no further test may be necessary, particularly when the polycythemia is due to acute plasma volume contraction (see below).

4. Is it necessary to perform red cell mass and plasma volume studies?

    These parameters will usually need to be measured to clearly establish whether the polycythemia is due to a true increase in the red cell mass or a contraction in the plasma volume. Until this has been established there is little point in proceeding with extensive investigations, unless there are clinical features indicating the cause.

Red Cell Mass (RCM) and Plasma Volume (PV) Measurements

There are well-standardized and accurate radioisotopic methods available for the measurement of these parameters and both these measurements should be performed in patients with unexplained polycythemia. The main problems relate to reference ranges, which are unacceptably wide, in order to allow for variations in body dimensions. Red cell mass and plasma volume are not independent variables and a patient may have significant polycythemia due to a combination of plasma volume contraction and increased red cell mass, yet both parameters lie within the reference range. For these statistical reasons, the diagnostic sensitivity in any individual patient is limited and, without previous laboratory measurements, it is not possible for an individual patient's "set point" for hematocrit to be taken into account when interpreting red cell mass and plasma volume measurements.

Venous and Whole Body Hematocrit

A peripheral venous blood hematocrit estimation is a simple and rapidly determined parameter providing some information regarding the ratio of red cell mass to plasma volume, but no direct indication of the red cell mass or plasma volume. There is generally a good correlation between the hematocrit and alterations in red cell mass and plasma volume. However, this is not a reliable enough relationship to allow the measurement of only one volume parameter to predict the other. This variation in the ratio is probably due to variations in red cell distribution in the body. The usual finding that the venous hematocrit is higher than the total body hematocrit is due to the normal hemodilution of the microcirculation. Assuming no changes in red cell mass, the hematocrit is in general an acceptable laboratory indicator of alterations in plasma volume.

POLYCYTHEMIA DUE TO INCREASED RED CELL MASS

If the red cell mass and plasma volume studies indicate an increased red cell mass, further investigation is directed towards finding the cause. As a general rule the cause will be apparent from the outset in that the clinical findings or initial laboratory findings are diagnostic. Under these circumstances any further tests are purely confirmatory or of a base line nature. On the other hand, the cause may not be obvious in which case the causes are excluded in a systematic fashion. In most circumstances the cause readily becomes apparent, but occasionally the clinician is left with the rather unsatisfactory diagnosis of idiopathic erythrocytosis.

Figure 4.6 outlines a practical approach to polycythemia secondary to increased red cell mass. Basically three questions are being addressed and the diagnosis is usually straightforward. However, the recalcitrant diagnostic case is where the red cell mass is clearly elevated and there are no clues in the initial clinical and laboratory findings. Under these circumstances the more specialized investigations listed below are warranted.

Are There Any Clinical or Laboratory Features Clearly Pointing to the Cause?

Classical polycythemia rubra vera, severe lung disease, intracardiac shunt and smokers polycythemia are relatively easy diagnoses to make in the majority of patients.

Is Erythropoiesis Autonomous?

This is seen in polycythemia rubra vera where erythropoietin is suppressed or in the inappropriate erythropoietin production syndromes.

Is the Increased Red Cell Production Due to Erythropoietin Stimulation of the Marrow? Is the Erythropoietin Response Appropriate (i.e., Tissue Hypoxia) or Inappropriate (i.e., Autonomous Erythropoietin Production)?

Laboratory Investigations

There are numerous investigations, some more complex and time consuming than others, available for the investigation of polycythemia, but in most circumstances it is only necessary to perform specific tests to confirm a provisional diagnosis made from the initial clinical and laboratory assessment. The concept of a "polycythemia screen" results in inappropriate usage of laboratory services.

Bone Marrow Aspirate and Biopsy Examination

As a general rule examination of the bone marrow is not a high-yield investigation, but the findings may assist in "swinging" the probabilities. Features of myeloproliferative disease, supporting the diagnosis of polycythemia rubra vera, may be found in chapter 9. Iron stores tend to be reduced in PRV, but normal or increased in secondary polycythemias.

Serum Assays for Vitamin B12, B12 Binding Capacity, Folic Acid, Ferritin, LDH, and Leukocyte Alkaline Phosphatase

Blood Gases

Reproducible arterial hypoxemia supports the diagnosis of a secondary polycythemia due to cardiac or respiratory disease. However, a normal arterial oxygen tension does not exclude these diagnostic possibilities. Carboxyhemoglobin may be elevated in smokers or in others exposed to carbon monoxide and sleep apnea syndromes may also cause polycythemia.

Oxygen Dissociation Curve Analysis

This investigation is carried out in specific circumstances for the diagnosis of an abnormal high affinity hemoglobin. The estimation of the P_{50} is important in the differential diagnosis. This measures a single point on the curve where hemoglobin is 50% saturated, but is only a crude measure of hemoglobin affinity. If a high affinity hemoglobin variant is a possibility, a full oxygen dissociation curve analysis should be carried out.

Erythropoietin Assay

Biological and immunoassays for erythropoietin, the hormone that regulates red cell production, have been available as a research procedure for some years. With this assay becoming technically easier and more reproducible it is likely to become an important test in the investigation of polycythemia. Its role will mainly be to assist in answering the questions outlined above in the initial directing of investigations in a patient with an increased red cell mass, in whom the cause is not immediately apparent.

Specific Investigations to Identify Underlying Pathology

When the initial investigations indicate the basic pathophysiology of the polycythemia, more detailed and sometimes invasive, investigations may be necessary. Consultation with the appropriate specialty is usually the correct course of action. Investigations may include cardiac examination, respiratory function tests and a search for an occult erythropoietin-producing tumor.

POLYCYTHEMIA RUBRA VERA (PRV)

Polycythemia rubra vera is a myeloproliferative disease in which there is autonomously increased activity of erythropoiesis with varying degrees of granulopoietic and megakaryocytic proliferation. It has a variable natural history gradually progressing to a "spent" phase with myelofibrosis and myeloid metaplasia in the majority of patients (see Fig. 9.9). The disease is clonal in nature and has the potential for acute leukemic transformation in as many as 25% of patients.

Clinical Features

History

PRV typically occurs in patients over the age of 40 years. Clinical features include hyperviscosity and hypervolemia, hemostatic impairment (epistaxis, GIT hemorrhage), pruritus (especially after heat exposure), thrombotic events and gout.

Examination

Patients are typically plethoric with signs of hyperviscosity, hypertension (30%), splenomegaly (75%) and hepatomegaly (35%).

Laboratory Features

Full Blood Examination

Polycythemia is present with normocytic normochromic red cells unless iron deficiency has supervened, leukocytosis in 75% of cases, thrombocytosis in 50% and reduced ESR is usual.

Bone Marrow

Bone marrow aspirate and biopsy may help by demonstrating hypercellularity with pan-hyperplasia, reduced iron stores and increased reticulin.

Other Hematological Investigations

Leukocyte alkaline phosphatase score (LAP), vitamin B12 and B12 binding proteins are elevated, ferritin and folate are commonly low. Abnormal platelet function may be found.

Biochemistry

Hyperuricemia is common and LDH may be elevated due to ineffective erythropoiesis.

Management

With treatment, the mean survival of patients with polycythemia is 10 to 15 years. In the past the majority of patients died from thrombotic events secondary to the hyperviscosity and factors inducing hypercoagulability. Initial treatment must be directed towards correcting hyperviscosity followed by a program for long-term control of the disease. Therapy must be individualized as some patients can be controlled with minimal therapy whereas others require more definitive, regular marrow suppressive medications.

Initial Control of Hyperviscosity

Polycythemia has always been the classical disease for which phlebotomy has been the mainstay of therapy. As the red cell mass may be markedly increased, large volumes of blood may need to be removed before the hematocrit is reduced to an acceptable level. The importance of adequate intravascular volume replacement to maintain normovolemia, especially in elderly patients, is crucial. Any sudden reduction in perfusion pressure may have additional detrimental effects on microcirculatory flow in the presence of hyperviscosity or large vessel stenosis. If only a single unit of blood is being removed at any one time crystalloid is usually adequate for volume replacement, but if larger volumes are being removed colloid replacement is desirable. The use of low molecular weight dextran is commonly advocated because of its rheological effects in improving microcirculatory flow.

Thrombocytosis commonly occurs following venesection which may arouse considerable alarm. It is unlikely that this is a reactive thrombocytosis as the disease process is autonomous. It is more likely that the increase in circulating platelets is an indication of platelet mobilization from the microcirculation as sludging is relieved by the hemodilution. Antiplatelet therapy is desirable if the platelet count is elevated (aspirin and dipyridamole). If the platelets are markedly elevated specific suppressive therapy is necessary (*busulphan* or radioactive phosphorus).

Definitive Long-Term Therapy

As long as polycythemia and thrombocytosis are controlled what therapy is used probably matters little, although there is debate among hematologists on this point. Some patients with more indolent disease can be treated with phlebotomy alone. Iron deficiency develops in most patients, but is usually not symptomatic and may assist in limiting erythropoiesis. There are some patients who are troubled by the iron deficiency despite a normal circulating hemoglobin level. Iron is required for enzymes and proteins other than hemoglobin, possibly explaining the symptoms. The severely hypochromic microcytic red cells do not function as well as normal cells. Iron deficiency has also been noted to aggravate pruritus. Thus, if venesection is required too frequently, or the iron deficiency becomes too severe, marrow suppressive therapy is indicated.

Busulphan as intermittent or continuous therapy is usually an effective marrow suppressive treatment, but requires close supervision. Radioactive phosphorus is effective and has the advantage of prolonged control with infrequent dosaging.

SECONDARY POLYCYTHEMIAS

Polycythemia Secondary to Hypoxemia

Any condition causing intermittent or chronic reduction in arterial oxygen saturation will stimulate the erythropoietin system, resulting in a reactive erythroid hyperplasia in the bone marrow. It is not essential to demonstrate hypoxemia on a random blood sample to suspect this type of secondary polycythemia. The maximum hypoxic stimulus may occur at other times, especially at night and sleep studies may be necessary. The possible causes of hypoxemic polycythemia are:

- Low barometric pressure (altitude dwellers).
- Cyanotic heart disease and other right-to-left shunts.
- Pulmonary disease.
- Hypoventilation syndromes.
- Sleep apnea.

Polycythemia Secondary to Tissue Hypoxia

There are several conditions where there is defective release of oxygen to the tissues, in which erythropoietin production is stimulated. This can occur in chronic carbon monoxide poisoning either from smoking or environmental exposure. Not only does carbon monoxide make some hemoglobin unavailable for oxygen transport, but the remaining functional hemoglobin has increased oxygen affinity. Carboxyhemoglobin measurements should be made at the times of peak exposure. An uncommon cause of secondary polycythemia is seen in families with congenitally abnormal high affinity hemoglobins where the hemoglobin dissociation curve can be markedly left-shifted. These are sometimes called "Llama" hemoglobins as their oxygen dissociation curve is similar to that of these high-altitude-dwelling mammals.

Polycythemia Secondary to Inappropriate Erythropoietin Production

On rare occasions polycythemia may be the presenting symptom of an underlying erythropoietin-producing tumor or of renal pathology. Renal ischemia, cysts and hydronephrosis as well as hypernephroma may be responsible. Other non-renal erythropoietin-producing tumors include: hepatomas, uterine myomas and cerebellar hemangiomas. Certain endocrine diseases, such as Cushing's syndrome, pheochromocytoma and androgenizing states, may also be associated with polycythemia. A condition of essential overproduction of erythropoietin has also been identified, explaining some cases of "idiopathic erythrocytosis."

POLYCYTHEMIA DUE TO PLASMA VOLUME CONTRACTION: RELATIVE POLYCYTHEMIA

It is becoming increasingly recognized that in the majority of patients with mild polycythemia the underlying mechanism is a contraction of the plasma volume, either due to a salt and water deficit, capillary leak of protein-rich fluid or a contraction of the venous capacitance volume with associated compensatory reduction in plasma volume to maintain normal central cardiac filling pressures and volumes (Fig. 4.7).

Dehydration and Salt Deficit

Plasma volume contraction secondary to water and/or salt depletion is usually due to excessive losses with inadequate intake, but disorders of thirst control may be responsible. Therapeutic dehydration is commonly used in order to treat or prevent edema formation in vital organs, especially the central nervous system and lung. Such therapy will severely contract the plasma volume and hemoconcentrate the blood. A fine line may be walked with such therapy and the whole blood hyperviscosity induced by such therapy cannot be ignored. Young, in contrast to elderly patients, can tolerate quite extreme hyperviscosity with few detrimental effects. Constant maintenance of adequate peripheral perfusion pressure is essential in the presence of severe hemoconcentration.

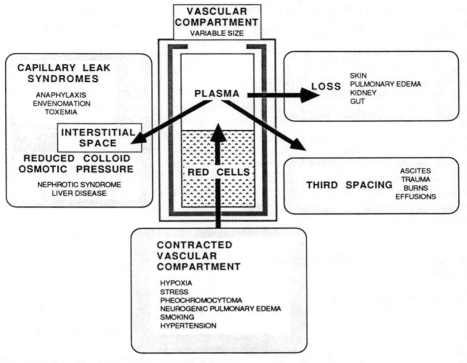

Figure 4.7. Causes and pathophysiology of contracted plasma volume syndromes

Chronic Disorders of Osmoregulation

Defects in the body's thirst mechanism classically occur in hypothalamic disease and its rarity would normally allow only passing mention. However, there is increasing interest in disorders of osmoregulation and the thirst mechanism which may cause severe dehydration, plasma volume contraction and polycythemia. The syndrome particularly occurs in elderly patients who may or may not have recognizable neurological disease resulting in chronic hypodypsia and dehydration. These patients have intact osmoreceptors and appropriate vasopressin responses, but the message is not communicated to the thirst center, so the patients will unknowingly allow themselves to become dehydrated despite the ready availability of water.

Diuretics

Acute and chronic diuretic therapy may both cause plasma volume contraction and polycythemia. The administration of diuretics to patients for the first time is particularly likely to result in sudden plasma volume reduction and associated hemodynamic consequences.

Hypoxic States

Rapid ascent to high altitude may be associated with the development of a syndrome of headache, insomnia, nausea, irritability, oliguria and sometimes life-threatening pulmonary edema and coma. This acute mountain sickness, although initiated by a low inspired oxygen tension, has a complex pathophysiology of which an important component is polycythemia with hyperviscosity and microcirculatory failure. The rise in hematocrit on ascending to high altitude is initially due to acute plasma volume contraction and hemoconcentration. As chronic adaptation occurs there is an increase in red cell production and red cell mass increases. When attempts are made to reach extremely high altitudes (e.g., conquering Mt Everest without the use of supplemental oxygen) further dehydration, hemoconcentration and hyperviscosity may become extreme. Maintenance of hydration in these rarefied and dry conditions is of crucial importance when undertaking such hazardous pursuits.

Acute hypoxic states from other causes, such as acute respiratory failure or carbon monoxide poisoning, produce varying degrees of plasma volume contraction. This is probably by the similarly poorly understood mechanisms responsible in acute mountain sickness. It is, however, logical that the only way to acutely increase the oxygen-carrying capacity of blood is to contract the plasma volume. Adequate filling of the heart is maintained by reducing the venous capacitance volume (probably via adrenergic mechanisms).

Anaphylaxis and Other Capillary Leak Syndromes

Any condition in which there is sudden release of large amounts of vasoactive amines will result in a sudden leakage of plasma into the interstitial space and acute hemoconcentration. The combination of acute hypovolemia in conjunction with hyperviscosity may lead to severe microcirculatory failure. Various forms of envenomation may also have acute capillary leak as a major manifestation.

Endocrine Disease

Acute diabetic hyperosmolar coma presents with severe hyperglycemia, dehydration, hyperosmolality and hemoconcentration, with minimal evidence of ketoacidosis. The syndrome occurs in elderly, maturity-onset noninsulin-dependent diabetics. The profound osmotic diuresis precipitated by severe hyperglycemia results in plasma volume depletion. The patients commonly present with cerebrovascular occlusive episodes. With early diagnosis of this syndrome followed by swift plasma volume expansion and more gradual correction of hyperosmolality, the patients commonly improve dramatically and are left with surprisingly little residual neurological deficit. This supports the concept that much of the cerebrovascular defect is microcirculatory in nature due to the severe hyperviscosity (from polycythemia) and low microvascular perfusion pressure due to the

systemic hypotension and artheromatous narrowing of the larger cerebral vessels.

Stress Polycythemia (Gaisbock's Syndrome)

It is not strictly correct to give this syndrome the status of a disease as many different disorders have been included under a multitude of different synonyms. Gaisbock originally described a group of patients with polycythemia and hypertension (polycythemia hypertonica) with splenomegaly. Some of these patients may have had polycythemia rubra vera. With the introduction of red cell mass and plasma volume measurements it became clear that there were patients with relative polycythemia due to plasma volume contraction and various terms were introduced to cover this entity, including chronic relative erythrocytosis, benign erythrocytosis, spurious polycythemia, pseudopolycythemia and stress polycythemia. To the associations of psychological stress and hypertension have been added obesity, vascular occlusive disease, excess alcohol intake and cigarette smoking. With all these common associations it is natural that there will be difficulties in elucidating causal relationships. Several theories have been proposed relating polycythemia to stress and the most tenable one at present is the increased venous tone theory. Catecholamines are known to cause venoconstriction and centralize the blood volume. In order to maintain normal cardiac filling pressures and volumes the plasma volume must contract.

Cigarette Smoking

The association between smoking and polycythemia has been recognized for many years, but it is only in the last decade that there has been a clearer understanding of the pathophysiology. Until recently it was assumed that pulmonary disease with arterial hypoxia was necessary for polycythemia to develop. The converse has been found, in that most heavy smokers with polycythemia have normal arterial oxygen tension. Red cell mass and plasma volume studies have revealed several different patterns. Some patients have clearly elevated total red cell mass, but the

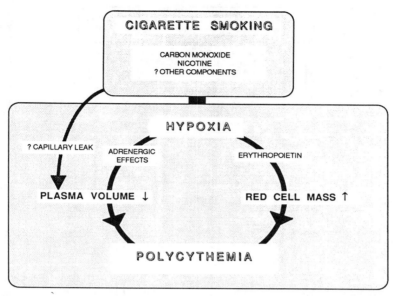

Figure 4.8. Hematological effects of cigarette smoking

majority have a significant plasma volume contraction with minimal or no increase in red cell mass. In some patients both parameters are within the normal range, but the plasma volume is at the lower limit and the red cell mass is at the upper limit (Fig. 4.8).

When plasma volume contraction is present, the effects of smoking on the hematocrit are relatively quickly reversible. Cessation of smoking may lead to the hemoglobin falling 10g/dL or more in a matter of 24 hours. It is a common observation in the coronary care unit that many patients are mildly polycythemic on admission with the hematocrit returning to normal in the days following admission to the unit. This is commoner in smokers, but recent diuretic therapy, dehydration or stress may also be incriminated.

Clinical Significance of Plasma Volume Contraction

The reduction in fluidity of the blood which occurs in association with plasma volume contraction may have detrimental effects on an already stressed circulation. This is not only likely to impair the oxygen transport chain, but may set up a series of vicious cycles within the microcirculation affecting all functions. The impaired microcirculatory flow

may ultimately culminate in thrombosis. Thrombosis may also be precipitated at other sites of vascular narrowing (e.g., atheroma or spasm). In any patient who develops a vascular occlusive episode close attention should be given to the possible precipitants including factors causing plasma volume contraction.

It is important to consider any alteration in the individual components of the blood as hemoconcentration from plasma volume reduction may have significant effects on microvascular rheology. Dysproteinemias, hyperfibrinogenemia, cryoproteins and elevation of acute phase reactants are important plasma factors which will affect the level at which a rising hematocrit begins to adversely effect whole blood viscosity. Red cell deformability, leukocyte numbers and platelet numbers are also important. Patients presenting for the first time with acute vascular occlusion of any vascular bed may have pre-existing plasma volume contraction or develop it soon after the vascular episode. Dehydration, smoking and diuretic therapy are the commonest reasons for depleted plasma volume in these patients. There is increasing recognition that a chronic hematological stress syndrome exists which has features in common with the hematological response to injury and infection. However, the reaction is probably inappro-

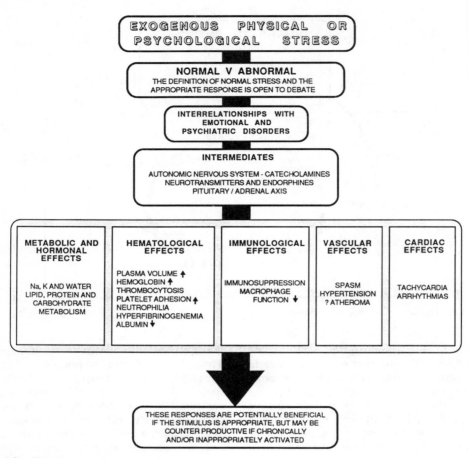

Figure 4.9. The stress syndrome

priate or excessive and reduced blood fluidity is a major feature, especially if polycythemia occurs (Figs. 4.9 and 4.10).

Management of Polycythemia due to Plasma Volume Contraction

The rate of onset of the plasma volume contraction will be important since it will be the main determining factors regarding the necessity for volume replacement to maintain effective circulating blood volume. It is in conditions such as anaphylaxis, where catastrophic sudden reduction in plasma volume occurs, with the development of hypotension, microcirculatory failure, and shock. Rapid colloid infusion may be life-saving in this group of patients.

Acute plasma volume expansion and he-modilution may be beneficial in the presence of vascular occlusive disease. Dextran is the commonly recommended plasma expander for hemodilution because of its additional flow-promoting and antithrombotic effects. The treatment of polycythemia due to chronic plasma volume contraction, if the cause is not apparent, is controversial. Identifiable contributory factors should be removed as far as possible. A persistently elevated hematocrit is a risk factor for vascular occlusive disease. At present there is no long-term therapy which effectively expands the plasma volume. Control of hypertension using alpha-adrenergic blocking agents such as prazosin may work in some patients. Most physicians resort to venesection to aid in controlling the polycythemia, which in most cases is successful, although on superficial analysis is illogical, therapy. However, it has been observed that

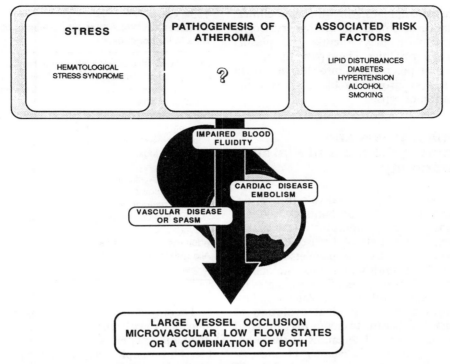

Figure 4.10. The stress syndrome and the multifactorial nature of vascular disease

the beneficial effects on hematocrit may persist for longer than can be clearly explained.

Prevention of blood fluidity crises must always be an integral part of management. Patients should be advised to maintain adequate fluid intake and to avoid dehydration. Careful attention to fluid balance in hot weather and adequate fluid replacement during times of intercurrent illness is important. Early recognition and treatment of sepsis will reduce the compounding effects of the acute phase reaction on blood fluidity. Careful attention should be given to avoiding iatrogenic factors which may acutely increase blood viscosity or reduce perfusion pressure. Diuretics, fasting for repeated investigative procedures, medication affecting autonomic function, radiocontrast media and blood transfusions are some of the factors which should be borne in mind as potential sources of this problem.

Leukostasis Syndromes

The hemorheological significance of extreme leukocytosis is variable. Leukocytes are less deformable than red cells and high counts may result in blood hyperviscosity affecting the microcirculation. The clinical importance of this probably relates to cell size and type. Cells of the granulocytic series are more likely to be associated with clinical evidence of hyperviscosity and microcirculatory failure. This occurs in its most dramatic form as the fulminant leukostasis syndrome. In this situation there appears to be a "chain reaction" in which the high count of primitive granulocytic cells leads to obstruction of the microcirculation, breakdown of lysosomes and local activation of the coagulation system. This results in sudden peripheral circulatory obstruction, particularly manifest in the cerebral and pulmonary circulations, and seen histologically as leukocyte-fibrin thrombi. This fulminant syndrome is usually irreversible and rapidly fatal and may be seen as the agonal event in untreated acute leukemias, especially those of myeloid origin, but may occasionally occur in extreme reactive leukocytosis.

There is a more common and less severe form of leukostasis which may be relieved by intensive leukapheresis in which the clinical presentation is similar to the hyperviscosity associated with polycythemia and plasma protein abnormalities. These patients may develop, or be precipitated into, the fulminant leukostasis syndrome by blood transfusion, dehydration or sepsis.

Thrombocytosis and Thrombocythemia and Platelet Hyperactivity

With the platelets central role in host defense and hemostatic mechanisms it is not surprising that it is important in the pathophysiology of a variety of diseases. Excessive numbers or overactivity of platelets may both threaten blood fluidity and thus microcirculatory flow. The spectrum of disease states resulting in part or solely from platelet pathology ranges from the gradual evolution of atheromatous disease to acute disseminated platelet aggregation. The causes of thrombocytosis are presented in chapter 11 and discussion will be restricted to those conditions in which thrombocytosis is the major problem. Space does not permit presentation of conditions in which hyperactivity of platelets is of pathophysiological importance. These are listed in Table 4.2.

ESSENTIAL THROMBOCYTHEMIA (ET)

In essential thrombocythemia there is overproduction of platelets and the characteristic symptoms of microvascular obstruction may occur. It is well recognized that peripheral ischemic lesions and gangrenous digits may occur in this syndrome. Impairment of the circulation in other vascular beds, e.g. mesenteric, splenic, hepatic, or cerebral, may occur. Headache, paresthesias and transient cerebral ischemic attacks are common. This condition should also be considered in the differential diagnosis of presenile dementia. Overlap with the other myeloproliferative disorders is common (see chapter 9), but strict differentiation is more of academic interest as therapy is similar. There is usually a qualitative defect in platelet function which may predispose the patient to bleeding, especially if invasive procedures or surgery are undertaken.

Table 4.2
Conditions in Which Platelet Activation May Play a Role in Pathogenesis

Arterial occlusive disease: atheroma formation, platelet aggregation, embolic phenomena, vascular spasm
Cerebrovascular disease: stroke and transient ischemic attacks
Coronary artery disease: angina, infarction, sudden death
Peripheral vascular disease
Amaurosis fugax
Diabetes
Raynaud's syndrome
Venous thrombosis
Renal glomerular disease
Heparin induced thrombosis thrombocytopenia syndrome
Adult respiratory distress syndrome
Allergic states
Migraine

Therapy is aimed at reducing platelet aggregability with antiplatelet therapy and reducing the platelet count as quickly as possible. Thrombopheresis offers a rapid method of alleviating the urgency of the situation. The long-term therapy of essential thrombocythemia usually involves marrow suppressive agents similar to those used in polycythemia rubra vera (busulphan, radioactive phosphorus, hydroxyurea).

REACTIVE THROMBOCYTOSIS

Reactive thrombocytosis is seen as part of the acute phase reaction and is probably of no rheological significance unless there are other factors affecting blood flow. Occasionally the thrombocytosis may be extreme ($>1000 \times 10^9$/L) and one must be concerned about the rheological significance. Antiplatelet therapy is the most appropriate therapy until the stimulus has resolved. Causes of marked reactive thrombocytosis ("platelet millionaires") include: postsplenectomy; malignancy; bacterial sepsis; inflammatory disease (e.g., rheumatoid arthritis). In some situations thrombocytosis may be a marker of disease activity, such as in rheumatoid arthritis.

PLASMA HYPERVISCOSITY

Hyperviscosity of the blood may result from several different plasma abnormalities.

In some, the presence of an abnormal protein or normal protein in excess is responsible, in others the particular characteristics of the protein lead to microcirculatory disease. In most patients plasma exchange is an effective mode of therapy, usually followed up with definitive therapy for the underlying disease.

MONOCLONAL IMMUNOGLOBULINS

Monoclonal IgM is one of the features of Waldenstrom's macroglobulinemia and is responsible for the hyperviscosity. Less commonly a similar picture may be seen with IgA multiple myeloma or occasionally with IgG. Details of the underlying hematological malignancies are described in chapter 9.

CRYOGLOBULINS

The various forms of cryoglobulinemia may manifest clinically as microcirculatory impairment with or without vasculitis. The cryoglobulin may consist entirely of monoclonal immunoglobulin produced by a malignant (e.g. myeloma) or benign (e.g. benign monoclonal gammopathy) immunoproliferative disease. In other patients it may be a mixed cryoglobulinemia in which one of the components may be a monoclonal immunoglobulin. Whatever the type of cryoglobulin, rapid removal by plasma exchange is a matter of urgency for some patients. This therapy may present technical difficulties as the cryoglobulin tends to precipitate in the extracorporeal circuit and obstruct flow. It is essential that the patient be kept warm at all times and that the plasma exchange procedure be carried out at a high ambient temperature, with prewarming of the cell separator and the infusion fluids.

COLD AGGLUTININS

Many patients with cold agglutinins are found to have a monoclonal IgM immuno-globulin in their plasma. If this is of high titer with a narrow thermal range the clinical manifestations are those of microcirculatory obstruction in the acral areas in relation to cold exposure. However, if the autoantibody has a wide thermal range and reacts above 30°C hemolysis is usually the clinical problem. Some patients with cold autoagglutinins may have an underlying immunoproliferative disease which will direct therapy.

HYPERFIBRINOGENEMIA AND CRYOFIBRINOGENEMIA

Fibrinogen, being an acute and chronic phase reactant protein, will be elevated in a range of reactive states. The development of mild anemia with the reaction usually offsets any hyperviscosity effects. However, there is increasing interest in the hematological stress syndrome and its relation to vascular disease. Any patient with vascular disease should have the basic hemorheological parameters measured and specialist opinion sought if significant abnormalities are found. Cryofibrinogenemia is uncommon and rarely causes major clinical problems. If present in large amounts the clinician should suspect an underlying malignancy or autoimmune disease. Hyperfibrinogenemia usually settles when the stimulus resolves but in the chronic state drugs such as metformin and arabolin (or stanazol) may have a role in therapy.

Further Reading

Cupps, TR, Fauci, AS *The vasculitides: major problems in internal medicine.* Vol. 21, Philadelphia: W.B. Saunders Company Ltd, 1981.

Firkin, BG *The platelet and its disorders.* Lancaster: MTP Press Limited, 1984.

Riezenstein, P *Haematological stress syndrome: the biological response to disease.* New York: Praeger Publishers, 1983.

Thompson, AR, Harker, LA *Manual of haemostasis and thrombosis. 3rd ed. Philadelphia: F.A. Davis Company, 1983.*

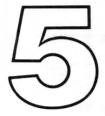

Hematological Aspects of Venous Thromboembolism

That surly spirit, melancholy,
Had bak'd thy blood and made it heavy, thick,
Which else runs trickling up and down the veins.

William Shakespeare (1564–1616) King John, III, iii, 42

Loss of blood fluidity is a constant threat to life and limb, however the continuing fluidity of blood is frequently taken for granted. In chapter 4 the problem of impaired blood fluidity in relation to arterial and microvascular disease is considered; in this chapter attention will be focused on the basic pathophysiological and therapeutic aspects of venous thrombosis. No branch of medicine is exempt from responsibility in relation to the prevention and diagnosis of venous thromboembolism. It remains the commonest cause of unexpected death in hospitals, particularly in the postoperative period. Venous thrombosis has a habit of presenting itself when least expected and when all else appears to be going according to plan. As the effects of venous thrombosis may present to the cardiologist or respiratory physician, as a pulmonary embolus, or to the vascular surgeon as a deep vein thrombosis, it is commonly not regarded as a hematological disease. The initial events leading to loss of blood fluidity in the veins and subsequent propagation of the thrombus are of a hematological nature and it is at this level that efforts to prevent and treat venous thrombosis should be directed. The basic principles are relatively straightforward and if applied in a logical fashion the prevention and management of venous thromboembolism would not be quite the confused and controversial subject it is today. Much work has been done in the last two decades to increase our understanding of this common disorder, but important aspects of this knowledge are not applied in day to day clinical practice. Old dogmas still tend to dominate practice.

Historical Background

Although venous thrombosis has been with us from early days it is only in the last century that our understanding has been placed on a scientific basis. There are basically three modern eras in our understanding of venous thromboembolic disease.

The Pathological Era of the Late 19th Century

The doyens of modern scientific medicine recognized venous thrombosis in autopsy studies from the mid 19th century. Rudolph Virchow's name is inseparably linked with this era and his triad of factors important in vascular occlusion remains as functional today as it was 100 years ago.

The Clinical Era and Introduction of Anticoagulants in the First Half of the 20th Century

During the 20th century clinicians became aware of the clinical entities of deep venous thrombosis and pulmonary embolism. Diagnosis was generally at an advanced stage and there was a lack of awareness of subclinical disease with little attention being paid to prevention. The introduction of anticoagulants for therapy of venous thrombosis improved the outcome of patients and the mortality from pulmonary embolism was considerably reduced. As a result of these successes certain dogmas and protocols were introduced into clinical practice, many of which still "hang

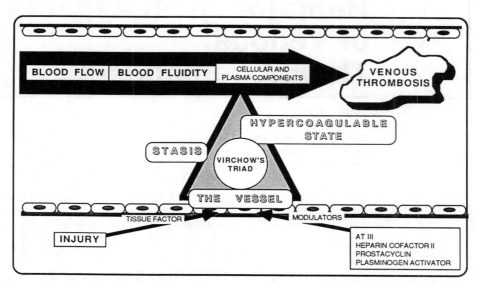

Figure 5.1. Virchow's triad in the etiology of venous thrombosis—AT III = antithrombin III

in" today with very little scientific basis for them.

The Laboratory Era and Introduction of Prophylactic Measures in the Second Half of the 20th Century

During the last two decades there have been significant advances in methods for diagnosis of both deep vein thrombosis and pulmonary embolism. There is a clearer understanding of the natural history of small subclinical thromboses. Programs for prevention of postoperative venous thrombosis have been developed. Understanding of the hemostatic system and identification of the risk factors for venous thrombosis have altered our whole concepts of pathophysiology and therapy.

It may well be asked why there are so many difficulties in the management of a disorder which can be diagnosed using sophisticated techniques, treated with highly effective drugs and prevented with appropriate attention to risk factors and prophylaxis. Most experienced clinicians are more than aware of this "Achilles heel" of modern clinical medicine.

Pathophysiology

When consideration is given to the large volume of blood pooled in the venous system at any point in time one is more inclined to ask the question, how does it remain fluid, rather than why does it occasionally clot? The blood and the vascular system have complex methods for maintaining blood fluidity and flow, even under the most adverse conditions. It is rare that a single factor is responsible for the development of venous thrombosis and it is usually when a combination of variables come together that thrombosis results (Fig. 5.1). Whether the thrombus will lyse, propagate or embolize is further determined by a multitude of factors.

VIRCHOW'S TRIAD

The Vessel

In contrast to arterial disease, unless there has been direct trauma, the vessel wall seems to be less important as an initiating factor in venous thrombosis. There are numerous mechanisms in the vein walls to protect against thrombosis. These mechanisms mainly emanate from the endothelial cells and include prostacyclin, plasminogen activator and antithrombin III. It is only when the vessel wall is directly damaged and the subendothelium exposed, that a nidus for thrombosis is available. This may be seen in hip surgery, some pelvic surgery and in relation to intravenous cannuli.

The Fluid

The hemostatic system is in a delicate equilibrium, but is able to sustain quite "hard knocks" without inappropriately solidifying the blood. When one considers the number of activating insults to which the hemostatic system may be exposed (see section on risk factors) it is amazing that the circulation of blood continues under such adverse conditions. As well as the factors mentioned above, in relation to endothelial cells there are several components of the blood itself which are responsible for rapidly controlling any extension of thrombosis beyond the site at which it is intended. Included among these mechanisms are antithrombin III, the fibrinolytic system and protein C. A great deal of attention has been given to the hypercoagulable state where there may be measurable alterations in the blood suggesting the risk or presence of thrombosis (see below). As a generalization, the coagulation and fibrinolytic phases of the hemostatic mechanism are of greater importance in the propagation of venous thrombosis than the primary platelet-endothelial interactions. This is not to deny the role platelets may initially play in thrombi forming in venous valve pockets.

The Flow

It has often been said that in order to keep the blood fluid it should be kept flowing. The role of stasis in venous thrombosis is important due to the mere nature of this component of the circulatory system. The stagnant pockets of blood around the valves of the soleal veins appear to be the main "breeding ground" for venous thrombi. The subsequent propagation will again depend on Virchow's triad, but the flow of blood will be one of the major factors. The prevention of pooling and efficient functioning of the lower limb muscle pump system is crucial.

Risk Factors for Developing Venous Thrombosis

As venous thrombosis is a multifactorial disorder, it is not surprising that there has been difficulty in identifying single independent variables (Fig. 5.2). There are some iden-

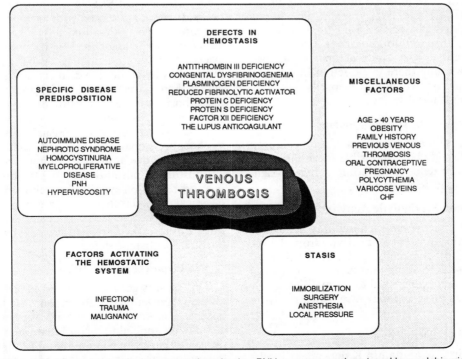

Figure 5.2. Risk factors for developing venous thrombosis—PNH = paroxysmal nocturnal hemoglobinuria

tifiable causal factors where specific defects are measurable in the hemostatic system, but in most circumstances it is the recognition of a risk factor without a satisfactory explanation for a causal relationship. In general, the current state of the art dictates that the clinician identifies risk factors and either takes steps to correct these or if not possible, takes appropriate prophylactic measures to reduce their likelihood of inducing thrombosis.

Identifiable Defects in the Hemostatic System

Control of the hemostatic system is discussed in chapter 1. There are now several clearly identifiable congenital and acquired defects predisposing to venous thrombosis.

Antithrombin III Deficiency

This is a rare quantitative or qualitative autosomal dominant deficiency of the key control protein of the coagulation phase of the hemostatic system. The patients are prone to venous thrombosis and tend to be resistant to heparin therapy. It can occur as an acquired disorder in the nephrotic syndrome, during pregnancy, with the use of oral contraceptives, with disseminated intravascular coagulation (DIC) and liver disease. The hemostatic system is more sensitive to reduction or dilution of the inhibitors of coagulation than of the active coagulation factors. In the postoperative state there is reduction in coagulation inhibitors which may be partly due to intravenous fluid dilution.

Congenital Dysfibrinogenemia

Congenital abnormalities of the fibrinogen molecule may be responsible for a variety of hemostatic defects, including a hypercoagulable state in some patients.

Reduced Fibrinolytic Activity

Some patients have a hereditary deficiency of plasminogen activator activity from the venous endothelial cells, a defect which may also be seen in some postoperative and traumatic states. Congenital abnormalities of the fibrinogen molecule may also occasionally be found.

Protein C Deficiency

Protein C is a vitamin K dependent inhibitor of coagulation which is activated at the endothelial surface. In its active form it is responsible for inactivation of factors V and VIII and activation of fibrinolysis. The full clinical significance of protein C deficiency is still being elucidated, but it appears more common than AT III deficiency and in its rare homozygous form is responsible for neonatal purpura fulminans.

Protein S Deficiency

Protein S is a cofactor for the action of protein C.

Factor XII Deficiency

As discussed in chapter 1 factor XII has a major role in the activation of fibrinolysis in the contact phase of coagulation activation and thus venous thrombosis is more of a problem in this group of patients than bleeding.

The Lupus Anticoagulant

The lupus anticoagulant, named because of its initial identification in association with systemic lupus erythematosus, has turned out to be a slight misnomer. The lupus anticoagulant should be suspected in patients with a prolongation of the APTT and is only associated with classical SLE in a minority of patients. It is not associated with an in-vivo hemostatic defect. Paradoxically, the lupus anticoagulant is associated with venous and arterial thrombotic tendency. A distinct syndrome has been identified in recent years in which there is recurrent arterial and venous thrombosis, recurrent abortion due to placental infarction, and thrombocytopenia. Venous thrombosis may occur in unusual sites, such as hepatic, renal, retinal and mesenteric veins. The lupus anticoagulant appears to be an anticardiolipin antibody, explaining false positive results on syphilis screening serology. Classical SLE serology in this group of patients often gives negative results. Specialized tests are necessary to further categorize this unusual hemostatic defect.

The Hypercoagulable State

This term is generally applied to individuals who have an increased tendency to thrombose. It is an unsatisfactory term as it has also come to be applied to a combination of laboratory investigations in an attempt to test for the prothrombotic state. Many of the changes measured are not directly relatable to the likelihood of venous thrombosis and are purely manifestations of the body's response to an invasive insult or stress. Except for the specific demonstration of an inhibitor deficiency state, these tests for the hypercoagulable state have not been of great assistance in the management of clinical problems or the prevention of venous thrombosis. Some of the tests may assist in the determination of the presence of active thrombosis and can be used as a relatively noninvasive screening test. Even so, the clinician will still need objective evidence of the presence of venous thrombosis or pulmonary embolism before committing a patient to continuing anticoagulant therapy. Table 5.1 lists the laboratory measures which may support the presence of a hypercoagulable state.

Table 5.1
Investigations Which May Be Helpful in Screening for the Hypercoagulable State

Full blood count
   Polycythemia
   Leukocytosis
   Thrombocytosis
   Elevated ESR
Elevated coagulation factors
   Fibrinogen and factor VIII
Dysfibrinogenemia
Presence of circulating activated coagulation factors
   Thrombin
   FDP's
   Fibrin monomer
   Fibrinopeptide A
Decreased inhibitors of coagulation
(biological and immunological assays)
   AT III
   Protein C
   Protein S
Defects in the fibrinolytic system
Prolonged euglobulin lysis time with poor inactivation following stasis
   Reduced plasminogen
   Reduced fibrinolytic activators
   Increased antiplasmins
   Defective plasminogen
Factor XII deficiency
Platelet and endothelial cell alterations
   Thrombocytosis
   Evidence of platelet activation (beta thromboglobulin, platelet factor 4 release)
   Hyperaggregability to collagen, ADP, adrenaline or spontaneous aggregation
   Reduced prostacyclin
Homocystinuria

Factors Which May Activate the Hemostatic System

There are numerous disease states and therapeutic interventions which may be responsible for activation of the hemostatic system. These include:

- Bacterial infection.
- Trauma—related to nature and extent, including surgery and labor.
- Malignancy—adenocarcinomas, leukemias.
- Blood transfusion—stored blood has some procoagulant activity.
- Excessive dilution with IV fluids.
- Intravenous lines and monitoring equipment.
- Cell destruction—tissue necrosis, hemolysis.
- Intravenous irritants and aggregating agents, e.g. radiological contrast media and sclerosing agents.

Factors Causing Stasis

- Immobilization in bed.
- Surgery—time-related.
- Anesthetic factors—including muscle relaxants.
- Local pressure.
- Pregnancy.

Disease States with Specific Predisposition

- Systemic lupus erythematosus.
- Lupus anticoagulant.
- Behçet's disease.
- Other autoimmune disorders.
- Nephrotic syndrome.
- Homocystinuria.
- Myeloproliferative disease.
- Paroxysmal nocturnal hemoglobinuria.
- Autoimmune hemolytic anemia.
- Hyperviscosity syndromes.
- Prosthetic vascular surfaces.

Miscellaneous Factors

- Age >40 years.
- Obesity.
- Family history.
- Previous venous thrombosis.
- Oral contraceptive.
- Pregnancy.

- Polycythemia.
- Blood group A.
- Varicose veins.
- Cardiac disease (especially congestive cardiac failure).

General Principles in the Diagnosis of Venous Thromboembolic Disease

From the "backing" of probabilities using relatively insensitive clinical assessment, the diagnosis of venous thrombosis and pulmonary embolism has moved into the arena of high-technology, high-cost medicine. It is now possible to establish a firm diagnosis in the majority of patients, either before, or soon after, therapy has been instituted. Despite this, the condition is commonly missed until late in its evolution or is found at autopsy. There are also numerous patients who are exposed to the hazards of anticoagulant therapy who do not have the disease. Why does this state of affairs exist? Is it due to ignorance or does venous thromboembolism remain the Achilles heel of even the most astute clinician? It is probably a combination of both. Pulmonary embolism, with sudden death, may be the initial presentation of venous thrombosis. Both pulmonary embolism and deep vein thrombosis may masquerade under several guises or be incorrectly blamed for the features of a totally unrelated condition.

The reader is referred to other texts for specific details of the diagnosis of deep venous thrombosis and pulmonary embolism, and only the essentials will be discussed. There are several questions which the clinician needs to address if he is to successfully prevent, diagnose and treat venous thromboembolism.

What Is the Risk of the Patient in Question Having a Venous Thrombosis, a Nonfatal Pulmonary Embolus or a Fatal Pulmonary Embolus?

It can be difficult to answer this question wtih any degree of accuracy. Information from some well controlled studies is available, and the clinician needs a level of awareness to keep the possibilities in mind. Classification of patients into low, moderate or high risk groups is usually adequate for clinical

purposes. The approximate risk of venous thrombosis detected by radiolabelled fibrinogen scanning is summarized in Table 5.2. The incidence of major deep vein thrombosis is considerably less; however, it is difficult to predict in which patients proximal propagation will occur.

Can Any of the Clinical Features in the Patient Be Explained on the Basis of Venous Thromboembolic Disease?

This question applies particularly at the outset of an illness where the diagnosis has not yet been established. It is of concern again if anything unexpected eventuates during the course of another illness.

If Venous Thromboembolism Is a Possibility, What Minimum Investigations Should Be Performed to Establish the Diagnosis and Should Heparin Therapy Be Instituted Initially?

This is probably the most difficult question and its answer depends to a large extent on the experience and skills of the clinician. It is difficult to lay down firm rules as to the need to proceed with invasive investigations. The clinician's predicament is similar to the old adage: "The science of medicine is knowing what to do, the art of medicine is knowing when to do it" (Fig. 5.3).

Points to Remember!

- The majority of venous thromboembolic phenomena go undetected and resolve whatever is done. This may give a clinician a false sense of security that thrombosis does not occur in his patients.
- Due to the falling autopsy rates the clinician is likely to be less aware of fatal pulmonary emboli.
- There is general preoccupation with the acute thrombotic or embolic episode to the neglect of prophylaxis and the possible long-term sequelae.
- There is evidence that the incidence of clinically severe disease and its sequelae is decreasing, but, when sensitive screening methods are used, the overall incidence may be increasing.
- A careful clinical history is essential when

Table 5.2
Recommendations for Prophylaxis Against Venous Thromboembolism

These guidelines are based on personal preferences from experience and review of the literature.

Patient group

Surgery

High risk	—General surgery 30% to 60%	Continuous low/moderate dose heparin (IV or SC) or low-dose SC Heparin + pneumatic compression
	—Surgery in which bleeding would be hazardous, e.g., neurosurgery	External pneumatic compression
	—Hip replacement Hip fracture	Postoperative oral AC or dextran
	—Major knee surgery	Pneumatic compression
	—Major lower limb trauma	Pneumatic compression or dextran or delayed oral AC
Moderate risk		
	—General surgery 10% to 40%	LD SC heparin 5000 units eighth or twelfth hourly or pneumatic compression
	—Surgery with hazards from bleeding	Pneumatic compression or graded compressive stockings
Low risk	—All surgery <3%	Early ambulation and graded compressive stockings.

Medical

High risk	—General medical	LD SC heparin eighth or twelfth hourly
20% to 40%	—Myocardial infarction	Variable all depending on ambulatory status LD SC heparin, or oral AC graded compressive stockings.
60%	—Stroke	LD SC heparin or pneumatic compression

Individualized therapy for high-risk patients

Some patients are in an ultra-high-risk group with up to 100% chance of venous thrombosis and most of these patients need individualized therapy, usually with full anticoagulation soon after the initial surgical or medical event

High risk	Age >40 with extra risk factor (especially previous *DVT or PE*)
Moderate risk	Age >40 with no extra risk factors
Low risk	Age <40 with no extra risk factors

LD = Low Dose
AC = Anticoagulants
SC = Subcutaneous
IV = intravenous
DVT = deep vein thrombosis
PE = pulmonary embolism
As a general rule, graded compression stockings should be used whenever possible.

assessing the probabilities. Most of the clinical presentations of venous thrombosis and pulmonary embolism have a long differential diagnosis and there is nothing absolutely specific in the clinical features.

- If pulmonary embolism is a strong possibility, it is safe to instigate anticoagulation therapy with heparin if there is no bleeding or defect in the hemostatic system. Bleed-

ing caused by heparin is rare during the first 48 hours of therapy.

- Venography remains the reliable and reproducible method for demonstrating venous thrombosis in the lower limbs.
- At least 30% of patients with pulmonary embolism do not have a demonstrable origin for the thrombus.
- Between 30% and 50% of patients present-

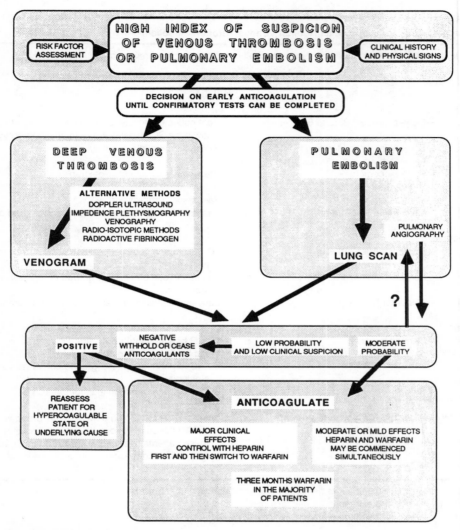

Figure 5.3.   The diagnosis of venous thromboembolic disorders

ing with a provisional diagnosis of deep vein thrombosis in the legs are subsequently proven on objective methods to have the disease. Not only will an incorrect diagnosis lead to inappropriate therapy and its associated hazards, but the label of venous thrombosis can be a difficult one to remove and can become an unfortunate "stigma" in a patient's medical history. "Thromboneurosis syndrome" is a term applied to patients who have been incorrectly labelled where there is no objective evidence to support the diagnosis in the past or at present. The patient may have been living under the constant "threat" of major thrombosis, not an insignificant psychological burden to bear.

● Isotopic perfusion lung scanning is the most widely available method for the exclusion of pulmonary embolism. Its reliability in confirming the diagnosis is variable, but is enhanced if a ventilation scan is performed at the same time. Although pulmonary angiography is the "gold standard" for diagnosis, it is an invasive procedure and not without risk.

Unusual Forms of Venous Thrombosis

Most patients with venous thrombosis develop obstruction of lower limb or pelvic veins. There are, however, several organ veno-occlusive syndromes which occur in specific disease states or in which the precipitating factors cannot be identified. Unusual veno-occlusive syndromes may affect portal, hepatic, retinal, axillary, renal, mesenteric and intracranial veins. In each of these conditions it is important to seek out any local or systemic factors which may be contributory. In many of these patients a hypercoagulable state can be identified and in some patients corrected. The clinical effects of some of these organ-specific veno-occlusive disorders may be considerable with severe end-organ dysfunction.

Treatment of Venous Thromboembolism

It is generally accepted that patients with a confirmed diagnosis of deep vein thrombosis should receive full anticoagulation therapy if there are no absolute contraindications. There is no doubt that immediate heparinization will prevent propagation of thrombus and markedly reduce the mortality from pulmonary embolism. Most of the early trials were based on patients with gross clinically obvious disease, known to have a high mortality or major postthrombotic sequelae. With the sophisticated diagnostic armamentarium available today the clinician is not always able to predict the natural history of any individual patient's disease, but still feels committed to a full anticoagulation regimen and its associated risks. At times the clinician is in an invidious position and his therapy may be dictated by traditional dogma rather than careful consideration of the risks and benefits of therapy, or no therapy, in the individual patient. It should again be emphasized that initial heparin therapy until all diagnostic information is available is in general a wise policy. As the coagulation cascade is an amplifying system, it is important that thrombin generation be controlled as soon as possible, firstly to prevent thrombus propagation and

secondly, to reduce the risk of a fatal pulmonary embolism.

The following questions should be considered when making therapeutic decisions in relation to patients with a confirmed diagnosis of venous thrombosis and/or pulmonary embolism.

What Are the Objectives of Therapy?

The clinician must always have a clear idea in mind as to the priorities and objectives at each point during a patient's illness, allowing for flexibility and changes which may occur throughout. In the overall plan the following are the objectives in the management of venous thromboembolism:

- Avoid life-threatening pulmonary embolism.
- Relieve leg symptoms as soon as possible.
- Avoid inappropriate use of anticoagulants.
- Minimize the risk of recurrence in the short and long term.
- Minimize the risk of postphlebotic syndrome.
- Keep anticoagulant side effects to a minimum.

What Is the Role of Medications Acting on the Hemostatic System?

To instigate anticoagulation therapy in a patient with venous thrombosis seems a logical decision to make and relatively simple to carry through. This could not be further from the truth, and it is probably at this point in the decision process that most errors are made and subsequently perpetuated. An extensive arsenal of drugs is available for the therapeutic manipulation of the hemostatic system and there is no question about their efficacy in increasing or decreasing action of the system at several points. These are all agents which have potentially fatal effects on a complex, integrated host-defense system. Figure 5.4 schematically summarizes anticoagulant therapy of acute venous thrombosis and pulmonary embolism.

Initial Therapy

The aim of initial therapy is to arrest thrombin generation and thus "switch off"

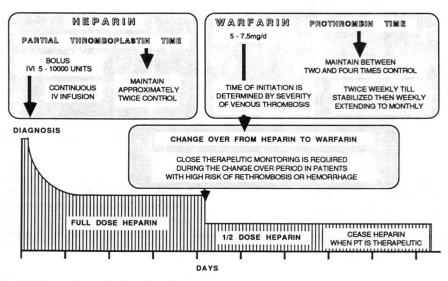

Figure 5.4. Initiation and control of anticoagulant therapy—PT = prothrombin time

the coagulation mechanism. The only immediately acting drug available for this purpose is heparin which should be given as an initial bolus dose to achieve a high initial blood level. In most circumstances thrombus generation will be controlled in the short term and a more definitive plan of management can be organized. Venous thrombi are normally lysed over a variable number of days by the body's own fibrinolytic system, but there is some evidence that heparin may potentiate this process. Under some circumstances, such as life-threatening pulmonary embolism or extensive deep venous thrombosis, the use of drugs which activate the fibrinolytic system may be considered (e.g. streptokinase, plasminogen activator).

Intermediate Therapy

Most patients with significant venous thromboembolic disease will be confined to bed in the initial phase of therapy. The logic for this is questionable and based more on theoretical considerations than clinical observation or therapeutic trials. The "standard" 10 days of heparin therapy and bed rest is inappropriate for the majority of patients and in itself may have inherent risks. Initial bed rest in patients with significant respiratory compromise and in patients with a painful swollen leg is wise. Early mobilization of patients

in whom the symptoms have resolved following heparinization is probably beneficial and has not been shown to be associated with any increased risk of pulmonary embolism. Early commencement of oral anticoagulant therapy will reduce the time spent in hospital and allow better stabilization before discharge from hospital.

Long-Term Therapy

Unless contradicted any patient committed to full heparin therapy should have continued anticoagulation therapy following discharge from hospital for a variable period of time. The need to continue anticoagulation beyond 3 months will be determined by the following considerations:

- Continuing presence of the initial thrombotic stimulus or other complications increasing the risk.
- Mobility.
- Age.
- Past history.
- Risk of anticoagulation.

As a general rule, the increased risk of recurrent *thrombosis* is in the first 3 months, and all things being equal, there is usually little to gain by continuing long-term anticoagulant therapy beyond this time.

How Should the Patient Be Managed in the Long Term?

A firm diagnosis of venous thromboembolic disease "marks" a person for life. This is not to say they will have a further thrombosis, but rather to alert the patient and future medical advisers to the proven risk. The main points in long-term management include:

- Decisions regarding anticoagulant medications and control.
- Advice regarding prevention of the postphlebotic syndrome.
- Advice in relation to future situations where there may be a risk of further thrombosis.

Some Unresolved Issues in the Management of Venous Thromboembolism

- Natural history of untreated calf vein thrombosis remains *sub judice*.
- There are problems in diagnosis and management of recurrent thrombosis.
- How long should heparin therapy be continued in management of the acute episode?
- What is the incidence of heparin-related complications?

- Are there better methods of monitoring anticoagulant therapy?

Prevention of Venous Thrombosis

With a disease in which the initial presentation may be sudden death or irreparable venous damage it is obvious that early detection or prevention is essential. There are several methods of prophylaxis of proven benefit, but these are associated with increased risks of bleeding or present economic problems. Although logical, the early detection and therapy of subclinical disease is associated with prohibitive costs and cannot be justified on cost benefit analysis. Identification of high-risk, moderate-risk and low-risk patients is necessary in order to apply appropriate intensities of prophylaxis. Figure 5.5 schematically summarizes the problems of venous thromboembolic disease and its prevention. Table 5.2 summarizes various categories of patients and their risk of thrombosis and an attempt is made, in general terms, to recommend various types and levels of prophylaxis. Methods of prophylaxis remain controversial and are only summarized. There are several important questions to address in deciding the type of prophylaxis.

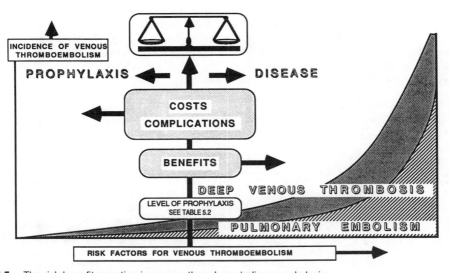

Figure 5.5. The risk-benefit equation in venous thromboembolism prophylaxis

Table 5.3
Methods for Prevention of Venous Thrombosis

Pharmacological
    Low dose Heparin
    Dextran
    Dihydroergotamine
    Oral anticoagulants

Physical
    Early ambulation
    Graded elastic stockings
    Pneumatic calf compression
    Electrical calf stimulation

Attention to anesthetic and operative technique
    Time
    Relaxants
    Intravenous therapy, including blood transfusion

Attention to reversible preoperative risk factors
    Cease estrogen-containing medications
    Reduce weight
    Correct polycythemia and other hyperviscosity
factors

What Is the Risk of Thrombosis in This Patient?

What Is the Risk of Venous Thrombosis in This Particular Clinical Setting? (i.e. Type of Surgery of Underlying Disease).

Will the Site of Surgery Affect the Type of Prophylaxis?

In surgery where bleeding is likely to result in serious complications, pharmacological agents should be avoided.

What Prophylactic Method(s) Should Be Used?

See Tables 5.2 and 5.3.

Further Reading

Goldhaber, SV ed. *Pulmonary embolism and deep venous thrombosis.* Philadelphia: WB Saunders Company, 1985.
Thompson, AR, Harker, LA *Manual of haemostasis and thrombosis.* 3rd ed. Philadelphia: FA Davis Company, 1983.

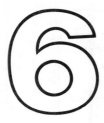

Hemostatic Failure

Have by some surgeon . . .
To stop his wounds, lest he do bleed to death.

William Shakespeare (1564–1616)
The Merchant of Venice, III, ii, 263

Failure of the hemostatic system can present the clinician with one of the most dramatic and challenging problems in clinical medicine. Not only is immediate action frequently required, but decisions may be necessary in the context of minimal laboratory data. Many bleeding disorders are eminently treatable as it is not only possible to achieve a definitive diagnosis, but a wide range of blood components are available for specific therapy. As hemostatic failure can present to any branch of medicine it is important that certain basic information is common medical knowledge so that appropriate action can be taken before specialist help is available. Hemostatic failure may complicate a wide range of medical, surgical and obstetric disorders, and its recognition is of crucial importance, particularly in the acute situation. Definitive therapy and factor replacement therapy may be major determinants of the outcome of the disease process. Complicated tests may be required for the definitive diagnosis, but therapy frequently cannot await the results of these investigations and must be initiated on clinical evidence and the minimum of laboratory results.

Presentation of Hemostatic Failure

The clinician is likely to be confronted with a hemostatic defect in several different contexts.

1. In relation to an acute hemorrhagic setting where inappropriate bleeding is occurring for which there is no obvious mechanical cause.
2. When surgery or an invasive procedure is contemplated and one wishes to predict the likelihood of hemorrhage.
3. A patient initially presenting with symptoms or signs of unexplained bleeding, bruising or purpura.
4. Abnormalities detected on laboratory screen.
5. Where there is a family history of hemostatic failure and investigation of an asymptomatic relative is requested.
6. Genetic counselling or antenatal diagnosis in a family with a known defect.

Assessing the Likelihood, Nature and Severity of a Systemic Hemostatic Defect

If certain basic principles are followed, it is possible to predict the likelihood of a systemic hemostatic defect being responsible for excessive bleeding. Figure 6.1 outlines the decision tree for the investigation of hemostatic failure.

Is There a Past History or Family History of Excessive Bleeding?

A detailed history should be taken from the patient, and from any available relatives, in relation to excessive bleeding from trauma in either the patient or relatives. If a negative history is obtained, specific questioning about teeth extraction, circumcision, tonsillectomy,

127

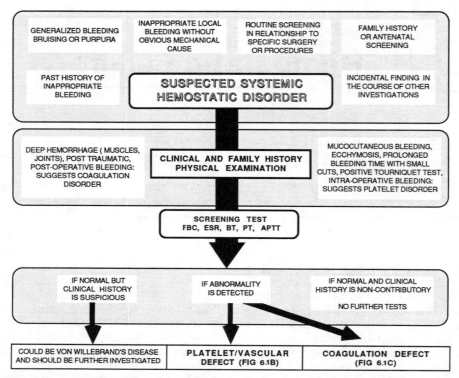

Figure 6.1A. Investigation of hemostatic failure: *A.* initial investigation; *B.* investigation of platelet/vascular defects; *C.* investigation of coagulation defects. BT = bleeding time; CBC = Complete blood count; PT = prothrombin time; APTT = activated partial thromboplastin time. TT = thrombin time; N = normal; VWF = von Willebrand's factor; VWD = von Willebrand's defect; DIC = disseminated intravascular coagulation

appendectomy and childbirth should be sought. History of blood transfusions is important.

Is There Any Underlying Medical Condition Which May Be Associated with Hemostatic Failure?

There are several conditions which may be complicated by hemostatic failure, including:

- Primary hematological disorders.
- Conditions associated with DIC.
- Liver disease.
- Uremia.
- Anticoagulant therapy.
- Antiplatelet drugs.
- Endocrine disorders (hypercortisolism).
- Nutritional (vitamin K or C) deficiency.
- Malabsorption syndromes.
- Massive blood transfusion.

What Signs Suggest Systemic Hemostatic Failure?

The characteristics of hemorrhage may point towards the presence of systemic hemostatic failure including:

- Inappropriate local hemorrhage.
- Bleeding from multiple sites.
- Unexplained bruising.
- Purpura, ecchymoses, buccal or retinal hemorrhages.
- Oozing from wounds or venipuncture sites.

Are There Features in the Patient's History and/or Clinical Findings Which Assist in Differentiating between a Disorder of Primary or Secondary Hemostasis?

Failure of primary hemostasis due to a platelet disorder is suggested by:

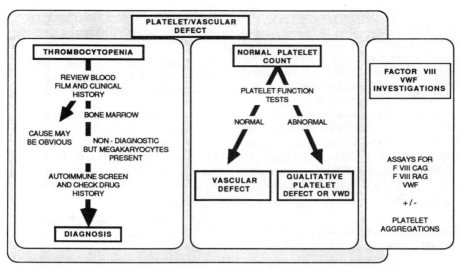

Figure 6.1*B.*

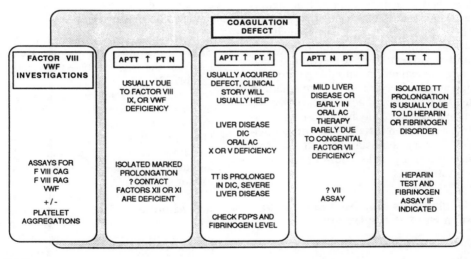

Figure 6.1*C.*

- Mucocutaneous hemorrhage—skin, nose, gums, vagina, GIT.
- Purpura and cutaneous ecchymoses.
- Bleeding intraoperatively or immediately postoperatively.
- Positive Tourniquet test.

Failure of the coagulation phases of hemostasis is suggested by:

- Deep hemorrhage—muscles, joints.
- Palpable ecchymoses.

- Delayed posttraumatic and postoperative hemorrhage.

How May Observation of the Blood Clot Assist in Diagnosing Systemic Hemostatic Failure?

Simple observation of a blood clot, although crude, may give helpful information in the initial assessment for hemostatic failure. Blood should be placed in a glass tube and kept at body temperature until clotted (under the arm if necessary). The approximate time to clot formation and subsequent clot dissolution can be measured. The size of the clot can be observed as can evidence for clot retraction. It is important that the blood be placed in a glass tube as leaving blood in a plastic syringe or siliconized glass syringe will result in delayed activation of the intrinsic system. Correctly collected blood will not clot in a plastic syringe and this does not reflect hemostatic failure. In contrast, traumatically collected blood may be activated by tissue factor and clot rapidly despite the presence of a coagulation defect.

What Screening Test Will Predict the Presence of a Defect in Hemostasis?

Reliance on screening tests to exclude a defect in the hemostatic system is fraught with problems. With such an approach a significant defect can be missed leaving the clinician with a false sense of security. The clinical history always remains of paramount importance and if suggestive of a bleeding defect, laboratory investigation should go beyond screening tests. Relying on a coagulation "profile" for detection of hemostatic defects is a common and potentially hazardous misconception. Coagulation tests will not detect disorders in primary hemostasis which require a bleeding time and platelet count as the minimum investigations.

What Medications May Be Important in Causing a Hemostatic Defect?

A careful drug history should always be taken. Besides obvious drugs such as anticoagulants and specific antiplatelet therapy, the nonsteroidal antiinflammatory drugs are most important in this respect. The patient may not immediately recollect having taken such agents (especially aspirin), and close, repeated inquiry and examination of hospital medication charts may be necessary.

What Is the Degree of Urgency?

It is important to establish the degree of urgency, priorities in diagnosis and therapy and the potential severity of the defect. Is the patient at risk of spontaneous fatal hemorrhage

(e.g., cerebral hemorrhage in association with severe thrombocytopenia)?

Are There Any Identifiable or Potentially Reversible Aggravating Factors Which May Increase the Risk of Bleeding?

Although there may be one major defect in hemostasis, it is common for other aggravating factors to be overlooked, such as antiplatelet therapy, anticoagulants and physical therapy (Fig. 6.2). One bleeding defect may be well tolerated, but two in association will not.

What Type of Invasive Procedure is Contemplated?

Concern regarding the significance or clinical severity of a bleeding disorder may be determined by the nature of the invasive procedure. The following factors warrant consideration in answering this question.

- Is bleeding likely to be hazardous to the patient as a result of the volume likely to be lost, or the site of bleeding (e.g., intracerebral)?
- Is it possible to achieve local surgical hemostasis even though there is a defect in the hemostatic system?
- How difficult will it be to establish whether bleeding is occurring? With needle biopsies and aspirations, the bleeding may be occult for some time.
- What other methods are available to assist with hemostasis? There are various surgical and anesthetic techniques which may be used to minimize blood loss, such as controlled hypotension, tourniquets, vasoconstrictors, and local thrombin application.

Accepting that a Hemostatic Defect Is Present, How Important Is the Performance of the Invasive Procedure in Question, and Do the Risks Outweigh the Likely Benefits?

Investigation for a Systemic Hemostatic Defect

The laboratory investigation of a patient who may be suffering a hemostatic defect will

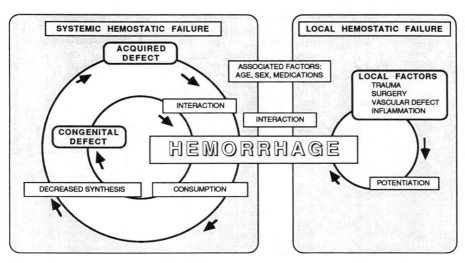

Figure 6.2. Interacting factors in hemostatic failure

vary depending on the degree of urgency. In many clinical settings it may be necessary to administer blood component therapy without a definitive defect in hemostasis having been proven. In elective settings the defect can be accurately identified and specific blood component therapy requested and given prophylactically or therapeutically. It is the responsibility of the clinician to delay any elective invasive procedure or operation until a suspected hemostatic defect can be properly investigated. The management of an undiagnosed hemostatic defect is more difficult in an emergency; and all too often, a potentially dangerous situation or real disaster could have been averted if a careful clinical history had been taken before elective surgery was initiated. There are few areas in clinical medicine where a brief history and simple laboratory investigations could be more cost effective. There are several principles which must be observed in the collection of blood samples for hemostatic investigations. All samples (except FDP determinations) are usually collected into citrated (sodium citrate) plastic or siliconized glass tubes. The amount of anticoagulant in the tube is related to the intended amount of blood which should be placed in the tube, which is usually indicated by a line on the label. Although there is slight leeway, it is important that the correct amount of blood be added to the tube and

mixed gently. The amount of citrate in the tube determines the amount of calcium added during the performance of the test. The samples for coagulation tests should be placed on ice, and those for platelet function tests should remain at room temperature. Rapid transportation to the laboratory is important. Careful attention to venipuncture technique is crucial. Any contamination of the sample with tissue factor, due to traumatic venipuncture, will activate the sample and invalidate the results (especially the APTT). It is best to avoid arterial lines for sample collection as heparin contamination is possible, even if the first sample withdrawn is discarded. Collection from any vascular access line may result in a diluted sample and should be avoided. If blood for hemostatic tests is not collected with due attention to these details, there is little point in doing the tests at all; the results are uninterpretable and may lead to incorrect or potentially dangerous clinical conclusions.

LABORATORY INVESTIGATIONS OF RELEVANCE FOR THE CLINICIAN

The investigations which may be carried out on the hemostatic system are complex and require considerable expertise in their performance and interpretation (Fig. 6.3). However, the clinician does require a basic understanding if he is to correctly utilize the

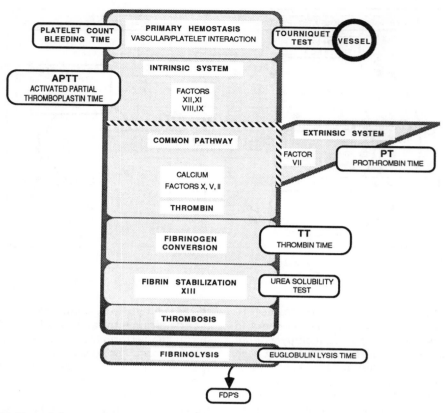

Figure 6.3. Hemostatic screening tests—FDP's = fibrin degradation products

laboratory and interpret the results. Table 6.1 summarizes the results of the standard hemostatic tests in different hemostatic defects.

TESTS OF PRIMARY HEMOSTASIS

The Bleeding Time (BT)

This is the most basic, but valuable, test in assessing primary hemostasis, the vascular phase and platelet plug formation *in vivo*. It is usually performed by the Ivy method (tourniquet applied to 40mmHg using a template to make a standard incision). Disposable units are commercially available for its performance. The incision is made on the flexor surface of the forearm and the accumulating blood is absorbed with blotting paper from the side. The normal range is 3 to 9 minutes. The BT is progressively prolonged when the platelet count falls below 75 to 100 × 10⁹/L assuming platelet function is normal. The BT is also prolonged when platelet function is de-

fective, or in capillary/vascular disease or certain coagulation defects (e.g., severe factor VII deficiency).

Platelet Count Normal Range (NR) 150 to 400 × 10⁹/L

The counting of platelets is usually performed as part of the complete blood count (CBC) by automated cell counters. In emergencies when a count is not immediately available, examination of the blood film by an experienced observer will usually give an approximation. It is not possible to perform accurate platelet counts on fingerprick blood.

Platelet Function Tests

Fresh citrated platelet-rich plasma is used for platelet aggregation tests. A platelet aggregometer is used to examine the response of platelets to aggregating agents, including collagen, adrenaline, ADP, arachidonic acid and

Table 6.1
Laboratory findings in coagulation disorders

Coagulation Defect	Bleeding Time (BT)	Prothrombin Time (PT)	Activated Partial Thromboplastin Time (APTT)	Thrombin Time (TT)
I	↑	N	N	↑
II	N	↑	↑	N
V	N or ↑	↑	↑	N
VII	N or ↑	↑	N	N
VIII	N	N	↑	N
vW Factor	↑	N	N or ↑	N
IX	N	N	↑	N
X	N	↑	↑	N
XI	N	N	↑↑	N
Contact factors	N	N	↑↑↑	N
XIII	N	N	N	N
Thrombocytopenia	↑↑	N	N	N
Qualitative platelet defects	↑↑	N	N	N
Liver disease	N	↑	N or ↑	N or ↑ (severe)
Vit K deficiency and oral anticoagulants	N or ↑ (if severe)	↑	↑	N
DIC	↑	↑	↑	↑
Heparin	N	N or ↑	↑	↑↑
Massive transfusion	↑	N or ↑	↑	N or ↑

ristocetin. From these studies it is possible to examine the primary and secondary aggregation responses, the release reaction and abnormalities suggesting von Willebrand's disease. Platelet adhesion can be measured through a glass or plastic tube, but the test is relatively crude and not of great clinical value.

TESTS OF THE COAGULATION SYSTEM

Thrombin Time (TT) or Thrombin Clotting Time (TCT) (NR of Control = 10 to 15 Seconds)

This is a test of the final conversion of fibrinogen to fibrin and bypasses the intrinsic and extrinsic systems as thrombin is added to the test system. Diluted thrombin is added to citrated plasma in a concentration which will clot normal plasma in 10 to 15 seconds. A prolongation of the time is caused by:

- Deficient substrate—hypofibrinogenemia.
- Defective substrate—dysfibrinogenemia.
- Inhibitors—antithrombin action of heparin; inhibition of fibrin polymerization due to FDP's; high levels of protease inhibitors in the acute phase reaction (e.g., alpha-2-macroglobulin).

The sensitivity of the test is adjusted by altering the dilution of the thrombin. With more dilute thrombin the test will become highly sensitive to heparin and will detect minor and clinically insignificant alterations in fibrin polymerization (especially in liver disease). There are several techniques available to test for the presence of heparin as the cause of a prolonged TT, including protamine sulfate reversal or reptilase time. Reptilase is a snake venom which can clot fibrinogen in the presence of heparin, confirming that hypofibrinogenemia is not the cause of the prolonged TT.

---

[1]NR varies considerably between laboratories.

Prothrombin Time (PT) (NR of Control = 10 to 14 Seconds)

The PT is a test of the extrinsic pathway where citrated plasma is recalcified at the same time as tissue factor (thromboplastin) is added and the clotting time recorded. The sensitivity of the test is dependent on the source of the thromboplastin as discussed in chapter 5. Thromboplastin of human brain origin is the most sensitive and widely standardized. Prolongation may be caused by:

- Factor VII deficiency—liver disease, vitamin K deficiency or oral anticoagulant therapy. Prolongation of the PT with a normal APTT is due to isolated factor VII deficiency. This may be caused by congenital deficiency, but more commonly is found early in oral anticoagulant therapy, before other factors have fallen.
- Common pathway deficiencies—APTT and PT are both prolonged due to factors X, V, II. The test is not sensitive to fibrinogen conversion because of the large amount of thrombin generated.
- Inhibitors—the PT is not particularly sensitive to coagulation inhibitors such as heparin unless there is also a factor deficiency.

Activated Partial Thromboplastin Time (APPT), (NR of Control = 25 to 35 Seconds)[1]

The APTT is a test of the intrinsic coagulation system in which the contact phase of the coagulation cascade is activated before the sample is recalcified in the presence of a platelet substitute. Prolongation of the APTT is caused by:

- Contact phase defect—if there is a defect in the contact phase (i.e., factors XI and XII) there is usually a marked prolongation of the APTT, but this prolongation does not correlate with the likelihood of hemorrhage.
- Factor VIII or IX deficiency—a mild to moderate prolongation of the APTT in the presence of a normal PT usually means that

one of the hemophilic factors is deficient or inhibited (i.e., factors VIII and IX).
- Common pathway defect—PT and APTT are both prolonged due to factor X, V, II deficiency.
- Inhibitors: acquired inhibitors of coagulation (e.g., factor VIII inhibitors and the lupus anticoagulant). The test is sensitive to the action of heparin for which it is a simple monitoring test.

Specific Coagulation Factor Assays

The clinical findings and the initial screening tests will usually give a strong guide to the likely defect in the coagulation system. The probabilities as to the exact defect can be narrowed further with the use of various mixing studies, and the subgroup of coagulation inhibitors can be identified. The next step in investigation is specific coagulation factor assay. All factors can be assayed but the following are the ones most commonly performed:

- Assays of the factor VIII components (see under hemophilia).
- Fibrinogen assay by functional, precipitation or immunological methods can be helpful in several of the acquired hemostatic disturbances, especially DIC, fibrinogenolysis and massive blood transfusion.
- Other individual factors.
- Coagulation inhibitor assays.

TESTS OF FIBRINOLYSIS

Fibrin Degradation Products (FDPs) (NR <10µg/ml)

When fibrin is lysed by the proteolytic activity of plasmin various cleavage fragments are released. These are usually measured immunologically on a serum sample. FDPs from primary fibrinogenolysis and secondary fibrinolysis are not differentiated by the standard test used in most laboratories. A specific test for D-dimer is necessary to identify that the lysis is a secondary phenomenon occurring after the formation of fibrin. Minor elevations of FDPs (20 to 40µg/ml or sometimes higher) may be seen in the postoperative state, in trauma, renal impairment, sepsis and venous thrombosis. It should not be concluded from

---

[1]Normal range must be determined for each laboratory depending upon reagents, procedure, equipment, and patient population.

such levels that an excess fibrinolysis is occurring. High levels of FDPs suggest excessive fibrinolysis as seen in DIC or a rare disorder of primary excessive fibrinolysis.

Euglobulin Lysis Time (ELT) (NR >90 Minutes)

In this test the acetic acid precipitated fraction of the plasma (euglobulin fraction) which is deficient in fibrinolytic inhibitors is clotted and the time to lysis recorded. The test mainly measures for the presence of plasminogen activators and a shortened time is indicative of systemic fibrinolytic activation (i.e., fibrinogenolysis).

ELECTIVE ASSESSMENT OF HEMOSTATIC FUNCTION

Elective assessment of the hemostatic system may be indicated under the following circumstances.

1. In patients in whom the history is negative no further investigations are usually necessary. Despite this, the clinician may require reassurance that the hemostatic system is functioning normally, especially if bleeding into a vital organ or occult bleeding is a worry. It is thus not unreasonable in certain clinical settings to perform the screening investigations outlined below.
2. In patients in whom the clinical findings are suggestive, only screening investigations should be performed and followed up with appropriate tests. Screening tests include:

   - Full blood examination, including platelet count, ESR and film examination. The presence of thrombocytopenia and any hematological disorders, such as myeloma or leukemia, should be detected or suspected.
   - APTT and PT will detect most significant coagulation defects.
   - Skin bleeding time will detect qualitative platelet defects as well as von Willebrand's disease.

3. In patients with a highly suggestive clinical history of a hemostatic defect or an abnormality on initial screening tests. It is important that patients with a strong history

of bleeding be fully investigated for a hemostatic defect as the yield will be high. This involves proceeding beyond the screening test and carrying out more detailed platelet function tests and coagulation factor assays. Detailed hemostatic investigations include:

- Platelet function studies.
- Plasma mixing studies to determine whether a factor deficiency or inhibitor is likely to be the cause.
- Specific factor assays based on the results of the APTT, PT and mixing studies. As von Willebrand's disease is the commonest congenital bleeding disorder and may only show mild defects in the screening investigations it is usual to carry out specific tests for this disorder.

URGENT ASSESSMENT OF HEMOSTATIC FUNCTION

The question of systemic hemostatic failure is commonly raised in patients in whom medical or postoperative bleeding continues without obvious reason. It is tempting to "blame" the hemostatic system for bleeding which will not stop using conventional measures. However, it should never be forgotten that the commonest cause of continued bleeding, especially in the postoperative period, is a hole in a vessel. Frequently, complicated tests are required for diagnosis of acquired disorders of the hemostatic mechanism, but diagnosis and therapy frequently cannot await the results of these investigations and therapy must be initiated on the basis of clinical evidence and the minimum of laboratory results.

PITFALLS IN THE INVESTIGATION AND MANAGEMENT OF HEMOSTATIC DISORDERS

- Inadequate attention to the clinical history and physical findings and overemphasis on laboratory investigations in initial patient assessment.
- Incorrect blood sample collection.
- Incorrectly assuming that normal results on hemostatic screening tests exclude a major hemostatic defect.
- Failing to realize that disorders of primary

hemostasis will not be detected in coagulation screening investigations.

- Incorrectly assuming there is a good correlation between laboratory results and the clinical severity of a hemostatic defect.
- Failing to request laboratory investigations in a systematic and logical manner.
- Incorrectly attributing postoperative bleeding to a systemic hemostatic defect and delay in reoperation.
- Failure to identify and appropriately investigate a potential hemostatic disorder prior to surgery.
- Reluctance to delay elective surgery when a hemostatic defect may be present.
- Excessive and inappropriate administration of blood products without correct identification of the hemostatic defect, if any.
- Failure to recognize associated factors which may potentiate a hemostatic defect or precipitate hemorrhage.
- Performance of an elective invasive procedure on a patient with a known hemostatic defect without consultation and ensuring that the appropriate blood products are available.

Disorders of Primary Hemostasis: Vascular and Platelet Disorders

The primary phase of hemostasis may be defective secondary to vascular disorders or quantitative or qualitative platelet abnormalities.

VASCULAR BLEEDING DISORDERS

Major bleeding due to vascular defects is uncommon. The diagnosis is usually apparent from the clinical history and physical signs. The following is a summary of the vascular disorders which may cause bleeding.

- Hereditary telangiectasia: autosomal dominant, mucocutaneous and GIT lesions; iron deficiency is common.
- Marfan's and Ehlers-Danlos syndrome.
- Angiodysplasia of the gastrointestinal tract is a common cause of unexplained acute or chronic GIT bleeding, iron deficiency is

common, and it presents more of a bleeding problem when there is an associated defect in hemostasis.

- Simple easy bruising: benign disorder of females, commonly aggravated unwittingly by antiplatelet therapy.
- Senile purpura: results from atrophy of supporting tissues and is prominent on the dorsal aspects of the forearms and hands.
- Scurvy: due to vitamin C deficiency, perifollicular petechiae, bruising and mucocutaneous hemorrhage.
- Cushing's syndrome and therapeutic corticosteroid administration.
- Vasculitis: many factors may damage the endothelium of vessels and result in purpuric and ecchymotic lesions (palpable purpura).

  Immune complex vasculitis: Henoch-Schöenlein purpura and other microvessel vasculitis. In these the purpura is palpable due to the inflammatory reaction. Infections: e.g., meningococcemia, staphylococcal infection in which disseminated intravascular coagulation may be present.
- Psychogenic purpuras (e.g., autoerythrocyte sensitization syndrome).

PLATELET DISORDERS

Thrombocytopenia

Thrombocytopenia is a common cause of hemostatic failure with congenital and acquired causes on the basis of decreased production or increased consumption (see Table 6.2). The following questions should be addressed and in most patients the cause of thrombocytopenia quickly becomes apparent. Figure 6.1B summarizes the decision tree for the investigation of thrombocytopenia.

1. Is the Thrombocytopenia an Isolated Finding with the Remainder of the Blood Count Normal?

Blood count and film examination may immediately reveal the cause of a thrombocytopenia:

- Leukocyte abnormalities suggesting a hematological malignancy.
- Pancytopenia suggesting marrow failure.
- Microangiopathy suggesting DIC or TTP.
- Morphological abnormalities in the plate-

**Table 6.2
Causes of Thrombocytopenia**

Congenital or hereditary thrombocytopenias
  Fanconi's syndrome
  Amegakaryocytic thrombocytopenia
  Wiskott-Aldrich syndrome
  May-Hegglin anomaly
  Bernard-Soulier syndrome
Acquired thrombocytopenia
  Shortened platelet life span
    Idiopathic thrombocytopenic purpura (ITP)
    Immune thrombocytopenia associated with
    autoimmune diseases SLE, Evans's syndrome
    Immune thrombocytopenia associated with
    lymphoproliferative disease
    Drug induced thrombocytopenia
    Thrombotic thrombocytopenic purpura
    Sepsis
    Massive blood transfusion
    Posttransfusion purpura
    Disseminated intravascular coagulation
    Hypersplenism
  Reduced platelet production
    Aplastic anemia
    Marrow infiltration: hematological (leukemia,
    lymphoma, myeloma) or metastatic malignancy
    Myelofibrosis
    Megaloblastic anemia (especially of acute onset)
    Alcohol
    Myelodysplastic syndromes

lets suggesting congenital platelet disorders. Giant platelets are commonly seen in immune thrombocytopenia.

- Features of acute megaloblastosis.
- Leukoerythroblastic blood film.
- Atypical mononuclear cells suggestive of a viral infection.
- Features of liver disease suggesting alcoholism.

2. Are There Any Clinical Features Which May Assist in Elucidating the Cause of Thrombocytopenia?

Common features in the clinical history and examination include:

- Known hematological disease.
- Recent marrow suppressive therapy.
- Lymphadenopathy, splenomegaly, hepatomegaly.
- Drug history.
- Alcohol and nutritional history.
- Recent infection.

- Features suggesting an autoimmune disease such as SLE.
- Overwhelming sepsis.
- History of recent blood component therapy.
- Massive blood transfusion.

3. Is a Bone Marrow Examination Indicated?

Unless the cause of thrombocytopenia is apparent a bone marrow examination is generally indicated and may provide the following information:

- Presence of megakaryocytes in order to separate failure of production from peripheral destruction. There are, however, some disorders in which megakaryocytes may be present but megakaryocytopoiesis is ineffective. In these conditions in which the marrow is dysplastic the cause is usually apparent.
- Diagnosis of hematological malignancy, marrow dysplasia, preleukemic syndromes, aplastic anemia, malignant infiltration.

4. What Other Tests Need to Be Carried Out to Identify Associated Disease When Thrombocytopenia Appears to Be an Isolated Finding?

If after investigation for the cause of thrombocytopenia along the lines outlined it becomes apparent that there is no underlying cause which is readily identifiable, the diagnosis of idiopathic thrombocytopenic purpura (ITP) is probable. At this point certain investigations need to be performed in conjunction with reanalysis of the patient's history to exclude any other causes of immune-mediated thrombocytopenia including:

- Serological tests for SLE.
- Antiglobulin test.
- Careful check of the patient's drug, medication and dietary history (alcohol, quinine in bitter drinks).
- Platelet autoantibody and drug antibody tests if available.

5. If the Cause Cannot Be Found, Is the Patient Therefore Suffering from ITP?

When the clinicopathological findings all point to a peripheral destruction of platelets without obvious cause it is reasonable to conclude the patient has ITP. A response to steroids would further support this diagnosis. Occasionally it is not possible to completely exclude a drug-related or preleukemic etiology.

Idiopathic Thrombocytopenic Purpura (ITP)

Pathophysiology

ITP is an autoimmune disorder where autoantibodies (IgG) are directed against the platelets which are subsequently destroyed by the monocyte macrophage system predominantly in the spleen. In some cases (especially the acute form) the pathophysiology is less well established and an immune complex mechanism with the action of complement may be involved.

Clinical Features

ITP is typically a disease of children and young adults. The acute form is more common in children (90%) with the chronic form predominantly in adults (90%). The spleen is rarely palpable. A prior viral infection is commonly identified in the acute form and recovery over weeks to months is the usual course. The course of the chronic form is variable and may spontaneously resolve, but more commonly needs specific intervention.

Therapy

Therapy of ITP remains controversial, particularly in children. Corticosteroids are usually used in initial therapy. However, the natural history of the acute disease is probably unaffected by corticosteroids, which should generally be regarded as short-term therapy. There is some evidence that the incidence of bleeding may be reduced when severe thrombocytopenia is present. In adults the majority of patients respond with a rise in the platelet count. After an initial high dose, 50 to 75mg of prednisolone a day until response occurs, the dose is gradually reduced. There is little evidence that corticosteroids will raise the platelet count in the acute disease, however their role in the short term in reducing the incidence of bleeding, which is highest in the first weeks, may be important.

Patients should be warned of the risks of bleeding and avoid body contact sports and other potentially injurious activities. Avoid-ance of antiplatelet therapy (e.g., aspirin) should be specifically emphasized. Splenectomy is usually recommended if the disease is difficult to control with corticosteroids, or remission has not occurred. The timing of splenectomy is not standardized and should generally be delayed as long as possible in the hope of a spontaneous remission. It should be emphasized that the risk of life-threatening bleeding in a patient with mild bruising as the main symptom is low and patients can be closely observed for long periods of time before the decision to perform splenectomy need be made. Other approaches may be used in ITP, including immunosuppressive agents, vincristine, high-dose IV immunoglobulin, plasma exchange and danazol.

Drug-Induced Thrombocytopenia

The clinical presentation of drug-induced thrombocytopenia may be as variable as ITP. Some may have a dramatic and fulminant presentation with marked hemostatic failure. Drugs with a particular reputation for inducing thrombocytopenia include quinine (also in bitter drinks), quinidine, antituberculous drugs, heparin, thiazide diuretics, penicillins, sulphonamides, rifampicin and anticonvulsants. A full list appears in appendix 2.

Sepsis

Platelets play an important role in the inflammatory response and a reactive thrombocytosis is usually seen in infection. However, if there is overwhelming sepsis, associated with DIC or marrow suppressive influences, thrombocytopenia may be seen. The combination of sepsis, shock, DIC, alcoholism and nutritional deficiency are common factors contributing to thrombocytopenia in critically ill patients.

Qualitative Platelet Disorders

Whenever there is evidence of primary hemostatic impairment with a prolongation of the bleeding time, but a normal platelet count, a qualitative defect in platelet function should be suspected. Defective platelet function *in vivo* can be congenital or acquired and due to the lack of cell membrane glycoprotein (Glanzmann's thrombasthenia and Bernard-Soulier syndrome), reduced or absent cytoplasmic storage granules (storage pool disease), a platelet enzyme (prostaglandin synthetase deficiency) or a plasma factor deficiency (von Willebrand's disease or hypofibrinogenemia). These abnormalities usually require sophisticated laboratory investigation, commencing with platelet aggregometry.

Hereditary Qualitative Platelet Disorders

Glanzmann's Thrombasthenia

This is a rare autosomal recessive disorder with normal adhesion of platelets, but absent aggregation responses and absent clot retraction. The platelet membrane glycoprotein IIb and IIIa complex is abnormal.

Von Willebrand's Disease

(discussed below)

Bernard-Soulier Syndrome

This is a rare autosomal recessive severe bleeding disorder with large platelets, defective adhesion and markedly prolonged bleeding time. The platelet membrane glycoprotein I complex is abnormal.

Storage Pool Disease

In this group of platelet disorders there is a mild bleeding defect due to a defective storage pool of platelet nucleotides, resulting in impaired secondary wave on platelet aggregation studies.

Congenital Aspirin-Like Defect

This recently recognized syndrome is due to prostaglandin synthetase deficiency.

Acquired Platelet Defects

Acquired defects in platelet function are much more common than the hereditary ones listed above. Table 6.3 lists the conditions in which platelet function may be impaired. Most of these disorders are discussed elsewhere in the text.

Antiplatelet Drugs

Antiplatelet agents are being used increasingly for prophylaxis and therapy of arterial and microvascular disease and many of the nonsteroidal antiinflammatory agents are also platelet inhibitory drugs. Aspirin has an irreversible effect on platelet function and platelet function tests may show abnormalities for up to 10 days after aspirin medication. Most of the other antiplatelet agents have a revers-

Table 6.3
Causes of Acquired Disorders of Platelet Function

Nutritional
19- or 21-chain fatty acids (salmon oil)
Mo-Er herb
Garlic and onions
Deficiency of folic acid, vitamins B12, C or E
Alcohol

Drugs
Nonsteroidal anti-inflammatory agents (see chapter 5)
Corticosteroids
Diuretics: furosemide
Serotonin antagonists
Anesthetic agents: lidocaine, cocaine
Antibiotics, especially penicillins
Antidepressants
Alpha and beta adrenergic blocking agents

Uremia

Dyshemopoiesis
Myeloproliferative diseases
Myelodysplastic and preleukemic syndromes
Leukemias: acute and chronic granulocytic
Megaloblastosis

Autoimmune disorders
Idiopathic thrombocytopenic purpura
Systemic lupus erythematosus

Exhausted platelet syndromes
(Acquired storage pool disease)
Disseminated intravascular coagulation
Massive blood transfusion
Extracorporeal circuits e.g., cardiac bypass
Sepsis

Infections
Viral, bacterial, protozoal and rickettsial
Parasitic: Eosinophilic purpura

Paraproteinemia

Metabolic and endocrine disease
Uremia
Liver disease
Hypothyroidism

ible effect lasting a matter of hours, or occasionally days. Aspirin is now one of the commonest causes of postoperative bleeding. The bleeding is usually mild and of nuisance value, but occasionally the effects may be serious, depending on the nature of the surgery (e.g., neurosurgery or cardiac surgery) and in some situations, a platelet transfusion may be necessary to arrest the bleeding. In other cases, the patient may already have a mild hemostatic defect (e.g., von Willebrand's disease) and aspirin may have a synergistic effect leading to major hemostatic failure.

Uremia

Hemostatic failure is a common manifestation of renal failure, its mechanism is not fully elucidated, but high levels of guanidinosuccinic acid and hydroxyphenylacetic acid are implicated and can be substantially corrected by dialysis. Prolongation of the bleeding time, defects in aggregation responses, diminished adhesion and reduced platelet factor 3 availability have all been demonstrated. Diminished prostacyclin synthesis may also be important. Factor VIII abnor-

malities have also been demonstrated which may be corrected by 1-deamino,8-*d*-arginine vasopressin (DDAVP) or cryoprecipitate infusions. A relationship between the degree of anemia and prolongation of bleeding is usually demonstrable; increasing the hemoglobin level reduces the bleeding time.

PLATELET TRANSFUSION THERAPY

Platelet transfusion therapy has made considerable advances in the last decade and most patients with platelet deficiency or dysfunction may benefit by such therapy. As a general rule in patients in whom the problem is related to increased platelet consumption, platelet transfusions are likely to be of mini-

Table 6.4
Characteristics and Therapy of the Various Coagulation Factor Deficiencies

Factor[a]	Deficiency States	Hemostatic Level	Half-Life	Source of Treatment
I	Afibrinogenemia Dysfibrinogenemia Defibrination syndromes Severe liver disease	10–25%	4–6 days	FFP Cryoprecipitate
II	Hereditary Liver disease Vitamin K deficiency Coumarin therapy	40%	3 days	FFP Supernatant plasma Prothrombin complex
V	Hereditary Massive blood transfusion DIC	10–15%	12 hours	FFP
VII	Hereditary Liver disease Vitamin K deficiency Coumarin therapy	5–10%	4–6 hours	Supernatant plasma FFP Prothrombin complex
VIII	Hemophilia A Von Willebrand Massive blood transfusion DIC	10–40%	12 hours	VIII concentrate Cryoprecipitate FFP
IX	Hemophilia B Liver disease Vitamin K deficiency Coumarin therapy	10–40%	18–24 hours	IX concentrate Supernatant plasma FFP Prothrombin complex
X	Hereditary Liver disease Vitamin K deficiency Coumarin therapy	10–15%	2 days	Supernatant plasma FFP Prothrombin complex
XI	Hereditary	variable	3 days	Supernatant plasma FFP
XII	and other contact factors are not associated with a bleeding abnormality			
XIII	Hereditary Liver disease	1–5%	?1 week	FFP XIII concentrate

[a]For completeness it should be mentioned that factor III is platelet factor III, factor IV is calcium and factor VI has not been assigned.

mal or no benefit. In some disorders, such as immune thrombocytopenia or alloimmunized patients, transfusions are usually ineffective and may even be deleterious. The role of platelet transfusion in various platelet disorders may be summarized as follows:

- Proven benefit
    - Aplastic anemia
    - Marrow suppression or infiltration
    - Hereditary and acquired qualitative platelet defects
- Probable benefit
    - Massive blood transfusion
    - Extracorporeal circulation platelet damage
    - Disseminated intravascular coagulation
- Doubtful, no benefit or possibly harmful
    - Immune thrombocytopenia
    - Alloimmunized patients
    - Posttransfusion purpura
    - Extrinsic platelet defects: hypersplenism, uremia,
    - Paraproteinemia

Coagulation Disorders

One of the most exciting, interesting and scientifically elucidating stories in medicine has been the unfolding of our understanding of blood coagulation disorders. The complex coagulation system has been dissected into its numerous individual proteins, their molecular structure elucidated, amino acids sequenced, and with some coagulation factors, the genes of origin mapped. "Experiments of nature" such as hemophilia, have commonly been the "sign post" for researchers in this field. The groundwork which has identified

the components of the coagulation system has set the scene for current research which is directed towards an integrated understanding of hemostasis, outlined in chapter 1. Despite the spectacular discoveries in the field of coagulation, which have had major influences on other areas of medical science, only one Nobel prize has ever come the way of the coagulationists.

Table 6.4 summarizes the congenital and acquired defects of the hemostatic system and the blood components available for therapy.

CONGENITAL COAGULATION DISORDERS

It is now possible to identify a wide range of hereditary disorders of the coagulation system. Most of these are uncommon and only of concern to the specialist. Abnormalities of the factor VIII complex are responsible for the majority of congenital bleeding disorders as seen in hemophilia A and the various von Willebrand syndromes.

Hereditary Disorders of the Factor VIII Molecule

The Factor VIII Complex—Structure and Function

The factor VIII complex consists of two components which have distinctly different biochemical and immunological structures, different biological functions and are under different genetic control. The characteristics of these two components of factor VIII are summarized in Table 6.5. The smaller of the components, known as factor VIIIC, has antihemophilic factor coagulant activity and is

Table 6.5
The Factor VIII/von Willebrand's Complex

Factor VIII AHF Procoagulant Protein	von Willebrand's Protein
Factor required in the intrinsic coagulation system and corrects the defect in Hemophilia A plasma	Shortens the skin bleeding time, and necessary for platelet plug formation
F VIII C (functional)	F VIII R:RCo (ristocetin cofactor)
F VIII C:Ag (immunological)	F VIII R:Ag (immunological)
Isolated deficiency in Hemophilia A	Deficient or functionally abnormal in von Willebrand's disease
X-Chromosome inheritance	Autosomal inheritance (usually dominant)
M.W. 250,000–300,000	M.W. 1.12×10^4
(?triplet of 85,000, 88,000 and 93,000)	(?heterogenous population of multimers)
Synthesis site unknown (?Liver)	Synthesis in endothelium of vessel walls

measured by a functional clotting assay or immunologically as factor VIII CAg by defined antibodies. The larger moiety factor VIII R (von Willebrand factor) is factor VIII-related antigen protein and interacts with platelets in the primary phase of hemostasis measured as ristocetin cofactor (VIIIR:RCo) or VIIIR: Ag. Factor VIIIC is an X-chromosome linked inherited characteristic, while factor VIII R is autosomal. Factor VIII R is a high molecular weight glycoprotein produced by endothelial cells. The site of synthesis of factor VIII C remains *sub judice*. In classical hemophilia there is diminished production of normal factor VIII C with the synthesis of a nonfunctional precursor, while factor VIII R synthesis and function are normal.

Hemophilia A (Classical Hemophilia)

Hemophilia A is a sex-linked disorder due to a deficiency of factor VIII. It accounts for 85% of the hemophilias and has a population incidence of 20 per 100,000 males. The clinical severity may vary from severe disease (factor VIII C <1%) with spontaneous hemorrhage 2 to 4 times a month, to mild disease (factor VIII C >5%) when hemorrhages usually only occur in relation to trauma.

Clinical Features

Excessive bleeding occurs in relation to minor cuts or trauma. A wide range of spontaneous hemorrhages may occur including hemarthroses, musculoskeletal bleeding, hematuria, GIT intramural hematoma, retropharyngeal and retroperitoneal hemorrhage. Many of these hemorrhages lead to long-term disabling sequelae, especially arthropathy. Along with the medical problems there are numerous psychosocial, economic, vocational and genetic problems.

Laboratory Diagnosis

The APTT is prolonged and factor VIII coagulant activity reduced.

Therapy

Depending on the nature of the bleeding or type of surgery, specific factor VIII therapy should be given in the form of cryoprecipitate or factor VIII concentrate to increase factor VIII levels to the appropriate level. Local control of hemorrhage and good surgical hemostasis are essential components of therapy. It is not possible to lay down rigid therapeutic formula, as treatment must be tailored to the individual patient's needs, and will be influenced by the clinician's experience and preferences, the amount of factor VIII available and the form in which it is presented. The management of hemophilia has become specialized, requiring a team approach to the numerous potential problems which confront these patients. The recent problems in relation to the acquired immunodeficiency syndrome (AIDS) and its transmission by blood transfusion has created numerous practical and ethical problems in relation to the supply of factor VIII. The radical developments occurring in joint surgery in the recent past have now made definitive joint repair and/or replacement a practical proposition for many hemophiliacs. Synovectomy, osteotomy and arthrodesis of knee, ankle and elbow joints are now being documented, as is total hip replacement.

Carrier Detection

Assay of F VIII C, F VIII CAg and F VIII RAg have assisted in identifying carrier females, in whom F VIII RAg is normal and F VIII C or VIII CAg are reduced on average by 50%. Prenatal diagnostic measurements have been made possible recently by the technique of fetoscopy. More recently DNA technology is allowing more definitive prenatal diagnosis and carrier detection. The F VIII CAg/F VIII RAg detects 70% to 90% of carriers and more sensitive techniques are needed.

Hemophilia B (Christmas Disease)

Factor IX deficiency is less common than classical hemophilia A, but the clinical features are identical. Some patients do not synthesize any factor IX molecule whereas others make a nonfunctional protein. For therapy, frozen plasma, factor IX concentrates or Proplex T can be used. Due to the longer half-life of factor IX, therapy is given less frequently than factor VIII for hemophilia A.

Von Willebrand's Disease (VWD)

Von Willebrand's disease is the commonest of the hereditary hemostatic disorders and grouped under this diagnosis is a heterogeneous collection of phenotypic variants. It is an autosomal dominant disorder character- ized by a prolonged bleeding time associated with deficiency, or a qualitative defect, in von Willebrand factor function.

Clinical Features

This is a milder hemostatic disorder than hemophilia and is not associated with the crippling features of hemophilia. The bleed- ing is superficial skin and mucocutaneous hemorrhage. Excessive bruising, bleeding after dental extraction, postoperative bleed- ing and menorrhagia are common char- acteristics.

Laboratory Diagnosis

Prolongation of the bleeding time is a hall- mark in the diagnosis of von Willebrand's disease due to reduced platelet adhesion. The bleeding time may be variable in the milder forms. The APTT may be slightly prolonged, factor VIIIC and VIIIAg are reduced, and de- fective platelet aggregation to ristocetin is found in some patients. There are several types of von Willebrand's disease. In the clas- sical form (type I) there is a variable decrease of factor VIIIC, factor VIIIR:Ag and VIIIR: CoF to 10% to 40% of normal. In the milder forms one or more of the factors may be in- termittently or consistently normal, especially during stress or pregnancy. In type II disease there is a specific absence of the high molec- ular weight multimers of VIIIR:vWF in both the plasma and platelets (type IIa) or solely in the plasma (type IIb).

Treatment

In general, management is not dictated by the variant of the disorder, with cryoprecipi- tate or fresh frozen plasma being used. The rise in factor VIII level achieved in patients with von Willebrand's disease is greater and more prolonged (12 to 24 hours) than would be expected from the amount of infused fac- tor VIII, but the von Willebrand component of the molecule will show the expected post- transfusion decay. This allows doses to be spread more widely than with hemophilia A. A characteristic feature of von Willebrand's disease is the continued rise of factor VIIIC beyond 12 hours because of in-vivo synthesis. The bleeding time may be more difficult to correct with therapy than the factor VIII de-

ficiency and the effect short-lived. A twice- daily dosage is usually required if hemostasis is crucial (e.g., surgery). In mild cases, the use of 1-deamino-8-D-arginine vasopressin (DDAVP) in conjunction with local measures may be sufficient therapy.

Afibrinogenemia and Dysfibrinogenemia

This rare group of disorders is well catego- rized and is being identified with increasing frequency as a result of preoperative hemo- static testing. The hemostatic defect in both afibrinogenemia and dysfibrinogenemia is mild in most cases, although wound healing may be poor. Therapy is with fibrinogen con- centrates or cryoprecipitate.

Other Coagulation Factor Deficiencies

Hereditary deficiencies of factors II, V, VII, X, XI, XII and XIII are all rare and when de- tected, should be treated with the appropriate plasma component (see Table 6.4).

ACQUIRED HEMOSTATIC DISORDERS

The acquired abnormalities of coagulation are usually more complex and multifactorial than the hereditary disorders. For most, spe- cific therapy apart from blood component in- fusion is indicated. This is discussed in other texts. However, a unified approach is essen- tial for the successful management of these potentially life-threatening situations and transfusion therapy cannot be discussed in isolation from other treatment.

Massive Blood Transfusion

The nature and management of hemostatic defects when massive blood loss has occurred are not completely understood. Further aggra- vation of the complications of massive blood transfusion can be avoided or minimized if attempts are made to identify correctable de- fects in the hemostatic system. The following are the factors which may contribute to he- mostatic failure following massive blood transfusion.

- Preexisting hemostatic defect.
- Loss of coagulation factors, platelets and inhibitors.

- Dilution of coagulation factors, platelets and inhibitors.
- Impaired synthesis due to effects of shock on liver and bone marrow function.
- Effects of trauma: disseminated intravascular coagulation and fibrinolysis.
- Effects of storage lesion: depletion of coagulation factors and platelets, aggravation or precipitation of DIC.
- Depletion of modulators of hemostasis (e.g., antithrombin III, fibronectin and protein C).
- Incompatible transfusion reaction: DIC.
- Citrate toxicity.

The relative importance of the different possible mechanisms responsible for hemostatic failure is difficult to determine and may vary from patient to patient. If hematological investigations indicate a specific quantitative or qualitative defect in the hemostatic system, it is logical to transfuse that particular component. If a patient requires continuing blood transfusion, it is inevitable that some degree of hemostatic failure will result if stored blood more than a week old is used for resuscitation. The labile factors V and VIII are not well preserved beyond a week; platelets are aggregated and nonfunctional after a few days, if not sooner; some coagulation factors may be activated during cooling and storage; and microaggregates and degenerate cells may be responsible for aggravating or initiating disseminated intravascular coagulation (DIC).

Assuming normal hemostasis before the massive blood loss, coagulation deficiency is usually confined to factors V and VIII. Coagulation screening tests (APTT, PT and TT) should be performed, but the urgency of the situation does not usually allow the performance of specific factor assays, and fresh frozen plasma should be infused if the test results are abnormal. Thrombocytopenia is a common feature following massive blood transfusion and, as with coagulation defects, loss, consumption, dilution and reduced production are all contributory factors. Quantitative platelet defects may be present. When a patient has exceeded transfusion of 10 units of stored blood and there is clinical evidence of hemostatic failure, there is a strong case for obtaining fresh blood.

Hemostatic Failure Associated with Liver Disease

The liver is the production site of nearly all the coagulation and inhibitory factors involved in hemostasis. There are numerous reasons why hemostasis may be disturbed in patients with liver disease, including (see Fig. 6.4):

- Deficiency of vitamin K dependent clotting factors.
- Deficiency of fibrinogen and factor V.
- Dysfibrinogenemia.
- Disseminated intravascular coagulation.
- Excessive fibrinolytic activity.

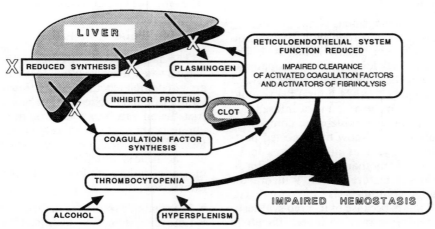

Figure 6.4. Pathophysiology of hemostatic failure in liver disease

- Circulating anticoagulants.
- Platelet abnormalities.

Bleeding in association with liver disease can be devastating and difficult to manage. Not only is the diagnosis of any specific defect difficult, but one may be dealing with a combination of excessive consumption of coagulation factors, impaired synthesis of coagulation factors, coagulation inhibitor proteins and activators of fibrinolysis. To add to the problems, the effects of massive blood loss, shock and transfusion must also be considered.

In the case of deficiency in vitamin K dependent coagulation factors in patients with predominantly cholestatic liver disease, the defect may be rapidly reversed with vitamin K. If the abnormality is not reversed, it is likely that hepatocellular damage is present. When a patient with liver disease is to undergo an elective procedure, prophylactic replacement of vitamin K dependent factors, and possibly factor V, is usually all that is necessary. The method by which this is achieved depends on the blood products locally available. Fresh frozen plasma, supernatant plasma or factor concentrates may be used. Unfortunately the transfused factors, particularly factor VII, disappear rapidly from the circulation so that patients must be repeatedly transfused if there is continuing bleeding or risk of bleeding. Low fibrinogen levels in liver disease usually indicate advanced disease with a poor prognosis, or the presence of disseminated intravascular coagulation. The diagnosis of disseminated intravascular coagulation in the presence of liver disease may be extremely difficult.

Disseminated Intravascular Coagulation (DIC)

DIC (consumption coagulopathy, defibrination syndrome) occurs when the finely balanced hemostatic and fibrinolytic systems become disturbed and inappropriately activated in several clinical situations. The causes of disseminated intravascular coagulation are:

- Shock (from any cause)
- Intravascular hemolysis
- Infection—septicemia, purpura fulminans, postsplenectomy sepsis, meningococcemia

- Obstetric complications
- Burns, electric shock
- Heat stroke
- Fat embolism
- Surgery—cardiac bypass surgery, lung, brain
- Envenomation
- Malignancies—acute promyelocytic leukemia, prostatic and GIT malignancies
- Pancreatitis
- LeVeen shunts
- Vascular disorders—hemangiomas, aneurysms, grafts, vasculitis

Pathophysiology

Figure 6.5 illustrates the pathophysiology of DIC, highlighting the stages of the process, modifying factors and therapy. It is characterized by the consumption of clotting factors and platelets within the circulation, resulting in varying degrees of microvascular obstruction. When significant platelet and coagulation factor consumption occurs, bleeding becomes a major feature. A secondary fibrinolysis occurs, which in some cases, may accentuate the bleeding. When it occurs in acutely ill patients with multisystem failure, the prognosis is poor. The essence of success in managing acute DIC is directed at both the initiating cause and the syndrome itself. It must, on the other hand, be remembered that DIC may, in some cases, be an agonal event and should not be treated. DIC may overlap with microangiopathy syndromes (e.g., TTP and HUS) or with DVT. Figure 6.6 attempts to represent the relationship between this spectrum of disorders.

Clinical Features

The clinical presentation of DIC varies, with patients showing thrombotic, hemorrhagic, or mixed manifestations in various organ systems. DIC is sometimes associated with the adult respiratory distress syndrome and acute renal failure following trauma. Some patients have the laboratory features of DIC without any clinical manifestations.

Laboratory Findings

- Prolongation of the TT, APTT, PT
- Hypofibrinogenemia, thrombocytopenia, low factor VIII
- Elevated fibrin degradation products

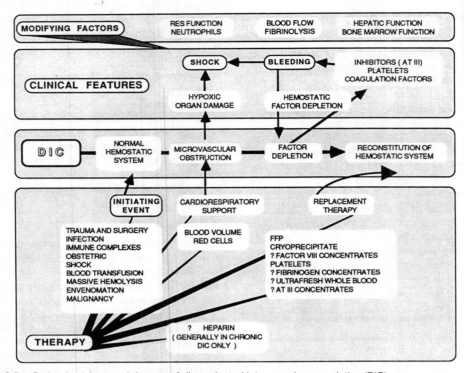

Figure 6.5. Pathophysiology and therapy of disseminated intravascular coagulation (DIC)

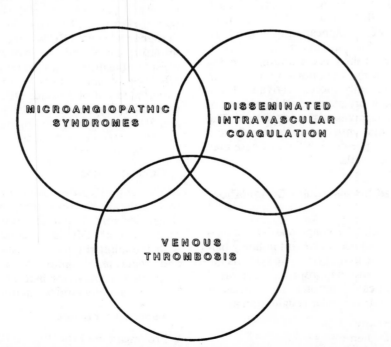

Figure 6.6. Relationships between microangiopathic hemolytic anemia, venous thrombosis, and disseminated intravascular coagulation

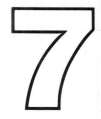

Host Defense Failure

As it takes two to make a quarrel, so it takes two to make a disease, the microbe and its host.

Charles V. Chapain (1856–1941)

The contribution of the hemopoietic and immune systems to host defenses is summarized in chapter 1. Failure of the host defenses may be the first clue to hematological and immunological disease. This may be in the form of recurrent infections with common organisms in a previously healthy person or a single episode of an unusual infection (opportunistic) in a healthy person. The history and type of infection will commonly give a clue to the nature of the defect in the host defense system. As self-limiting infections are a part of day to day life it is only occasionally that a patient will turn out to have an underlying hematological or immunological problem. The challenge is to identify, among a "sea" of coughs, colds, sores and fevers, those patients requiring further investigation. In view of the expanding field of host defenses, immunology and microbiology it is only possible to present a succinct conceptual approach to host defense failure. The reader is referred to other texts for further information.

Clinical Assessment for Host Defense Failure

The following questions should be addressed in order to identify patients with underlying hematological disease. Figure 7.1 outlines the decision tree approach to the investigation of host defense failure and Table 7.1 the congenital and acquired host defense defects.

What Is the Infectious Organism and Nature of the Infection?

- A single infection with a common organism is likely to be a unifactorial disease which will follow an expected natural history.
- Common infections may arouse suspicion of host defense failure if there are recurrent episodes, delayed resolution, unexpected natural history, multiple sites of infection, unusual sites of involvement, incomplete clearance of infection or systemic spread.
- Unusual organisms should always arouse suspicion of an opportunistic infection (see Table 7.2).
- Multiple infections with different organisms should always cause concern.

Is the Patient Already in a Risk Group for Having a Host Defense Defect?

The patient's past or present medical history may be relevant to the likelihood of a defect being present.

- Nonhematological disease—diabetes, uremia, liver disease, malnutrition, alcoholism, drug addiction, age, prematurity, malignancy, rheumatoid arthritis.
- Hematological disorders—splenectomy, hematological malignancy, known host defense defect, chronic atypical mononucleosis syndromes.
- Family history—immunodeficiency, allergy, autoimmune diseases, malignancy.
- Medications—immunosuppressive therapy, cytotoxic therapy, corticosteroids, antibiotics.

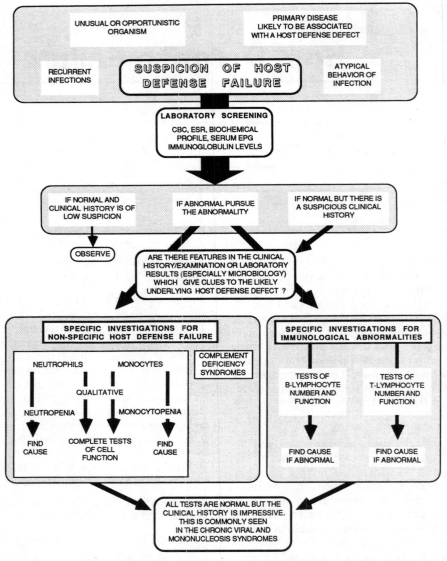

Figure 7.1. The investigation of host defense failure—CBC = *complete* blood count; EPG = serum electrophoretogram

Are There Any Clinical or Simple Laboratory Findings Which Suggest an Underlying Disease?

- If the patient has previously been well and there has been a change in susceptibility to infection, an acquired defect is likely.
- Clinical evidence of bone marrow failure: associated hemostatic failure or anemia.

- Historical information suggestive of immune deficiency or defective immunoregulation—allergies, unexplained transfusion reactions, autoimmune disease, recurrent infections, chronic diarrhea.
- Physical findings suggestive of hematological or other disease: lymphadenopathy, organomegaly, skin rash, retarded growth, autoimmunity.

Table 7.1
Congenital and Acquired Host Defense Defects

Congenital phagocytic and opsonic function defects
    Chronic granulomatous disease
    G6PD deficiency
    Myeloperoxidase deficiency
    Chediak-Higashi syndrome
    Job's syndrome
    Tuftsin deficiency
    Lazy leukocyte syndrome
    Complement deficiency syndrome
Primary Immunodeficiency diseases
(WHO classification)
A. Predominant antibody defects
    1. X-linked agammaglobulinemia
    2. X-linked hypogammaglobulinemia with growth hormone deficiency
    3. Autosomal recessive agammaglobulinemia
    4. Immunoglobulin deficiency with increased IgM (and IgG)
    5. IgA deficiency
    6. Selective deficiency of other immunoglobulin isotypes
    7. k-chain deficiency
    8. Antibody deficiency with normal gammaglobulin levels or hypergammaglobulinemia
    9. Immunodeficiency with thymoma
    10. Transient hypogammaglobulinemia of infancy.
    11. Common variable immunodeficiency with predominant B-cell defect
    12. Common variable immunodeficiency with predominant immunoregulatory T-cell disorder
        (a) Deficiency of helper T cells
        (b) Presence of activated suppressor T cells
    13. Common variable immunodeficiency with autoantibodies to B or T cells
B. Predominant defects of cell-mediated immunity
    14. Combined immunodeficiency with predominant T-cell defect
    15. Purine-nucleoside phosphorylase deficiency
    16. Severe combined immunodeficiency with adenosine deaminase deficiency
    17. Severe combined immunodeficiency
        (a) Reticular dysgenesis
        (b) Low T-cell and B-cell numbers
        (c) Low T-cell and normal B-cell numbers (Swiss)
        (d) "bare-lymphocyte syndrome"
    18. Immunodeficiency with unusual response to Epstein-Barr virus (Ducan's syndrome), or X-linked lymphoproliferative syndrome
C. Immunodeficiency associated with other defects
    19. Transcobalamin 2 deficiency
    20. Wiskott-Aldrich syndrome
    21. Ataxia telangiectasia
    22. Third- and fourth-pouch/arch (DiGeorge's) syndrome
Acquired
  Neutropenic syndromes (see below)
  Acquired immune deficiency syndrome (AIDS): T and B-cell
  Hematological malignancies
    Acute leukemias: bone marrow failure
    Chronic lymphocytic leukemia: B-cell +/− T-cell
    Hodgkin's disease: T-cell
    Non-Hodgkin's lymphoma: B-cell
    Hairy cell leukemia—neutropenia and monocytopenia
    Multiple myeloma—impaired B-cell function and increased suppressor T-cells
  Immunosuppressive therapy—marrow failure, T-cell depression
  Plasma exchange—hypogammaglobulinemia

Table 7.1 *continued*

Miscellaneous conditions—multifactorial host defense defects
   In the course of common viral and bacterial infections
   Burns/multiple trauma
   Shocked patients
   Malnutrition and protein losing states
   Consumption opsinopathy
   Alcoholism
   Uremia
   Drug addicts
   Aging
   Malignancy
   Hyposplenism
   Diabetes
   Corticosteroids
   Liver disease
   Antibiotic therapy
   Anesthesia

- Abnormalities on initial or "routine" complete blood count and film: anemia, leukocyte abnormalities, thrombocytopenia.

Does the Clinical Picture Assist in Defining the Nature of the Host Defense Defect?

- Does the clinical presentation suggest a primary hematological or immunological failure without underlying disease? This should not be assumed until primary disease has been excluded.
- Does the clinical picture clearly indicate that the hematological and/or immunological failure is a manifestation of underlying disease or its therapy?

Table 7.2 outlines the types of infections which occur as a result of specific host defense defects. In some diseases there may be multiple host defense defects. This especially applies to hematological malignancy and its associated therapy.

Who Should Be Investigated?

1. In patients in whom there is no clinical suspicion of a defect in host defenses, only a complete blood count is necessary. This is a simple, low-cost investigation where the incidental detection of an unexpected hematological disorder may be important.

2. In patients in whom there is a moderate suspicion of host defense failure, complete blood count, biochemical profile and serum electrophoresis should be performed initially. If these are noncontributory, there is no underlying disease detected and the infection is resolving, no further investigations need to be performed.

3. In patients in whom the suspicion of host defense failure is high, more detailed investigations of hematological and/or immunological function need to be carried out. The nature and extent of the investigations will depend on the clinical picture, type of infection), age of the patient and the nature of abnormalities detected on initial screening.

What Screening Investigations Are Indicated?

- Complete blood count will detect quantitative and morphological defects in cellular elements (neutropenia, lymphopenia, leukemia) but not, in general, qualitative disorders.
- Biochemical profile will assist in the diagnosis of acquired disorders such as multiple myeloma, uremia, liver dysfunction.
- Serum electrophoresis is a good screening test for multiple myeloma, severe hypogammaglobulinemia, polyclonal hyper-

based on the individual doctor's or parent's experience. In the case of the elderly, "immunological dementia" inevitably sets in and memory is lost without there necessarily being a major immunological defect present (e.g., shingles). In general the clinician should allow greater latitude in children and the elderly before referring the patient for complex investigations, assuming that the initial simple screening tests outlined above show normal results.

- One of the commonest problems is the story of the child, adolescent or young adult suffering from a chronic glandular fever-like syndrome who is prone to recurrent infections and recrudescence of symptoms. This syndrome is not well understood and is discussed in chapter 8.

General Principles of Therapy in Host Defense Failure

To this point the reader has probably, correctly, gained the impression that the investigation of host defense failure may be complex, frustrating, expensive and frequently unrewarding. When turning to therapy the situation is similar and on the one hand can be scientific and specific, whereas on the other, borders on "quackery." With better understanding of the host defense system it is becoming increasingly possible to satisfy the long-held desire of both patients and medical practitioners to administer specific potions to reconstitute or augment the body's response to disease. An integrated approach to the management of patients with host defense failure should include:

- Accurate identification and sensitivity testing of pathogenic organisms.
- Identification of the host defense defect and the diagnosis of any underlying pathology.
- Early institution of antimicrobial therapy.
- Close attention to supportive care, including nutrition, fluid therapy, local therapy to the site of infection.
- Administration of specific replacement therapy.

The following is a brief summary of therapeutic replacement options for individual host defense defects. It should be emphasized that this remains a complex, evolving and specialized area of medical therapy and advice should be sought in individual patients.

REPLACEMENT THERAPY FOR DISORDERS OF THE HOST DEFENSE SYSTEM

Agranulocytosis and Severe Neutrophil Defects

Granulocyte transfusions may have a role in specific circumstances.

B-Cell Disorders and Hypogammaglobulinemia

Human gammaglobulin is used for the prevention and treatment of bacterial infections. Hyperimmune gammaglobulins are utilized when exposure to specific infections occurs, e.g., varicella, hepatitis B.

T-Cell Defects

This is a more complex area of immunotherapy where promising advances are occurring. Modes of therapy which may be used include: bone marrow, fetal liver or thymus transplants; transfer factor; interferons; interleukin II; thymosin and red cell transfusions (for enzyme deficiencies).

Opsonic Defects

Fresh frozen plasma or fresh blood may have a part to play in the consumption syndromes (e.g., fibronectin deficiency, DIC), complement deficiency and malnutrition.

Some of the More Common and Important Host Defense Defects

NEUTROPENIA

Neutropenia is one of the most common and important leukocyte abnormalities seen in clinical practice. With severe agranulocytosis the patient is at risk from overwhelming bacterial sepsis. If associated thrombocytopenia is present the combination of sepsis and hemorrhage is poorly tolerated. The neutrophil count needs to fall below 1×10^3/cu mm before there is an increased incidence of spontaneous infection, however, it is not until the count drops below 0.2×10^3/cu mm that the risk rises exponentially. Early microbiological investigation and empirical antibiotic therapy is mandatory if death from septicemia is to be avoided. When neutropenia is due to margination or peripheral destruction the incidence of infection is less, and correlates poorly with the peripheral blood level. Mild neutropenia is a common finding, especially in females, for which no cause can be found, but bacterial infections are not a major problem. Clinically insignificant neutropenia is a normal finding in some people of Negro extraction.

The following factors should be considered when managing a patient with neutropenia.

Is There Infection Present?

Mouth, perianal, urogenital, skin, IV sites, respiratory.

Is the Cause of Neutropenia Readily Apparent?

If so, management of the disorder is a high priority (e.g., hematological malignancy, cytotoxic therapy, aplastic anemia).

If the Cause Is Obscure What Investigations Need to Be Performed?

In many patients there are associated clinical conditions which are known to be complicated by neutropenia and detailed investigations may be avoided e.g., SLE, rheumatoid arthritis (in particular Felty's syndrome), viral infections. In other patients a bone marrow examination is usually warranted in order to separate failure of production (including possible marrow pathology) and peripheral destruction or margination. The causes of neutropenia include:

    Decreased production
        Aplastic anemia
        Drug induced agranulocytosis (see appendix 2)
        Chemotherapy and radiation
        Hematological malignancies, especially acute leukemia
        Myelodysplastic and preleukemic syndromes

        Bone marrow replacement with metastatic malignancy
        Immune mediated suppressions of marrow production
        Megaloblastosis
        Paroxysmal nocturnal hemoglobinuria
        Familial and cyclical neutropenia
    Increased destruction or margination
        Hypersplenism
        Acute and chronic viral infections
        Tuberculosis, brucellosis and typhoid
        Drug-induced antibody mediated destruction
        Familial causes
        Autoimmune disorders e.g., SLE, rheumatoid arthritis
        Acute consumption with sepsis, DIC

In unexplained neutropenia, a careful drug and toxin history should be taken and immunological investigations (antinuclear antibody (ANA), rheumatoid factor, Coombs' test) performed.

BRUTON TYPE X-LINKED AGAMMAGLOBULINEMIA

Congenital agammaglobulinemia is one of the longest-recognized immunodeficiency syndromes and presents with severe pyogenic infections. The patients are unable to make any antibodies due to the absence of plasma cells, resulting from a block in maturation between the pre-B cell to B cell differentiation. Persistent viral and parasitic infections are also a problem. Chronic diarrhea and a sprue-like syndrome may occur which may be associated with giardia infestation and rotavirus infections. The mainstay of therapy in agammaglobulinemia is gammaglobulin replacement therapy which is best given intravenously in high dose.

SELECTIVE IgA DEFICIENCY

A selective reduction or absence of IgA is probably the commonest congenital immune deficiency syndrome, occurring in as many people as 1 in 700. The majority of cases detected by screening of blood donors do not have significant clinical disease, but on the other hand IgA deficiency may be associated with a surprisingly wide range of allergic and autoimmune disorders. Recurrent infections,

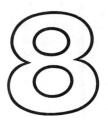

Organomegalies: Lymphadenopathy and Disorders of the Spleen and Thymus

More is missed by not looking than not knowing.

Thomas McCrae (1870–1935)

Clinical Investigation of Organomegaly

Enlargement of the organs of the hemopoietic system or extranodal lymphoid tissue is commonly found in both primary hematological diseases and as a reactive response to diseases of other systems. The organomegaly may come to clinical attention in several different ways:

- The patient may notice a swelling or localized pain.
- Lymphadenopathy or splenomegaly may be found on routine physical examination.
- Obstruction of a vein, bronchus, gut, renal tract or lymphatics.
- Extranodal mass lesion, e.g., spinal cord compression, proptosis, skin lesions.
- Incidental finding as a result of an organ imaging investigation such as chest or abdomen x-ray, CT scans.
- Organomegaly may be specifically sought on physical examination in the light of the clinical history or laboratory findings.

The evaluation of patients with *hemopoietic* organomegaly must be individualized, but there are general guidelines to assist in making important clinical decisions.

What Clinical Features May Assist in Diagnosis?

Distribution

If the lymphadenopathy is localized to a single nodal region the drainage areas should be carefully examined for evidence of infection or malignancy. With generalized lymphadenopathy systemic disease or hematological malignancy is more likely.

Pain

Painful nodes are usually due to an infectious or inflammatory cause. The same principle applies to splenomegaly unless there has been a splenic infarct or hematoma.

Size and Consistency

As a generalization, the larger and firmer the organomegaly the more likely it is due to malignancy. Fixation of lymph nodes to underlying tissues is highly suggestive of metastatic malignancy. Large "matted" lymph nodes are commonly found in non-Hodgkin's lymphoma in contrast to rubbery, mobile nodes which are typical of Hodgkin's disease.

Clinical History

The length of history, the presence of systemic symptoms (e.g., malaise, weight loss, fever, sweats, pruritus), infectious contacts, historical or physical findings in other systems, recent travel and drug history are important.

Hemopoietic Failure

Clinical features of anemia, hemostatic failure or immune deficiency may be important.

What Initial Investigations Should Be Carried Out?

The plan of investigations in a patient with organomegaly can only be determined after the initial clinical assessment to establish the probabilities as to the likely causes. There are, however, certain essential relatively inexpensive investigations, though nonspecific, which may yield valuable information. These include the following:

Complete Blood Examination

The presence of morphological and/or quantitative leukocyte abnormalities may point towards hematological malignancy or an atypical mononucleosis syndrome. Varying degrees of cytopenia may be due to marrow failure, hypersplenism or autoimmune abnormalities.

Erythrocyte Sedimentation Rate

An elevated ESR may be a clue to infectious, inflammatory or malignant disease. In the case of malignant hematological disease, a markedly elevated ESR suggests the possibility of a monoclonal protein, Hodgkin's disease or cold agglutinins.

Biochemical Profile

Abnormalities such as hyperuricemia, hypercalcemia, abnormal liver function test results, impaired renal function and elevated LDH may all be helpful.

Chest X-ray

Evidence of mediastinal or bronchial lymphoid enlargement is significant.

Serum Electrophoresis

Evidence for the acute or chronic phase reaction due to systemic infectious or inflammatory disease may be present. Hypogammaglobulinemia and hypergammaglobulinemia should be detected, and in the case of hypergammaglobulinemia monoclonal proteins should be apparent.

Serological Screening Tests

Test for infectious mononucleosis, CMV and toxoplasmosis should be performed.

When and What Biopsies Should Be Performed?

This is commonly a pivotal decision in the investigation of hematological organomegaly and will usually reveal a definitive diagnosis in the case of malignancy, some infectious diseases, granulomatous disease and some atypical lymph node reactions. If biopsy is indicated, an adequate sample of tissue should be obtained. Needle aspiration, although simple, rarely yields the information required and may in some patients confuse rather than clarify the issue. The architecture of the tissue is frequently as important as the cellular morphology in diagnosis.

Lymph Node Biopsy

The decision to biopsy lymph nodes is usually not difficult. In cases where malignancy is likely from the criteria outlined above, node biopsy is essential unless the pathological diagnosis is apparent from other investigations (blood examination or bone marrow). In cases where there are features or confirmatory tests for an infectious or inflammatory disease, node biopsy is rarely necessary. It is in circumstances where the diagnostic possibilities lie between these two examples that the clinician may be in a quandary. The main reason for biopsy is to confirm or exclude a diagnosis of malignancy and if in doubt it is better to biopsy as the procedure is safe and vital organs are not being removed.

There are certain generalizations which may assist the clinician in the decision-making process. With increasing age, the likelihood of malignancy increases. If generalized lymphadenopathy is present and the patient is reasonably well, procrastination is justified, especially as delayed diagnosis is not usually relevant to the outcome. Lymph nodes in the neck in young patients in association with recent ear, nose or throat symptoms are almost certainly reactive, as are inguinal nodes in many circumstances.

Bone Marrow

Bone marrow aspiration and *biopsy* is usually performed as a staging procedure, but in some patients it may yield diagnostic information. This is commonly the case when there are abnormalities in the peripheral blood suggesting a lymphoproliferative disease.

Spleen

It is generally too hazardous to biopsy the spleen, although fine needle aspiration in experienced hands may be helpful. If it is important to establish a definitive diagnosis, and the spleen is the only likely source of material, a splenectomy may be warranted, but this is unusual and observation without therapy is usually more appropriate.

Other Organs

Under some circumstances, a definitive diagnosis is made following examination of other tissues either by design or as a result of surgical intervention for a complication. Gut, pulmonary, hepatic and cutaneous tissue are the common sources from which diagnosis of hematological disease is established.

What Organ Imaging Investigations Should Be Performed?

The range of organ imaging procedures available to search for occult organomegaly or masses has expanded in recent years, and careful selection of appropriate investigations is necessary. Few would debate that the most valuable technique for the investigation of patients with hematological organomegaly is computerized tomography, and this investigation stands out from all other radiological and nuclear medicine techniques. The method is ideal for identifying intrathoracic, intraabdominal and pelvic disease. Ultrasound and liver/spleen isotope scanning may help in analysis of intraorgan defects and in the sizing of organs. Skeletal surveys, bone scanning and gallium scanning may have a role in specific situations. However, in general radioisotope techniques are unhelpful and are only occasionally indicated.

Lymphadenopathy

Table 8.1 lists the causes of lymphadenopathy and Figure 8.1 the investigative decision tree; the different diseases are discussed in the appropriate chapters.

DISORDERS OF THE SPLEEN

Splenomegaly

The spleen is not normally palpable on physical examination and it usually enlarges to twice its normal size before becoming palpable. A palpable spleen usually requires explanation, but its enlargement is more commonly an associated clinical finding, or of diagnostic assistance rather than of direct clinical or therapeutic assistance. The cause of splenomegaly is readily apparent in most patients either as a feature of primary hematological disease or secondary to systemic inflammatory or infectious disease. Asymptomatic splenomegaly requires investigations, but if a cause is not uncovered with relatively noninvasive investigations, observation is the appropriate course of action in most patients.

Splenic enlargement or disease may present in the following ways:

- Splenomegaly on physical examination.
- Incidental finding on radiological or organ imaging investigation.
- Symptomatic splenomegaly—abdominal

Table 8.1
Causes of Lymphadenopathy

Localized lymphadenopathy
Local acute infections
Local chronic infection: TB, cat-scratch disease, lymphogranuloma venereum
Metastatic solid tumor
Hematological malignancy: Hodgkin's disease
       High grade non-Hodgkin's lymphoma
       Low grade lymphomas (less common)

Generalized lymphadenopathy
Acute and chronic infections: TB, brucellosis, syphillis, mononucleosis, HTLV-associated lymphadenopathy syndrome, toxoplasmosis, fungal and rickettesial infection, CMV
Hematological malignancy: Lymphoproliferative disease
Granulomatous diseases: Sarcoidosis
Immune mediated diseases: Serum sickness, rheumatoid arthritis, SLE
Drug reaction: Pseudolymphoma (Dilantin)
Dermatopathic lymphadenopathy

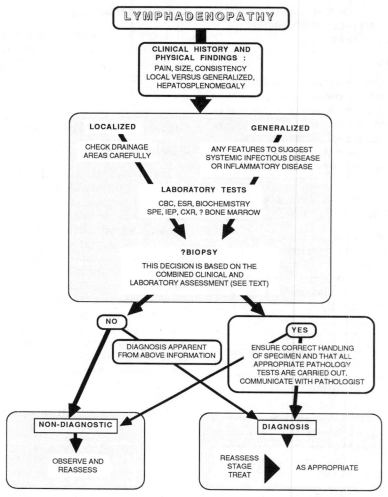

Figure 8.1. The investigation of lymphadenopathy—CBC = Complete blood count; EPG = serum electrophoretogram; ESR = erythrocyte sedimentation rate; CXR = chest x-ray

enlargement, GIT fullness, dull left hypochondrial pain, self-palpation of the mass.

- Splenic infarction—acute left hypochondrial pain, pleuritic pain, left shoulder tip pain.
- Splenic rupture—traumatic or spontaneous.
- Peripheral blood abnormalities—features of hypersplenism.
- Primary disease of which splenomegaly is a feature, e.g., portal hypertension and malaria.

Investigation of Splenomegaly

For practical purposes, enlargement of the spleen (measured from the costal margin) can be broadly divided into "just palpable" (1 to 2cm), moderate splenomegaly (3 to 10cm) and massive splenomegaly (enlargement beyond 10cm to the umbilicus and below). Table 8.2 lists the causes of splenomegaly. Diagnosis is made along the lines outlined in Figure 8.2. In the majority of patients, a diagnosis can be made on the basis of the clinical findings in conjunction with the peripheral blood. If the cause is not apparent early in the investigations, consultative assistance is usually necessary. It is most uncommon to require splenectomy for diagnosis; and under these circumstances, the operation is being performed for therapeutic reasons and the establishment of a diagnosis is usually a secondary consideration.

Table 8.2
Causes of Splenomegaly

Hyperplasia of lymphoid tissue
Infectious: Infectious mononucleosis, CMV, AIDS-associated virus
Autoimmune: SLE, rheumatoid arthritis (Felty's syndrome), serum sickness
Neoplastic: Lymphoproliferative diseases—
          Lymphoma, primary splenic lymphoma*
          Chronic lymphocytic leukemias*
          Hairy cell Leukemia*

Hyperplasia of Monocyte-macrophage tissue
Infection: Viral: Viral associated hemophagocytic syndrome (VAHS)
          Bacterial: Endocarditis, septicemia, TB
          Protozoal: Malaria and tropical splenomegaly syndrome,* Kala azar*
Chronic extravascular hemolysis: Autoimmune hemolysis, hereditary spherocytosis, sickle cell disease (early),
Storage diseases: Gaucher's disease,* sea blue histiocyte syndrome
Neoplastic: Histiocytic medullary reticulosis

Splenic hemopoiesis
Congenital disorders: Thalassemias*
Myeloproliferative disease: Myelofibrosis, myeloid metaplasia, polycythemia rubra vera
Neoplastic: Acute and subacute leukemias
          Chronic granulocytic and monocytic leukemias*

Splenic blood pooling (may also occur in association with the above)
Portal hypertension secondary to liver disease
Venous obstruction secondary to portal, splenic, hepatic presinusoidal, hepatic vein
Congestive cardiac failure

Miscellaneous
Amyloidosis, splenic cysts, hyperthyroidism
Idiopathic nontropical splenomegaly syndrome

---

*May cause massive splenomegaly.

Treatment of Splenomegaly

In general splenomegaly per se does not require therapy and usually reduces or disappears in conjunction with other therapy for the underlying disease. In certain circumstances specific therapy, usually a splenectomy, for the splenomegaly is necessary unless chemotherapy or radiotherapy is considered a feasible alternative.

Indications for Splenectomy

- Massive symptomatic splenomegaly.
- Splenic rupture.
- Recurrent splenic infarction.
- Symptomatic hypersplenism (severe thrombocytopenia, excessive transfusion requirements, recurrent infection).
- Splenectomy in relation to a staging laparotomy.

Protocol for Splenectomy

In the majority of patients, splenectomy is a relatively safe procedure as long as certain precautions are followed.

- Referral to a surgeon experienced in the technique in "hematological patients"; this is especially necessary if there has been recurrent splenic infarction and adhesions are likely, or there are host defense or hemostatic defects.
- Appropriate identification and correction of host defense defects; hypogammaglobulinemia, qualitative or quantitative platelet defects, coagulation defects, anemia.
- Immunization with polyvalent pneumococcal vaccine.
- Prophylaxis for venous thromboembolism.
- Appropriate instructions to the surgeon for the performance of any biopsy procedures—lymph node, liver.

Hazards of Splenectomy

Splenectomy may have short-term and long-term sequelae and the procedure should not be undertaken lightly.

Short-term. Hemorrhage in association with a hemostatic defect or capsular adhesions, subphrenic abscess, fulminant septi-

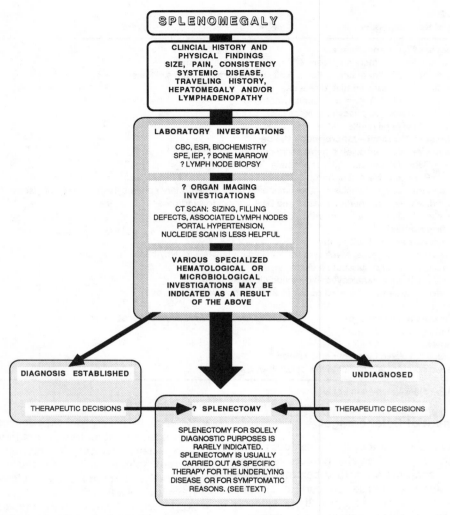

Figure 8.2. The investigation of splenomegaly—CBC = complete blood count; EPG = serum electrophoretogram; IEP = Immunoetechophoresis

cemia, venous thromboembolism and thrombocytosis are short-term problems.

Long-term. The main concern of the postsplenectomy or splenic atrophy state is the overwhelming postsplenectomy infection (OPSI) syndrome (see below).

HYPOSPLENISM

It is now well recognized that absence or atrophy of the spleen is not solely a cosmetic defect. In particular, there is enhanced sus-

ceptibility to overwhelming sepsis, but there is risk also of tropical diseases such as malaria when a person travels to areas of risk. The spleen need not be physically absent or even reduced in size for splenic hypofunction to occur. The minimal splenic function to produce the various defects is not known. The causes of hyposplenism are:

- Congenital absence/hypoplasia
- Splenectomy
- Splenic arterial occlusion (iatrogenic)
- Splenic arterial or venous thrombosis
- Splenic irradiation

- Splenic atrophy
   sickle cell disease
   celiac disease
   dermatitis herpetiformis
   ulcerative colitis
   hyperthyroidism
   thrombocythemia
   thorium dioxide induced SLE
- Transient hyposplenism
   colitis
   hemolysis
   blood transfusion
   myeloproliferative disease
   incomplete splenic infarction
   sepsis
   malaria and other tropical diseases

The Hyposplenic Blood Film

There are characteristic changes in the blood film indicative of hyposplenism:

- Howell-Jolly Bodies
- Pappenheimer Bodies
- Target cells
- Spiky spherocytes
- Irregularly contracted cells
- Hypochromia (due to excess membrane to volume)
- Thrombocytosis (variable)
- Atypical monocytic and lymphoid cells
- Heinz Bodies (supravital staining)

Under stress, the film may become leukoerythroblastic, and marked thrombocytosis, neutrophilia and monocytosis may occur.

OVERWHELMING POSTSPLENECTOMY INFECTION (OPSI) SYNDROME

This fulminant syndrome is more common in children and within 5 years of splenectomy; but may occur at any time in a patient with no splenic function. The rapid onset of a febrile shock state with associated disseminated intravascular coagulation characterizes the syndrome. Early diagnosis and the rapid institution of antibiotic therapy is crucial, as the syndrome has a greater than 50% mortality rate, increasing if the diagnosis is delayed. The pneumococcus is usually responsible, but other organisms may be implicated (Hemophilus, staphylococcus). Immunization with pneumococcal vaccine does not always protect against pneumococcal OPSI, as the vaccine may not contain all the capsular serotypes or immunization may not be effective due to immune deficiency. Penicillin prophylaxis is effective, but OPSI may be due to penicillin-resistant organisms and has occurred in patients receiving penicillin.

HYPERSPLENISM

In hypersplenism there is usually marked splenomegaly and hyperfunction of the spleen. The resultant effects include selective cytopenia or pancytopenia, hypercellular bone marrow and correction of the changes following splenectomy. Besides splenomegaly and cytopenias, there is pooling of blood in the spleen, varying degrees of hemolysis, increased plasma volume and a hypercellular bone marrow. The effects of the various cytopenias in hypersplenism are not as great as may be seen in similar cytopenia from other causes, and cytopenia alone should not be regarded as an indication for splenectomy. There is not a good correlation between the degree of splenomegaly and the peripheral blood features of hypersplenism. Any of the conditions listed in Table 8.2 may have associated hypersplenism.

Disorders of the Thymus

Disorders of the thymic gland are uncommon and very much in the realm of the specialist in hematology and immunology. The thymus may be implicated in disease states in the following ways:

- Enlargement detected because of compression symptoms or as a result of radiological investigations.
- Functional deficiency manifest as congenital failure of delayed hypersensitivity.
- Implicated in relation to other diseases
   Autoimmune disease—myasthenia gravis, pure red cell aplasia, pancytopenia, SLE and other connective tissue diseases
   Neoplastic disorders—leukemia and lymphoma (especially T-cell), Hodgkin's disease, myeloma
   Endocrine disorders—thyroid and adrenal disease
   Hypogammaglobulinemia

THYMOMA

Thymomas are epithelial neoplasms with varying degrees of lymphoid proliferation. It is not possible to predict the malignant nature of these tumors from the histology alone. The tumors are locally malignant and rarely metastasize.

Other Hematological Mass Lesions

Malignant hematological mass lesions may present in almost any part of the body and are usually established as hemopoietic or lymphoid in origin as a result of a biopsy procedure. The commonest presentations would include: abdominal mass, hepatomegaly, mediastinal mass, skin infiltration, spinal cord compression, pulmonary nodule or infiltrate and gastrointestinal obstruction. The management of hematological disease diagnosed in this manner is determined by the pathology.

Further Reading

Jaffe, ES *Surgical pathology of the lymph nodes and related organs.* Major problems in pathology Vol. 16. Philadelphia: WB Saunders and Company, 1985.

Lewis, SM *Clinics in haematology: the spleen.* June 1983. Vol. 12 No. 2. Philadelphia: WB Saunders Company Ltd.

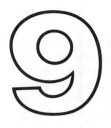

Hematological Malignancy

It is difficult to say what is impossible, for the dream of yesterday is the hope of today and the reality of tomorrow.

Robert H. Goddard

The heterogeneous nature of the *hemopoietic* and lymphoid cells, their individual kinetic characteristics and the disseminated nature of hemopoietic and lymphoid tissue explains the complexity of hematological malignancy. The nonspecialist can be excused for finding this area of hematology difficult to comprehend. The numerous classifications advocated to clarify our understanding have in many cases increased the confusion. It is not the aim of the author to present a comprehensive summary of the subject nor to discuss therapy in detail, but rather to outline the important principles which will assist in diagnosis and understanding of hematological malignancy. If these principles are elucidated, in most cases based on understanding of the normal physiology, the nonspecialist should be better able to interrelate where necessary.

Introductory Overview

BASIC CONCEPTS

Cell Kinetic Characteristics

The cells of the hemopoietic (including lymphoid) system are continuously replicating cells, similar to gut mucosa and skin. This is in contrast to cells which are intermittent replicators (e.g., renal tubular cells, hepatocytes) and nonreplicators (e.g., neurones, muscle cells, glomerular cells). Their potential for malignancy is thus greater and hemopoietic cells will be more susceptible to toxic therapeutic agents such as chemotherapy and radiotherapy. Lymphoid cells are unique in that they have the ability to pass from a resting state to an actively dividing state (blast transform) in order to perform their normal immune function. The site at which this normally occurs depends on the nature and localization of the particular lymphoid cell, as it does with malignant counterparts of these normal cells.

Cell Developmental Characteristics

In the adult the hemopoietic and lymphoid systems have their origins in the bone marrow. In the fetus blood elements are formed in the liver and spleen. There are some hematological malignancies, such as myeloproliferative disorders, in which hemopoiesis comes to resemble that in the fetus (myeloid metaplasia).

Except for the basophil and its tissue equivalent the mast cell, of which the developmental sequence remains controversial, erythrocytes, platelets and granulocytes undergo their full development in the bone marrow and carry out their function in the peripheral blood as end cells with no reproductive potential. Malignancy of these cell lines, such as the various types of leukemia, generally originate in the bone marrow. In contrast, the monocyte, as discussed in chapter 1, undergoes further development after it leaves the bone marrow. The monocyte populates all the tissues of the body to form the monocyte-macrophage system known as the reticuloendothelial system (RES). Monocyte-macrophage malignancy may thus be bone marrow or tissue based.

The primitive leukemic cells are probably arrested in their maturation and an abnormal clone accumulates, ultimately suppressing or compromising normal marrow function. The marrow is hypercellular and in the acute leukemias it is not until the blastic proliferation is advanced that leukemic cells appear in the peripheral blood. Disease outside the bone marrow is truly metastatic, but is referred to as extramedullary leukemia. In the chronic leukemias the cells are arrested later in their development and are more likely to leave the bone marrow and accumulate in extramedullary sites where the normal counterparts of the cells may be found (e.g., lymph nodes, spleen) and are thus not metastatic in the true sense of the word. Under these circumstances bone marrow failure occurs late in the disease when there may be a considerably larger tumor burden than will be found in the acute leukemias.

The lymphoid arm of the hemopoietic system also originates in the marrow, undergoes development into T and B cells in the primary lymphoid tissue (thymus and bone marrow) and is subsequently distributed throughout the secondary lymphoid areas (lymph nodes, gut-associated lymphoid tissue, spleen, skin, bronchial-associated lymphoid tissue). With the lymphocyte's blast transforming ability, malignant change may occur anywhere lymphoid cells are normally located. If the malignant cells are at a stage in their development when they may be relatively mobile they are likely to recirculate and accumulate in sites determined by their "homing" characteristics. In contrast, more primitive lymphoblastic cells proliferate locally and behave more as solid tumors, with dissemination being a late and sinister occurrence. The

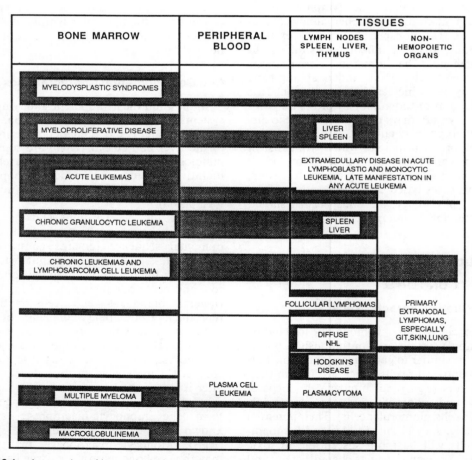

Figure 9.1. An overview of hematological malignancies—NHL = non-Hodgkin's lymphoma

term lymphoma is applied to hemopoietic malignancy (usually lymphoid) originating in the extramedullary lymphoid tissue. Because of the biological nature of the cells it is logical that there will be overlap syndromes where bone marrow, peripheral blood and extramedullary sites are involved. Under these circumstances it is generally a semantic problem whether the disease is called a leukemia or lymphoma. Figure 9.1 is a schematic representation of the localization of the various hematological malignancies.

Functional Defects

The hematological malignancies are primary diseases of the body's host defense system in contrast to the solid tumors where the specific host defense system is usually intact. Failure of the host defense system is likely to be a feature of *hemopoietic* malignancies. Bone marrow infiltration will lead to marrow failure as manifest by anemia, neutropenia and thrombocytopenia. This particularly occurs in the acute leukemias as a feature at presentation. Lymphoid malignancies may lead to specific immune deficiency syndromes and be complicated by opportunistic infections (see chapter 7). Failure of immunoregulation may be responsible for the development of autoimmune syndromes. Inappropriate phagocytosis of hemopoietic elements may be seen in the malignancies of the macrophage-monocyte system.

The Spectrum of Hematological Malignancy

Figure 9.1 summarizes the complex spectrum of hematological malignancies. The biological and clinical behavior of most of these malignancies can be predicted if the normal function of the cell involved is analyzed.

ETIOLOGY

Hematological malignancy has for decades led the way in the unfolding of our understanding of the basic pathophysiological processes involved in malignant disease. Although there is a long way to go we do appear to be identifying the factors involved in the evolution of malignancy. The geneticists, molecular biologists, virologists and immunologists have all contributed their insights. As with most unsolved diseases of today the etiology is unlikely to be unifactorial and research efforts are now directed towards the multitude of etiological factors and how they interact to initiate malignant change. The recent recognition of a human T-cell leukemia retrovirus (HTLV) and insights into the oncogenic potential of the EB virus have been major steps forward. The wide application of in-vitro cell culture techniques has allowed study of the various growth requirements of cells and the identification of numerous growth stimulation and differentiation factors essential in normal, orderly cell turnover.

The ultimate origins of any cellular changes during the development of a malignancy must reside in the cell genome. The concept of malignancy being simply the result of rapid, disorderly cell proliferation is now being replaced by the hypothesis that it is a highly logical, coordinated process in which certain cells acquire a unique combination of specialized abilities. The sequence of events leading to malignant transformation involves many of life's most fundamental processes. Malignancy appears to subvert processes normally aimed at ordered cell growth or repair. The process of malignant transformation begins when the DNA of the genome is altered in some way. Exposure to chemical carcinogens, oncogenic viruses, radiation or chromosomal rearrangements may alter the genome with the defects being passed on to cell progeny. To counteract some of these environmental insults there are DNA repair mechanisms to detect and splice out alien molecules attached to DNA before they can be immortalized into cell progeny.

Some viruses have been known to have oncogenic potential since Rous' landmark work in 1910, but it was 56 years before he was awarded a Nobel Prize and 65 years before it was discovered that the Rous sarcoma viruses oncogenic potential could be traced to a single gene (i.e., sequence of DNA) which could convert a cell to malignant growth. The concept of oncogenes was thus born. It was soon realized that these viral oncogenes have a counterpart in normal cells (proto-oncogenes) which may have crucial roles in cell replication, differentiation and regulation of cell growth. Their relative constancy throughout evolution strongly suggests that proto-oncogenes play basic and vital roles in the physiology of cells and organisms as a whole, possibly in proliferative processes such as embryogenesis, hemopoiesis and tissue healing. Many of the known oncogenes code for proteins vital in cell proliferation. Those identified to date include:

- Protein kinases necessary for anchorage of cells.
- Protein kinases as a component of surface receptors for epidermal growth factor (EGF), but is defective in that it is incapable of binding EGF and the oncogene product could mimic the receptor activity without the appropriate signal.
- Growth factors such as platelet-derived growth factor, which may result in autostimulation of cells.
- Proteins with possible activity in the cell nucleus.

These oncogene products could conceivably be involved in regulating the expression of specific cellular genes; possibly in switching them on or off. They could also bind directly to nuclear DNA and physically block the transcription of genes.

From the recent research in oncogenesis, it is thus likely that oncogenes are a necessary component of the oncogenic process. Proto-oncogenes may be activated to oncogenes by several possible mechanisms (Fig. 9.2).

- The normal proto-oncogene may be mutated by one of the carcinogens mentioned above. The mutant gene may not subserve its role as a repressor of a second gene encoded for a growth factor. Uncontrolled cell proliferation may thus result.
- The oncogene may encode directly for a growth factor and be expressed in excess (gene amplification).
- Chromosomal translocations may remove a proto-oncogene from its normal genomic environment and place it into a position where it may become activated by adjacent genes.
- Oncogenes may be activated directly by viruses. The retroviruses, which are RNA viruses replicating by reverse transcribing through the host cell's genome, owe trans-

forming ability to their potential to acquire modified genes from the host cell (i.e., oncogenes), a process known as transduction. Other viruses such as the EB virus may directly insert into the genome and possibly alter the functioning of a proto-oncogene.

It can thus be seen that there are many complex mechanisms which may come together under certain circumstances to initiate malignant transformation in cells. Under some circumstances there may be a premalignant phase of a disease where predominantly excessive proliferation of the cells is seen with varying degrees of differentiation and disordered cell function. Under other circumstances, the cell may immediately undergo blastic transformation and unregulated growth, in this case differentiation is arrested at an early stage.

The body's host defense systems are normally primed for the recognition of abnormal cell division and elimination of abnormal cells. However, it is well recognized that when there are disorders of immunoregulation, malignantly transformed cells are able to escape the normal host defenses.

These exciting insights into oncogenesis have placed oncology on the threshhold of a molecular biology revolution, and many tantalizing questions are now being addressed. In the short term, oncogenic research may be providing us with highly specific markers for the diagnosis of various malignancies. In the future, it may be possible to better understand the processes of oncogenesis and thus evolve therapeutic initiatives that are more directed at processes rather than the "shotgun" approach which is used with cytotoxic drugs today. In the even more distant future, it may be possible using the techniques of molecular biology to identify risk groups and introduce gene control or gene prophylaxis to prevent the development of malignancy.

Presentation of Hematological Malignancy

From the discussion above and in chapters 2, 8 and 11, it is clear that hematological malignancy may present in a wide variety of ways and commonly via specialities other than hematology.

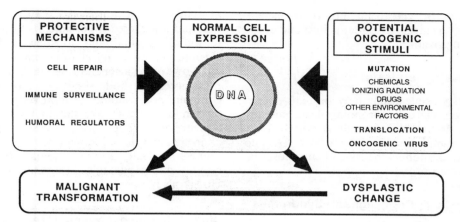

Figure 9.2. Potential oncogenic mechanisms

1. Hemopoietic failure
   - Anemia, bleeding or infection.
2. Hemopoietic system organomegaly
   - Lymphadenopathy: detected because of symptoms, physical examination, organ imaging or compression (e.g., superior or inferior vena caval obstruction, ureteric obstruction).
   - Thymic enlargement.
   - Splenomegaly: detected because of symptoms, physical examination or organ imaging techniques.
   - Hepatomegaly.
3. Infiltration or organomegaly in nonhemopoietic systems
   - Skin—diffuse or localized infiltration.
   - GIT—obstruction, malabsorption, other symptoms.
   - Neurological—discrete lesions or diffuse infiltration.
   - Pulmonary—solid lesion, diffuse infiltrate or pleural effusion.
   - Other system involvement less common: thyroid, renal, pericardial.
4. Autoimmune disease due to immunoregulatory failure
   - Autoimmune hemolytic anemia, thrombocytopenia, neutropenia.
   - Glomerulonephritis.
   - Vasculitis.
   - Miscellaneous skin eruptions.
5. Tumor products or biochemical effects
   - Monoclonal immunoglobulin production in immunoproliferative disorders.
   - Procoagulant activity—DIC, venous thrombosis.
   - Hyperuricemia.
   - Hypercalcemia.
6. Systemic effects of malignancy
   - Fever, night sweats.
7. Non-neoplastic manifestations
   - Neurological disease—peripheral neuropathy, multifocal leukoencephalopathy, myopathy.
   - Endocrine syndromes—e.g., hypercalcemia.
8. Laboratory presentation
   - Abnormality on peripheral blood count
     Leukocytosis—abnormal differential leukocyte count
     Evidence of hemopoietic failure
     Leukerythroblastic blood film.
   - Biochemical abnormalities
     Hypercalcemia
     Hyperuricemia
     Elevated LDH
     Elevated globulins
     Abnormal liver function test results
     Uremia.
9. Incidental radiological finding
   - Chest X-ray abnormality
     Mediastinal mass
     Pleural effusion
     Intrapulmonary lesion.
   - Skeletal abnormality
     Osteoporosis
     Lytic bone lesions.
   - CT scan.

Investigations

As with any malignant disease the definitive diagnosis of hematological malignancy is dependent on the morphological demonstration of tissue abnormalities. As the malignant hemopoietic cell has its normal counterpart, it may at times be difficult to establish a categorical diagnosis unless there are pathognomonic features in cell morphology, tissue architecture or cell behavior. It is usually possible to categorize patients into one of the following groups:

Reactive Hyperplasia

A responsible agent may or may not be identified. The cell morphology is normal, tissue distribution of the cells is normal (e.g., normal lymph node architecture), there is no evidence of monoclonality and chromosomal studies are normal.

Dysplastic (? Premalignant) Syndromes

There may be evidence of functional impairment. Dysplastic morphology, chromosomal defects and evidence of monoclonality may be found. Included in this group are some of the myeloproliferative syndromes, preleukemic syndromes, abnormal lymphoproliferation and benign monoclonal gammopathies.

Hematological Malignancy

Clinical and laboratory features establish a pathognomonic diagnosis of malignancy.

In establishing a diagnosis of hematological malignancy the following investigative sequence is usually followed.

What Investigations Are Likely to Establish a Definitive Diagnosis?

In the case of leukemia and myeloma the peripheral blood in conjunction with the bone marrow is usually diagnostic. With the lymphomas, a lymph node or other involved tissue needs to be biopsied. It is important that the specimen is processed correctly as fixation of the sample may be crucial. When the diagnosis of lymphoma is suspected before biopsy, it is desirable to communicate with the pathologist to check how the sample should be handled. Most pathologists are reluctant to make a firm diagnosis of lymphoma on a frozen section. However, frozen sections do play a role in confirming that adequate tissue has been obtained for diagnosis, that excision of a primary lymphoma has been adequate, or to indicate that definitive surgery should be postponed until a confirmatory diagnosis is available. The site of biopsy may be important and if a choice is possible, it is desirable to avoid inguinal and tonsillar nodes as chronic inflammatory changes may be present, however as a general rule, the largest and most accessible node should be biopsied. A complete node should be removed and distortion of the material should be avoided. The important questions addressed when an abnormal lymph node is biopsied include: benign versus malignant; lymphoma versus carcinoma and Hodgkin's disease versus non-Hodgkin's lymphoma.

What Other Investigations Are Necessary to Further Categorize the Malignancy?

When a firm diagnosis of hematological malignancy has been established further investigation is usually in the hands of a hematologist. As will be seen later, each of the malignancies requires detailed classification in order to determine prognosis and therapy. Special investigations include the following:

Cytochemical Stains

Each of the leukemias has cytochemical characteristics which assist in cell identification and classification. Stains used include: peroxidase; esterase; PAS; Sudan black; acid phosphatase and oil red O.

Cell Marker Studies

It is now possible to study cell surface characteristics to establish the lineage of the malignant cells. More recently with the introduction of monoclonal antibodies, there are a wide range of reagents available for cell identification. Antibodies are not only available to identify cell type but also the stage of development. There are several methods available for the use of the monoclonal antibodies, including immunofluorescence and cytochemical enzyme linked assays. These studies not only assist in classification of the malignancies, but have added considerably to our knowledge of the pathophysiology. This has become a highly complex and specialized area of laboratory medicine and the reader is referred to specialized texts on the subject for further information.

Electron Microscopy

Detailed ultrastructural features may be helpful in some cases of hematological malignancy.

Chromosomal Analysis and Molecular Biological Techniques

For many years chromosomal investigations were of academic interest and had little role in the management of patients with hematological malignancies except in chronic granulocytic leukemia where the Philadelphia chromosome is a marker of the disease. In recent years, this situation has changed due to the development of more sophisticated techniques for the identification and analysis of chromosomes, such as banding and DNA probes. It is likely that the role of chromosomal and DNA analysis will increase in the forthcoming years.

Cell Culture Studies

Culture of peripheral blood and bone marrow cells has added significantly to our understanding of the kinetic behavior and development of normal and malignant hemopoietic cells. It is likely that these studies will establish a role in patient management especially in decisions regarding therapy.

What Staging Investigations Need to Be Performed?

After the establishment of a diagnosis of malignancy, complete staging of the disease is usually the next step in deciding prognosis and therapy. Although this is true for solid tumors the application of staging to hematological malignancy has always been controversial. As already highlighted the hemopoietic and lymphoid systems are normally disseminated and malignancies are likely to behave in a similar fashion. In most hematological malignancies the prognosis depends more on the pathobiology of the malignant cell rather than the staging of disease. A patient with stage I lymphoma with highly malignant histology is likely to have a worse prognosis than a patient with stage IV disease and a more favorable histological picture. In patients with favorable morphological appearances, such as some of the chronic leukemias or follicular lymphomas, may have extensive disease and a high tumor load, but prognosis may not be much affected by therapy. This is in contrast to patients with a highly blastic stage I lymphoma where aggressive therapy may be curative in a significant percentage of patients. The main role of staging in hematological malignancy is to determine, firstly, whether there are any complications which may require specific therapy, such as metabolic derangements and compression syndromes. Secondly, staging may be important in therapeutic decision making and thirdly, may help in assessing prognosis. Fourthly, it is desirable to know the extent of the disease in order to monitor response to therapy and as a "baseline" for comparison when restaging after relapse. Figure 9.3 illustrates the main lymph node regions and organs which should be assessed. Depending on the disease in question the following investigations may be indicated:

Clinical Pathology Investigations

- Hematological investigations—
  Full blood examination
  Bone marrow aspiration and biopsy or trephine biopsy
  Appropriate cell marker studies
- Biochemical profile—
  Renal and liver function
  Serum calcium, uric acid, alkaline phosphatase
  Lactic dehydrogenase
- Histological and cytological examinations—
  Diagnostic biopsy
  Aspiration cytology: e.g., CSF

Organ Imaging

- Radiological investigations—
  Chest X-ray, skeletal survey, IVP
  Computerized tomography of appropriate regions
  Lymphangiogram
- Ultrasound investigations—
  Liver, spleen.
- Radionucleide scans—
  Liver, spleen, bone, gallium scan.
- Nuclear magnetic resonance.

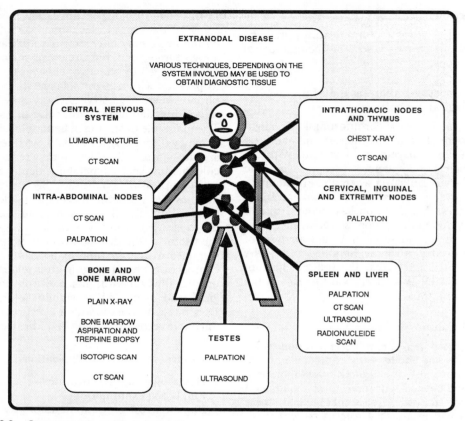

Figure 9.3. Organomegaly and its investigation

General Principles of Management

The therapy of hematological malignancy has been one of the evolving success stories in modern medicine. With better understanding of the pathophysiology and the discovery of effective modes of therapy, the life expectancy of many patients has been improved. In some diseases the potential for cure has been realized, including Hodgkin's disease, childhood acute lymphoblastic leukemia and some aggressive lymphomas. In recent years bone marrow transplantation is offering some adults with acute leukemia long-term survival and possible cure. The impressive chemotherapeutic advances in hematological malignancy, firstly with single agent therapy, and subsequently multiple agent therapy, has paved the way for their general use in other malignancies and the evolution of oncology as a speciality in its own right.

QUESTIONS IN THE THERAPY OF HEMATOLOGICAL MALIGNANCY

Figure 9.4 outlines a general approach to the management of hematological malignancy. Patients with hematological malignancy can usually be classified in relation to one of the following questions.

Can the Disease Be Cured?

(Childhood ALL, Hodgkin's disease, some aggressive lymphomas, occasional adult leukemias.)

If a malignant disease can be cured, the suffering and complications of therapy can usually be justified. If the patient and relatives can expect a high probability of cure they will be prepared to accept the apparent paradox that the treatment seems worse than the disease. Intensive support may be necessary and constant encouragement and understanding

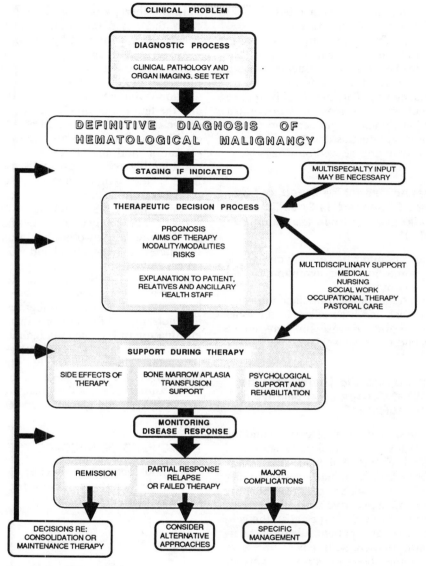

Figure 9.4. An overview of the management of hematological malignancy

provided. Attention to psychological needs (e.g., alopecia, feelings of dehumanization, infertility, concern about death), physical effects of therapy (e.g., nausea and GIT upsets and other toxic effects of therapy) and nutrition are essential.

If the Disease Cannot Be Cured Can Life Expectancy Be Extended?

(Adult leukemias, aggressive lymphomas, multiple myeloma.)

In many diseases it is possible with specific therapy to control the disease and prolong life. However, the operative word is life in the fullest sense of the word. The clinician must constantly be aware of the possibility that he may be prolonging death. There is increasing awareness of quality of life when considering therapy for malignant disease. It is sometimes difficult for the patient and relatives to understand that unpleasant specific therapy is justified on the basis that a remission may be induced with a good quality of extended life provided. It should be emphasized that, as functional failure (e.g., severe pancytopenia) may be a feature of hematological malignancy, a patient may be acutely ill at presentation and in the remission induction period, yet return to normal health as soon as a remission is achieved. This particularly applies to acute leukemia, a disease in which most people find it difficult to understand how a patient can be at "death's door" one day and suddenly recover and be well only days later.

If the Disease Cannot Be Cured, or Life Expectancy Prolonged, Is Specific Therapy Likely to Improve the Patient's Quality of Life?

(Chronic granulocytic and lymphocytic leukemia, some follicular lymphomas and splenic lymphomas.)

In several hematological malignancies specific therapy has had little effect on the long-term outcome of the disease, but may relieve symptoms and improve wellbeing.

If There Is No Specific Therapy for the Disease What Nonspecific Palliative Therapy Is Indicated?

Full discussion of this subject is beyond the scope of this text, but it suffices to say that if the clinician is unable to offer specific therapy for a patient's disease he has a responsibility to ensure that appropriate palliative therapy is provided and supportive services utilized.

It is important that the specialist, the general practitioner and patient all fully understand the aims of therapy. It may be necessary to readdress the above questions at various points during the clinical course of the patient's disease. The patient should be aware of these questions and receive a full explanation of the decision process. It is only with the full understanding and cooperation of the patient and his or her relatives that the physical and psychological needs of the patient can be correctly managed. As many of the malignancies in question are likely to shorten a patient's life and result in significant pain and suffering, the clinician should not shy away from his overall responsibility to the patient as a person and not just a disease.

In the therapy of most hematological diseases there is a remission induction phase which may be followed by consolidation and subsequent maintenance therapy. In diseases which are curable or in which life can be significantly prolonged the initial remission induction is the most significant part of therapy and the first major hurdle before other therapeutic questions can be addressed. After the establishment of remission, the role of consolidation and maintenance therapy varies considerably from disease to disease. In childhood acute lymphoblastic leukemia, and probably in some adult patients, maintenance therapy and CNS prophylaxis have been shown convincingly to have significant affects on the cure rate. In other hematological malignancies it is the initial induction therapy which decides the long-term result. In most malignancies this therapy is carried out over a six-month period and may be multimodal (e.g., chemotherapy, radiotherapy, surgery). The current belief is that cure depends on the elimination of the "last malignant cell." This is not to deny that the body's own nonspecific or specific defenses may be important in achieving this end. All stages of the therapeutic decision process will be affected by the patient's age, general physical and mental state.

PRINCIPLES OF SPECIFIC THERAPY

Certain general principles govern the choice of modality of therapy and these warrant summarizing.

Surgery

Surgery has little role to play in the management of hematological malignancy after the diagnosis and staging has been completed. However, in certain circumstances surgical consultation and operation may contribute to management:

- Removal of bulk disease—GIT lymphoma, splenectomy.
- Therapy of specific complications—spinal cord compression, GIT or renal obstruction, abscess drainage, anorectal complications, acute abdomen, management of pleural effusions.

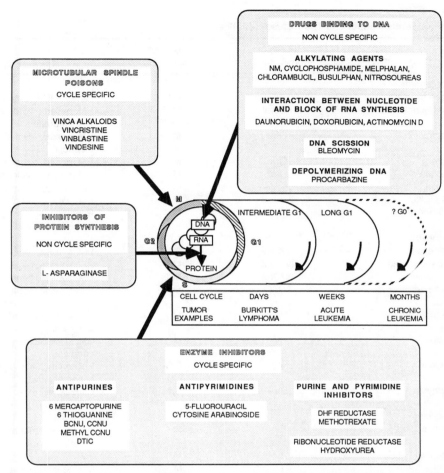

Figure 9.5. Mechanisms of action of chemotherapeutic agents. NM = nitrogen mustard; BCNU = 1,3,-bis-(2-Chloroethyl)-1-nitrosourea; DTIC = 5-(3,3-Dimethyl-1-triazeno) imidizole-4-carboxamide; CCNU = 1-(2-Chloroethyl)-3-cyclohexyl-1-nitrosourea; DHF = Dihydrofolate.

● Insertion of venous and CNS access devices.

Radiotherapy

Radiotherapy may be used in several ways:

● Primary control of disease—local, half-body, total body, radioactive phosphorus.
● For CNS prophylaxis.
● For therapy to sites of bulk disease after initial control with chemotherapy.
● For management of localized disease or pain relief when chemotherapy may not be effective or the dosage required may be too toxic—spinal cord compression, venous or lymphatic obstruction, intracranial disease, cutaneous infiltration.

Chemotherapy

Chemotherapy is the mainstay of therapy for hematological malignancy. Figure 9.5 illustrates the sites of action of the commonly used chemotherapeutic agents and Table 9.1 lists the drugs and their side effects. Cytotoxic chemotherapy may be used in the following ways:

● Single-agent low dosage, with or without corticosteroid: such therapy is generally

Table 9.1
Chemotherapeutic Agents and Their Characteristics

Drug	Route of Administration	Route of Elimination	Toxicity
Alkylating agents			
Nitrogen mustard	IV	M[a]	Nausea, BM, gonads
Cyclophosphamide	IV/oral	M/R	BM, nausea, bladder, gonads, fluid retention
Chlorambucil	Oral	M	BM, gonad, myelodysplasia, alopecia
Melphalan	Oral	M	BM, gonad, nausea
Busulphan	Oral	M	BM (may be prolonged), gonad, pulmonary, hyperpigmentation
BCNU & CCNU	IV/Oral	M	BM, nausea, renal, pulmonary
CIS-platinum	IV	R	Renal, nausea, neurological, hypersensitivity
Antimetabolites			
Methotrexate	IV/Oral	R	BM, nausea, renal, neurological
6-mercaptopurine	IV/Oral	M/R	BM, nausea, hepatic, fever
6-thioguanine	IV/Oral	M/R	BM, nausea, hepatic, fever
Cytosine arabinoside	IV/SC	M	BM, nausea, hepatic, stomatitis
Antibiotics			
Daunorubicin	IV	M	BM, alopecia, cardiac, cutaneous
Doxorubicin	IV	M	BM, alopecia, cardiac, cutaneous
Bleomycin	IV	R/M	Pulmonary, skin, pyrexia, hypersensitivity
Mithramycin	IV	R/M	Nausea, skin, neurological, hemorrhage
Vinca alkaloids			
Vincristine	IV	M	Neuropathy (peripheral and autonomic)
Vinblastine	IV	M	BM
Vindesine	IV	M	BM, neurological
Hormones			
Corticosteroids	Oral/IV/IM	M	Metabolic
Miscellaneous			
Procarbazine	Oral/IV	M/R	Nausea, BM, neurological
Hydroxyurea	Oral/IV	R	BM, nausea, skin
L-asparaginase	IV/IM	?M	Hypersensitivity, nausea, neurological
VP 16 (etoposide)	Oral/IV	R/?M	BM, alopecia, stomatitis, nausea
VM 26 (teniposide)	IV	R/M	BM, hypersensitivity, nausea, stomatitis, alopecia

M = Metabolic, R = Renal, BM = Bone marrow suppression
For dosages, interactions and administration instructions the reader is referred to the major texts and the drug information. These drugs should only be used by practitioners cognizant of the indications and complications. Close monitoring of therapy is essential.

used in malignancies in which control and not cure is the aim of therapy.
- Multiple agent—in this type of therapy synergism is usually achieved by combined use of agents with different mechanisms of action, increasing the likelihood of eradicating disease.

Intermediate intensity therapy, multiagent therapy

Aggressive multiple agent therapy

Supralethal chemotherapy combined with bone marrow rescue
Intrathecal, intrapleural, intraperitoneal, cutaneous.

Other Less-Commonly Used Modalities

- Immunotherapy—stimulation, monoclonal antibodies.
- Heat, e.g., microwave.

Combined Modality Therapy

In many diseases a combination of the above modalities may be used.

MONITORING OF THERAPY

As with any therapy close clinical and laboratory monitoring is an integral part of patient management. When a patient enters a therapeutic program care must be taken to ensure that the original aims outlined in the above four questions are being achieved. In some circumstances there may be a high complication rate. This may be acceptable as long as there is good evidence that the malignancy is responding. If this is not the case, or the disease relapses after initial therapy, the four questions outlined above must be readdressed. The need for repeated investigations can be controversial and should be considered along the following lines:

What Tests Are Essential for Monitoring the Toxicity of Therapy?

Hematological and biochemical monitoring is essential for chemotherapy and most forms of radiotherapy. The investigations required are readily available and relatively inexpensive.

How Should Response of the Malignancy Be Monitored?

If there are simple clinical, laboratory or radiological parameters which can be followed, detailed and expensive organ imaging investigations are unnecessary in the initial phases of therapy, unless complications occur. It is not until important therapeutic decisions will be affected by the results of such investigations that their performance can be justified.

What Investigations Need to Be Performed to Detect Evidence of Relapse in Patients Receiving Maintenance Therapy or No Therapy?

The answer to this question depends on the importance of detecting early relapse in relation to the therapy and prognosis. As a generalization, unless complications have occurred (e.g., spinal cord compression, venous obstruction, metabolic disturbances), in most hematological malignancies the response to therapy and prognosis is determined by the biology of the malignant cell, rather than the extent of tumor.

The Hematological Malignancies

THE LEUKEMIAS

The leukemias are broadly divided into acute and chronic, generally according to the time span of their clinical course. In general, a leukemia which is blastic in appearance behaves in an acute and rapidly fatal manner, in contrast to the chronic leukemias where cells are more differentiated or mobile and the disease follows a more indolent course. There are exceptions in some patients where the morphological characteristics suggest acute leukemia but the patient has a more subacute or "smouldering" clinical course. In acute leukemia the blast cells and tumor load are predominantly confined to the bone marrow, and death of the patient occurs when the total leukemic burden exceeds 1×10^{12} leukemic cells (10^{12} cells = 1kg). This is in contrast to the chronic leukemias in which the cells are more widely distributed and surprisingly large tumor burdens of 10kg or more may be tolerated.

All leukemias are classified on the basis of their cell of origin (see Fig. 9.6). The broad division is into those of myeloid origin, in the broadest sense of the word (i.e., of hemopoietic marrow origin), and those of lymphoid origin, arising from the cells of the immune system. Within both these groups there are numerous subclassifications into cell types. Differentiation may have clinical significance

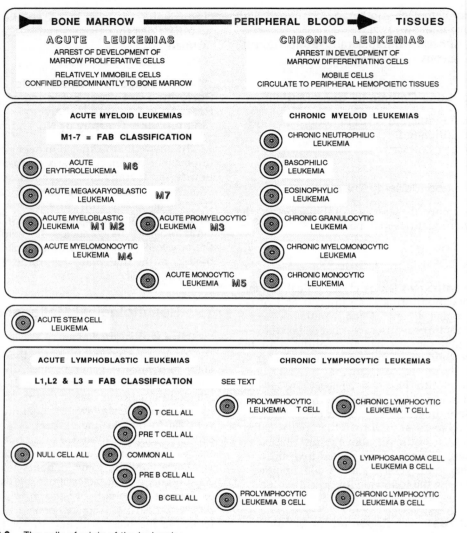

Figure 9.6.   The cells of origin of the leukemias

in terms of specific clinical features or complications, prognosis and therapy.

Acute Nonlymphocytic Leukemias

Acute myelogenous leukemia constitutes 25% of all leukemias, commonest in the middle-aged and elderly. Median survival in classical acute myeloblastic leukemia is approximately 1 to 2 months without therapy and approximately 12 months with therapy. A classification system called the FAB (French-American-British) is commonly used for subdividing this group of leukemias, into M1 to M7.

Acute Myeloblastic Leukemia—AML (M1 and M2)

The involved cell in AML is the myeloblast, the earliest cell committed to granulopoietic development. Patients usually present with features of bone marrow failure. It is rare to find extramedullary disease and organomegaly is uncommon. Leukocytosis is due to myeloblasts in the peripheral blood and >40% leukemic blast cells are found in the bone marrow. Morphologically the blast cells are large with several nucleoli, granules and Auer rods in the cytoplasm. Sudan black, peroxidase and chloracetate esterase stains are positive. M1 shows no morphological differentiation (20% of all AML), but is identified by the presence of occasional Auer rods, positive myeloperoxidase or Sudan black stains, or more recently with monoclonal antibodies, whereas M2 shows some features of granulocytic differentiation (37% of all AML).

Therapy consists of cytosine arabinoside and an anthracycline (adriamycin or daunorubicin) are the first line drugs for remission induction. Worthwhile survival usually depends on achieving a remission which occurs in approximately 70% of patients. Bone marrow transplantation should be considered in first remission if a compatible donor is available. Death is usually due to infection or bleeding from marrow failure from the disease or therapy. In untreated disease or resistant terminal disease, fulminant leukostasis from extreme leukocytosis may occur. There are no specific complications which are unique to this type of leukemia. Central nervous system disease may occur in advanced drug-resistant-disease. The short survival time is probably one factor contributing to the low incidence of CNS disease.

Acute Promyelocytic Leukemia—APML (M3)

The predominant cell involved in APML is the promyelocyte, the progenitor cell of all the granulocytic series of cells (i.e., neutrophil, eosinophil and basophil). Promyelocytes contain the primary granules which are then distributed to the progeny prior to the development of specific secondary granules. Hemorrhage is a major feature of this leukemia with cerebral hemorrhage commonly occurring at presentation. Bleeding is in part due to thrombocytopenia but the unique feature is the florid disseminated intravascular coagulation (DIC) caused by the release of granules from the cells, especially following chemotherapy. Marked fibrinogenolysis may also be seen. Peripheral blood leukocytosis is variable, but there are >40% leukemic blast cells in the bone marrow. Morphologically the leukemic cells are characterized by their hypergranularity, sometimes with numerous Auer rods (faggots), extremely strong peroxidase and Sudan black stains. APML makes up 7% of all AML.

Therapy can be difficult, not only due to the coagulopathy, but also because of resistance. Without therapy most patients die within a month. There is some evidence that if a remission is achieved (usually >50% of patients) extended survival may occur. Cytosine arabinoside and athracyclines are first line drugs, with specific therapy for DIC.

Acute Myelomonocytic Leukemia— AMML (M4) (Naegeli Type)

In AMML the common progenitor cell for granulocytic and monocytic development, in culture terminology known as the CFUc, appears to be arrested in development. This leukemia is usually clinically indistinguishable from AML, except that splenomegaly may be present. Both monocytic and myeloblastic blast cells are present in the peripheral blood and bone marrow. Peroxidase, chloroacetate esterase, nonspecific esterase and sudan black stains are positive. Serum and urine lysozyme (muramidase) may be raised. AMML makes up 23% of all AML. Therapy is similar to AML.

Acute Monoblastic Leukemia—AMoL (M5) (Schilling Type)

Arrest in development of the progenitor cell of the monocyte-macrophage system is responsible for AMoL. AMoL is a rare leukemia, more common in the younger age group, and usually follows an aggressive clinical course with extramedullary involvement a feature at presentation (gum hypertrophy, CNS disease, organomegaly). Fever directly due to the disease is common, and DIC may occur. Large, bizarre, monoblastic cells are present in the peripheral blood and marrow. Fine granules may be seen and nuclei convoluted. Nonspecific esterase stain (sodium fluroide sensitive) is strongly positive. AMoL is a difficult disease to control. Remissions may be rapidly achieved, but early relapse is common. Cytosine arabinoside and anthracyclines are first line drugs. Etiposide (VP16) seems also to be a valuable agent.

Acute Erythroleukemia—AEL (M6) (Di Guglielmo's syndrome)

Initially AEL involves the erythroid precursor, but as the disease evolves, dedifferentiation occurs and the leukemia becomes more blastic and primitive in appearance, similar to AML, and is no longer a pure erythroid leukemia. There may be a long prodromal period before the disease becomes a clearly blastic leukemia. The peripheral blood may show macrocytosis with abnormal red cell morphology and erythroblasts in the peripheral blood. The bone marrow is hypercellular with >50% abnormal megaloblastoid erythroblasts (PAS positive staining) with multinucleated cells and myeloblasts. In the advanced stages of the disease the marrow and peripheral blood findings may be indistinguishable from AML (M1 or M2). This form of leukemia may in some instances initially be followed without therapy. When acute blastic disease is present or evolves, it can be difficult to induce a remission, especially in elderly patients.

Rarer Forms of Acute Leukemia of Myeloid Origin

There are several rare forms of acute leukemia originating from the respective precursor cells. These leukemias include: acute megakaryocytic leukemia (M7), acute eosinophilic leukemia and acute basophilic leukemia.

Acute Lymphoblastic Leukemias—ALL

Acute lymphoblastic leukemia accounts for approximately 20% of all leukemias and is the commonest encountered in children. ALL is not preceded by a preleukemic phase such as may be seen in some patients with myeloid leukemia. The disease may originate from the bone marrow, thymus or lymph nodes, and although the clinical pictures and prognoses may vary, they are all essentially leukemias. ALL is classified on the basis of cell marker studies into T and B cell disease. On standard morphology the lymphoblastic leukemias are classified on an FAB classification. In L1 type the majority of the cells are small cells with scanty cytoplasm and regular round or clefted nuclei with indistinct nucleoli. In L2, the cells are larger with more cytoplasm, oval to round nuclei some with clefts and folds. The chromatin pattern is fine with prominent nucleoli. In the L3 type (also called Burkitt cell leukemia), the blasts are larger and homogeneous with finely stippled nuclei and deeply basophilic and vacuolated cytoplasm.

Organomegaly is more common in ALL than AML, bone pain being a common feature. Extramedullary disease is more common in ALL with musculoskeletal and neurological presentations. Cutaneous (especially in T-cell disease) and testicular disease are not infrequent. As with most of the leukemias there has been intense interest in cell marker studies to determine the origin of the malignant cell. These marker studies, in conjunction with chromosomal studies, are becoming increasingly important in determining prognosis.

Common Acute Lymphoblastic Leukemia—Common ALL (75% of Childhood ALL: L1 or L2)

ALL typically occurs in children, responds well to therapy and has the potential for cure in over 50% of patients when CNS prophylaxis and prolonged maintenance therapy is used. L1 morphology is usually found with block PAS positivity in the blast cells. Definitive identification is made using monoclonal antisera. Vincristine, Adriamycin, asparaginase and corticosteroids are the first line drugs for remission induction followed by 6 mercaptopurine and methotrexate for maintenance therapy. The prognosis in adult ALL does not appear to be as good as in children.

Null Cell Acute Lymphoblastic Leukemia

This form of ALL is morphologically similar to other ALL forms, but the cell markers are all negative. It is more common in adults and has a poor prognosis.

T-Cell Acute Lymphoblastic Leukemia— T Cell ALL

This type of ALL is suggested by the clinical picture of a mediastinal mass (thymus) and a high peripheral blast cell count. Definitive identification is made with the demonstration of acid phosphatase and nonspecific esterase staining of the blast with T cell marking characteristics. The disease most commonly occurs in the 10 to 20 years age group and has been regarded as having poor prognosis. However, in the light of recent experience with more aggressive chemotherapeutic protocols, 40% to 50% long-term survival may be possible.

B-Cell Acute Lymphoblastic Leukemia— B Cell ALL

This is the least common form of ALL, and has the worst prognosis of all types. On cytochemistry the vacuoles in the blast cells are positive with oil red O stain, and B cell markers are present. The disease commonly has the L3 morphology, and extramedullary (especially CNS) disease is common. Hyperuricemia may be a problem and tumor lysis syndrome may complicate therapy. In this syndrome there is a sudden breakdown of malignant cells with metabolic overload. Hyperphosphatemia and hypocalcemia may be a problem. It is essential that adequate hydration is maintained and the urine alkalinized.

The Chronic Leukemias

Almost half of the leukemias are classified as chronic. They are broadly divided into myeloid and lymphoid, with increasing subclassification in recent years. A common feature of the chronic leukemias is to enter a more aggressive phase of disease, and in some cases, to become frankly blastic, as commonly seen in chronic granulocytic leukemia. Except in specific circumstances, therapy offers little to improve the long-term survival of this group of leukemias. However, therapy has been beneficial in improving patients' quality of life. As patients may have a substantial tumor burden before they develop symptoms or evidence of bone marrow failure, diagnosis of the disease may be incidental. In the case of chronic lymphocytic leukemia, this occurs at times of elective surgery, during medical checks or when the patient is being investigated for an unrelated problem. This is in stark contrast to acute leukemia when the patient presents because of symptoms which are directly related to the leukemic process.

The maturation defect in the chronic leukemias occurs at a later stage in cell development in the case of chronic granulocytic leukemia. The granulopoietic cells have developed to the point where they are able to leave the bone marrow, circulate and accumulate in extramedullary sites, such as liver and spleen. In the early stages of chronic lymphoid leukemias, the malignant cell is relatively mobile as it is in a resting phase and, although primitive in its development along the B or T cell lineage, it is at a stage when it is "permitted" to move around the body along specified lymphoid "traffic lanes" and accumulate in sites characteristic for its normal counterpart at that stage of maturation.

Whereas marrow failure is usually the presenting feature of classical acute leukemia, in the chronic leukemias this is usually a late manifestation of the disease. Organomegaly is a common presentation of all varieties of chronic leukemia. With the chronic lymphoid leukemias failure of immune function may be the presentation with the development of infections. The specific immunodeficiency varies with the type of malignancy.

Chronic Granulocytic Leukemia—CGL

There is a clonal abnormality in CGL which is identified with the demonstration of the Philadelphia (Ph) chromosome in 90% of patients. This is demonstrable in all granulopoietic, erythroid and megakaryocytic lines where part of the long arm of chromosome 22 is translocated to chromosome 9. Normal hemopoietic cells are usually few or not demonstrated.

Patients may complain of generalized symptoms of lethargy, weight loss, sweats and anemia. Symptoms referrable to the spleen may occur. The disease is commonest in the middle age group. Peripheral blood examination reveals leukocytosis, which may be extreme, with a left shift in granulopoietic cells, ranging back to promyelocytes. Myeloblasts may constitute 5% to 10% of leukocytes without it representing an acute transformation. Basophils and eosinophils may be increased, leukocyte alkaline phosphatase (LAP) score is low. Thrombocytosis can be a feature in some patients. The bone marrow is grossly hypercellular with granluopoietic hyperplasia. Hyperuricemia, elevated vitamin B12 binding proteins and elevated LDH are found. Median survival of CGL is 3 to 4 years, and therapy has little effect on the long-term outcome. The main role of therapy is to control symptoms from the effects of tumor burden. Clinical problems may result from organomegaly (especially splenomegaly), leukocytosis, thrombocytosis, anemia and hypermetabolic effects of tumor load. Alkylating agents (busulphan) are the commonly used therapeutic agents. However the disease will respond to splenic irradiation, leukapheresis and other chemotherapeutic agents. The aim of therapy is to control symptoms without necessarily maintaining the leukocyte count at normal levels. Busulphan may be used in intermittent high dosage, intermittent low dose or continuous low dose.

Transformation of the disease to aggressive phase occurs in approximately 80% of patients. The transformation may take several forms. Acute blastic transformation (which may be myeloblastic or lymphoblastic in type) is usually fatal within 2 to 6 months. A slower myelofibrotic transformation may occur, mainly manifested by progressive anemia, thrombocytopenia and splenomegaly. The terminal phase of CGL can be particularly distressing and painful with bone pain, splenic infarction and bleeding. In rare circumstances, a splenectomy may be indicated for palliation or hypersplenism.

Rarer Chronic Leukemias of Granulocytic and Monocytic Origin

These are all rare varieties of chronic leukemia, including: chronic monocytic leukemia; chronic myelomonocytic leukemia; chronic eosinophilic leukemia and chronic basophilic leukemia, which are diagnosed from the laboratory findings and may evolve into more aggressive acute myeloid leukemia.

Chronic Lymphoid Leukemias

B-Cell Chronic Lymphocytic Leukemia— CLL

Classical CLL accounting for 25% of all leukemias involves the bone marrow based B lymphocytes. The patients are usually middle-aged or elderly, with males more frequently affected than females (2.5:1). There is usually generalized lymphadenopathy and splenomegaly in established disease. Patients are commonly asymptomatic with lymphocytosis and humoral immune defect. Presentation with bacterial infection is common, at which time a paradoxical lymphocytosis may occur and settle as infection resolves. In healthy people lymphocytes fall during bacterial infection.

Peripheral blood lymphocytosis, including smudge cells, is a *sine qua non* of CLL, with accompanying bone marrow lymphocytosis being essential for diagnosis. Anemia and/or thrombocytopenia may result from bone marrow failure in advanced disease, or on the other hand, may be secondary to hypersplenism or autoimmune mechanisms in some patients. Hypogammaglobulinemia is common, depending on the stage of disease and rarely a monoclonal paraprotein (usually IgM) may be found. Defects in cell-mediated immunity may also occur. Lymph node architecture is

effaced with a diffuse cellular proliferation of monomorphic well-differentiated lymphoid cells. In some patients there may be up to 10% of atypical lymphoid cells in the peripheral blood, but overall the morphology may be acceptable for CLL. Some authors refer to this as atypical CLL. If a greater percentage of the cells are large and atypical, differentiation from lymphosarcoma cell leukemia, prolymphocytic leukemia and lymphomas with circulating lymphoma cells may become difficult (see below).

CLL is the only leukemia in which clinical staging of the disease has been found useful in clinical practice (Rai classification.)

Stage 0: No organomegaly, peripheral blood and marrow lymphocytosis

Stage 1: Above plus lymphadenopathy

Stage 2: Stage 0 plus splenomegaly +/− hepatomegaly, nodes may also be palpable.

Stage 3: Stage 0 plus anemia due to the CLL, organomegaly may also be present.

Stage 4: Stage 0 plus thrombocytopenia due to CLL, organomegaly may also be present.

The overall median survival of all stages is approximately 5 years. Stage 0 and 1 may live for more than 10 years and stages 3 and 4 usually die within 2 years. The revised prognostic staging system proposed by the International Workshop on CLL is presented below.

Stage A Lymphocytosis without anemia or thrombocytopenia, and fewer than three areas of lymphoid involvement.

Stage B Lymphocytosis without anemia or thrombocytopenia but with more than three areas of lymphoid involvement.

Stage C Lymphocytosis with anemia or thrombocytopenia or both.

As therapy has not conclusively been shown to alter the long-term survival in most patients, treatment is directed towards symptoms and complications. The disease is responsive to corticosteroids and alkylating agents (chlorambucil or cyclophosphamide) as well as radiotherapy. Therapy needs to be individualized for each patient. Splenectomy may occasionally be indicated for hypersplenism or relief of local symptoms. Opportunistic infections are a common cause of death. Some patients enter an aggressive prolymphocytic type transformation while others gradually develop marrow failure from resistant infiltration which is not always related to progressive disease elsewhere in the body. Occasionally a large cell transformation may occur in lymph nodes, usually in the abdomen (Richter's syndrome).

T-Cell Chronic Lymphocytic Leukemia

A small number of patients with CLL have T-cell markers. The malignant lymphocytes may show nuclear indentations and cytoplasmic granules. Massive splenomegaly and cutaneous infiltration may be seen. Bone marrow failure may be out of proportion to the degree of lymphoid infiltration, suggesting lymphocyte suppressor effects on bone marrow function. Recently a syndrome of persistent T-cell lymphocytosis has been recognized in asymptomatic patients and in patients with autoimmune features. The relationship of this syndrome to chronic T-CLL remains to be determined. Due to the heterogeneous nature of the T cell lymphoproliferative disorders it is difficult to accurately prognosticate in individual patients, but in general, classical T-CLL follows an indolent course.

Prolymphocytic Leukemia—ProLL

This is a variant of CLL in which the predominant cell is a prolymphocyte which is a larger cell with a prominent nucleolus but well condensed nuclear chromatin. T and B cell types have been reported. The patients tend to have high peripheral blood lymphocyte counts, massive splenomegaly without major lymphadenopathy. The disease has a poorer prognosis than CLL and is resistant to conventional therapy. Leukapheresis and splenectomy may be helpful in control of the disease.

Chronic Lymphosarcoma Cell Leukemia—LSCL

The term lymphosarcoma cell leukemia has caused many semantic problems as it has been applied to several different types of lymphoproliferative disease. On occasions it has been applied to the terminal leukemic phase of any transformed lymphocytic lymphoma, the presence of circulating lymphoid cells in the follicular (nodular) lymphomas or to the leukemic presentations of lymphoblastic lymphomas. The term should be confined to the well-recognized chronic clinicopathological entity where there are large pleomorphic, clefted and folded lymphoid cells in the peripheral blood and lymph node histology demonstrates a follicular or diffuse, poorly differentiated histology. LSCL is a B cell malignancy which probably arises from a cell between the well-differentiated B cell from the bone marrow and the lymph node follicular center cell. Marrow, peripheral blood, lymph node and massive splenic involvement are characteristic. The disease has a variable natural history, but may be resistant to chemotherapy. As with ProLL, splenectomy and/or leukapheresis may be beneficial.

Hairy Cell Leukemia (Leukemic Reticuloendotheliosis)—LRE

This is a B-cell malignancy but the malignant cell has markers common to null cells, monocytes and T-cells. The disease presents with fatigue, weakness, weight loss and predominantly occurs in middle-aged males. Splenomegaly (90%) is common with hepatomegaly (50%) and lympadenopathy (25%) also found less frequently. Pancytopenia is usually present in the peripheral blood, hairy cells usually being found, but expert examination of the film is necessary for further identification. Bone marrow examination typically reveals a dry tap and trephine biopsy is necessary. Morphological features include a homogeneous population of cells with distinct cell borders, clear cytoplasm and monomorphous nuclei, small nucleoli with no mitosis, tartrate-resistant acid phosphatase and partial preservation of lymph node architecture.

The disease may have a long natural history with fluctuations in the clinical course. The patients appear to have specific quantitative and qualitative defects in monocyte-macrophage function which predisposes them to unusual opportunistic infections. Many modalities of therapy have been used but no standard therapies can be recommended at present. Recent experience with interferon has been most promising and it is likely to become the first line therapy in these patients. Splenectomy is helpful in many patients. Infection at times when the disease is relatively stable is a common cause of death. LRE is a most atypical lymphoproliferative disease about which much is to be learned.

THE LYMPHOMAS

Malignancies primarily arising in the lymph nodes or other lymphoid sites are broadly classified as lymphomas and arise from several different cellular origins at different stages of differentiation. Hodgkin's disease (HD) has its own characteristic clinical and pathological features which allow it to be specifically diagnosed and classified on its own. As a result of this separation of HD the term non-Hodgkins lymphoma (NHL) has evolved, mainly because of the difficulties in histological classification. In contrast to HD morphological criteria have been the mainstay of classification of the NHL, but traditional morphological dogmas are being increasingly challenged as our understanding of the lymphoid system unfolds. Cell marker techniques and functional studies are assisting in subclassification. There is a continuing debate as to whether a working classification should be based on cell of origin or on morphological features which correlate with a chronic, subacute or aggressive clinical course for the patient. Clinicians have found it difficult to understand and keep up with the many classification systems and prefer broad divisions into good, intermediate and poor prognostic groups in order to assist in therapeutic decision making. Such an approach is anathema to the mechanistic pathologist who desires the classification of a disease to have some relevance to the pathophysiology.

Hodgkin's Disease

Hodgkin's disease is one of the few malignant diseases in which therapy has undergone spectacular advances in the last three decades. An incurable disease in the 1940s, Hodgkin's disease can now be cured in nearly all patients with early disease and in the majority of patients with more advanced disease.

Clinical and Laboratory Features

Hodgkin's disease most frequently affects young and middle-aged people and presents with lymphadenopathy in the cervical region, or in the mediastinum (especially the nodular sclerosing histology). HD presenting in Waldeyer's ring or below the diaphragm is less common than in non-Hodgkins lymphoma. The lymph nodes are firm, but mobile, smooth and discrete. Hodgkin's disease is the lymphoma which commonly has marked systemic symptoms (B-symptoms) of weight loss, fever and night sweats and associated laboratory evidence of the hematological chronic phase reaction. Other less common presentations include: alcohol-induced pain, superior vena caval obstruction, splenomegaly, infective complications and rarely extranodal disease (hepatic, bone, pulmonary, spinal cord compression).

Histological diagnosis is usually established by biopsy of a lymph node or extranodal tissue (liver, bone, bone marrow). It is not uncommon for the initial node biopsy to be nondiagnostic and rebiopsy indicated. Most pathologists insist on the demonstration of Reed-Sternberg cells to make a diagnosis of HD. Despite its easily classifiable histological lesion, predictable prognosis and good response to therapy, the basic pathophysiology and cell of origin are poorly understood and the true neoplastic nature of the disease is sometimes questioned. The lineage of the Reed-Sternberg cells remains *sub judice,* macrophage and interdigitating reticulum cell being the main contenders. There are four histological types:

- Lymphocyte predominant (5%)—good prognosis.
- Nodular sclerosis (50%)—good prognosis, female > male, mediastinal involvement is characteristic.
- Mixed cellularity (40%)—intermediate prognosis.
- Lymphocyte depleted (5%)—poorer prognosis.

HD appears to be a unicentric disease which spreads predominantly via the lymphatics. Hematological and immunological features may include the following, depending on the activity and extent of disease:

- Normocytic normochromic (occasionally hypochromic) anemia, elevated ESR, neutrophilia, eosinophilia, lymphopenia, thrombocytosis, reactive bone marrow, defects in cell-mediated immunity, polyclonal hypergammaglobulinemia.

Staging

Accurate histological typing and staging are necessary to determine prognosis and decide upon effective therapy, but this was probably "overdone" during the 1970s. There is now less emphasis on the importance of accurate pathological staging unless it will affect therapeutic decisions in the management. It remains clear that lesser stage disease has a better prognosis, and the main reason for accurate staging has been to enable a decision to be made between the use of radiotherapy alone or chemotherapy alone. There has however been a reanalysis of combined modality therapy in recent years with the aim of using lesser amounts of radiotherapy and chemotherapy. Staging laparotomy has for some years been regarded as an essential part of staging patients who have clinical stage I or II disease. However, if laparotomy is not going to alter the ultimate decision for therapy, it is difficult to justify this procedure, especially in view of increasing awareness of the immunological defect induced by splenectomy, and the occasional deaths in cured patients due to postsplenectomy sepsis. This is not to say that staging laparotomy should be completely abandoned; however with modern methods of imaging, there appear to be very few cases where a staging laparotomy is indicated, particularly if combined modality therapy is going to be used on the majority of patients.

Stage I: Involvement of one lymph node region or a single localized site.

Stage II: Involvement of two lymph node regions or localized extra nodal disease with one or more lymph node regions, on the same side of the diaphragm.

Stage III: Involvement of lymph node regions on both sides of the diaphragm with or without splenic disease.

Stage IV: Disseminated involvement plus one or more extranodal regions.

The clinical staging can be qualified with A if there are no systemic symptoms, and B if there has been a greater than 10% weight loss in 6 months, fever or night sweats.

Therapy

Whatever the stage, HD at presentation should be regarded as a potentially curable disease. However, attempts should be made to identify subgroups of patients who may benefit from alterations to standard protocol. After staging and consideration of prognostic factors it is the remission induction therapy which is crucial as there is no good evidence that maintenance therapy further improves survival rates.

It is generally agreed that extended field radiotherapy is the treatment of choice for stages I and IIA without evidence of bulk disease, and that chemotherapy is optimal therapy for IIIB and stage IV disease. However, discussion continues as to the treatment of IIB and IIIA disease. If aggressive combined modality therapy is used, the incidence of complications rises. I and IIA with bulk disease are probably best treated with combined modality therapy, up to 3 cycles of MOPP (or equivalent) followed by extended field radiotherapy in reduced dose. The treatment of early disease with B symptoms remains debatable, unless a staging laparotomy has been done to confirm pathological staging of I and II. These patients should probably receive initial chemotherapy followed by radiotherapy to bulk disease sites. All patients with stage III and IV disease should receive full chemotherapy, possibly followed by reduced-dose radiotherapy to bulk disease sites.

The need for multiple agent chemotherapy has been well established and introduction of MOPP (mustine hydrochloride, vincristine sulphate, procarbazine hydrochloride and prednisolone) therapy has been one of the chemotherapy success stories of this century. However, it is a toxic regimen and unpleasant for the patient. There are several other drug combinations which have been well tested and have equal efficacy. It is likely that the standard chemotherapy for HD will change.

Prognosis

HD has moved from being an almost universally fatal disease without therapy to a curable one in the majority of patients. The overall 10-year survival is 60% to 70%; for stage I and IIA 90%+, stage IIIB and IVB 50%+, and IIB, IIIA intermediate between these figures.

It would clearly be desirable to select subgroups who may have a poor prognosis and require more aggressive therapy. If these could be identified, it would mean that less therapy could be given to the good prognosis groups. There is certainly a trend at the present time to give less therapy to patients for whom the prognosis is good. Indicators of a poor prognosis include:

- Lymphocyte depleted histological subtype, nodular sclerosing, and lymphocyte depleted Hodgkin's disease, B symptoms.
- Massive bulk disease especially in the mediastinum.
- Site of disease (extensive disease below the diaphragm, particularly involving the liver).
- Failure to achieve a complete remission with the first 3 cycles of chemotherapy.
- Increasing age (probably the effect of age not the HD).
- Immune status at the time of presentation (impaired, delayed hypersensitivity, lymphopenia).

The majority of relapses occur within the first 2 years of therapy and the majority of these respond well to further therapy and may still be cured.

Complications

Most of the early complications of therapy are acceptable. To the physician, these mainly consist of bone marrow suppression resulting in infections. For the patient, they mainly consist of the direct effects of chemotherapy (nausea, vomiting and hair loss). While clinicians often underrate the impact of these acute disturbances on patients, they are really tragic only in circumstances where therapy doesn't work. In cured patients, both they and their physician are able to put them into their proper perspective, even if the critics of chemotherapy do not.

In relation to late complications, while some people may consider it insensitive to say so, looking at long-term adverse effects is in fact a luxury that only follows successful treatment. There is now increasing concern about the long-term effects of treating Hodgkin's disease, particularly if excessive therapy is being given to patients who could be cured without such heavy therapy. The toxicity of greatest concern is the development of a second malignancy. In the majority of cases, this is acute myeloblastic leukemia which is resistant to therapy, but non-Hodgkin's lymphomas and various solid tumors may occur. It appears that the alkylating agents and procarbazine are the agents most commonly responsible, usually in combination with radiotherapy. Late infections can be a problem, particularly if a splenectomy has been per-

formed at the time of staging laparotomy. Longstanding defects in the immune system may also predispose the patient to infection. The production of sterility is also an increasing matter of concern, particularly as Hodgkin's disease occurs in the young.

Extranodal Hodgkins Disease

Hodgkins disease may rarely occur in several extranodal sites—skin, lung, pericardium, bone, soft tissue, thymus. Experience of most cases would indicate that survival of patients with extranodal disease is similar whether they receive radiation therapy alone or radiation therapy plus chemotherapy. It is thus suggested that extranodal disease should be staged in a similar fashion to nodal disease (subscript E being put after the staging).

Non-Hodgkins Lymphoma (NHL)

The nonspecialist has every reason to be perplexed and intimidated by this group of malignant disorders. There would be no other area of malignancy where, on the one hand there have been spectacular advances in our understanding of pathophysiology, yet on the other, confusion reigns supreme. This unfortunate state of affairs exists because of the cellular heterogeneity of the immune system resulting in the difficulties in establishing a logical and mechanistically based classification system which the clinican can understand and apply to the day to day care of patients. Therein lies our current dilemma, which is unlikely to be resolved while new knowledge accumulates at such a rate. However, patients still need to be treated and the clinician must be able to relate the pathological findings to the therapeutic decision process. The diagnosis of NHL is pursued along the lines outlined earlier in this chapter. In contrast to HD the management is almost totally dictated by the pathological diagnosis with staging of the disease being of secondary or little relevance.

Classification of Non-Hodgkins Lymphoma

Until recently pathological diagnosis and classification of NHL has been based solely on the microscopic findings on tissue sections. Rappaport's classification, because of its clarity and clinical applicability, has "held sway" in hematological practice for many years. It has even survived the recent on-slaught from immunologists, who have clearly exposed its flaws. It is not any inherent resilience of the Rappaport system, but rather the inability of workers to produce a lucid, logical and clinically useful alternative. The present author does not intend to list all the currently used classifications but rather to highlight the basic pathological and clinical concepts which are important in the diagnosis and management of NHL. The reader is referred to some key references in the vast literature on this fascinating area of malignancy. There is increasing use of the recently published Working Formulation (WF) on non-Hodgkins lymphomas which has been produced as a workable agreement from several major cancer centers (Table 9.2). This for-

Table 9.2
A Working Formulation of Non-Hodgkin's Lymphomas for Clinical Use, Compared with the Rappaport Classification

New Code	Working Formulation	Rappaport	Incidence
Low-grade lymphoma			
A	Malignant lymphoma, small lymphocytic Consistent with CLL Plasmacytoid	Lymphocytic, well differentiated with and without plasmacytoid features	4%
B	Malignant lymphoma, follicular small cleaved cell Diffuse areas Sclerosis	Nodular poorly differentiated lymphocytic	23%
C	Malignant lymphoma, follicular, mixed, small cleaved and large-cell Diffuse areas Sclerosis	Nodular mixed, lymphocytic and histiocytic	8%
Intermediate-grade lymphoma			
D	Malignant lymphoma follicular large-cell Diffuse areas Sclerosis	Nodular histiocytic	4%
E	Malignant lymphoma, diffuse small cleaved cell Sclerosis	Diffuse poorly differentiated lymphocytic	7%
F	Malignant lymphoma, diffuse mixed, small and large cell Sclerosis Epithelioid cell component	Diffuse mixed, lymphocytic and histiocytic	7%
G	Malignant lymphoma, diffuse large cell Cleaved cell Noncleaved cell Sclerosis	Diffuse histiocytic	20%
High-grade lymphoma			
H	Malignant lymphoma, large cell, immunoblastic Plasmacytoid Clear cell Polymorphous Epithelioid cell component	Diffuse histiocytic	1%
I	Malignant lymphoma lymphoblastic Convoluted cell Nonconvoluted cell	Lymphoblastic with and without convolutions	2%
J	Malignant lymphoma, small noncleaved cell Burkitt's Follicular areas	Diffuse undifferentiated Burkitt's and non-Burkitt's type	<1%

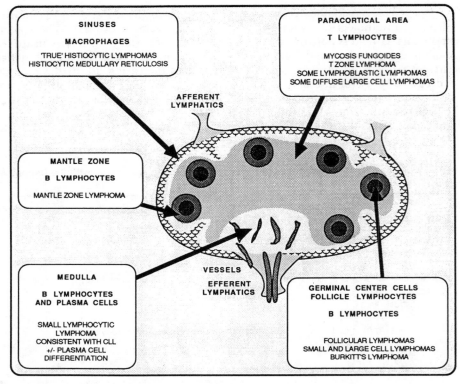

Figure 9.7.   The cells of origin of the non-Hodgkin's lymphomas

mulation is based on morphology alone and does not take into account the recent insights into cell origins of the NHLs and must thus be regarded as yet another interim classification. Figure 9.7 illustrates the cells of origin and localization of the different NHLs arising from the lymph node.

Pathological Concepts

The diagnosis of lymphoma depends on study of:

Lymphoid Tissue Architecture

The pattern of involvement may be helpful, follicular (nodular) versus diffuse being of prognostic significance in the small, cleaved cell and large cell NHLs. Follicular pattern correlates with a relatively good prognosis and diffuse with poor prognosis and diffuse/follicular being intermediate. This is not always absolute and must be interpreted in the context of the cell morphology and clinical findings. It is also not uncommon to find variable pathology in the same patient when

nodes from different sites are examined. As a general rule the prognosis of an individual patient correlates with the tendency to diffuse large cell disease even if a follicular pattern is noted, as the natural history of good prognosis disease is to undergo more aggressive transformation.

Cell Morphology

The degree of cell differentiation is also a determinant of prognosis. Small cells have usually been equated with well-differentiated disease, but this is now known not always to be the case as lymphoid cells may enter a resting phase and circulate to other lymphoid sites in the lymphoid system. Thus a disease with small lymphoid cells does not always mean the cells are well differentiated. The degree of blast transformation of the malignant cell usually correlates with cell size. The smallest lymphoid cells which are indistinguishable on standard light microscopy from normal mature lymphocytes are seen in chronic lymphocytic leukemia and well-differentiated lymphocytic lymphoma which have a diffuse pattern, but a good prognosis. The classical follicular small cleaved cell lymphomas have poorly differentiated lymphocyte morphology and the large cell types (histiocytic appearance of Rappaport) have a prognosis which is determined both by the cell size, and more importantly, by the degree of follicular pattern. Much is made of nuclear morphology in deciding the cell of origin with nuclear clefting, convolution, chromatin pattern and nucleolar appearance all being helpful.

Cell Markers

It is nearly always possible to establish the phenotypic characteristics of the malignant cells in a NHL. This can be done with various antibody reagents which react with cell surface antigens, cytochemistry and the study of functional characteristics. Many of these investigations are labor intensive, require specialized expertise and are usually only available in large institutions with an interest in lymphoma. Even so, they are likely to be of increasing importance in the decision making process in patient management.

Chromosomal Investigations

Initially of academic interest, chromosomal analysis in NHL is becoming of increasing practical importance.

Staging

The staging system used in HD is less helpful in the NHL and paradoxically, when NHL is considered as a whole, there tends to be an inverse relationship to the clinical stage and the prognosis. The aggressive large cell lymphomas tend to present as localized disease and behave as solid tumors, in contrast to the small cell follicular type which have circulating cells and behave as indolent "liquid tumors."

General Principles of Therapy

Therapy needs to be individualized for each patient after the following factors have been analyzed:

- Prognostic classification—good, intermediate or poor prognosis (see WF classification given earlier).
- Staging—more relevant in poor-prognosis disease.

- Bulk disease should be identified as follow-up radiotherapy may be indicated.
- Patient's symptomatology. Although therapy may not prolong life in the follicular lymphomas it may help with symptom control.
- Complications should be addressed early in management: venous compression, spinal cord compression, GIT or renal tract obstruction, biochemical abnormalities (e.g., hypercalcemia, hyperuricemia), marrow compromise, autoimmune disorders, monoclonal proteins.

Modes of therapy for different lymphomas will include:

- Good prognosis follicular or well-differentiated diffuse disease may not need therapy unless there is significant symptomatic disease. Local radiotherapy can be used for bulk disease or low-dose alkylating agents (chlorambucil or cyclophosphamide) with or without corticosteroids for disseminated disease. If resistant, combinations of pulse therapy may be used, e.g., alkylating agents, vinca alkaloids and high-dose corticosteroids.
- Intermediate prognosis disease usually requires high-dose pulse therapy using alkylating agents, vinca alkaloids and corticosteroids. As the disease becomes resistant other more potent, potentially toxic agents may be introduced (e.g., anthracyclines).
- High grade disease requires aggressive high-dose chemotherapy if there is to be any hope of cure. It is in this group where prolongation of life and possible cure are the stimulus to an optimistic approach to therapy, even though the protocols may be toxic. High-dose pulse chemotherapy with alkylating agents, vinca alkaloids, anthracyclines and corticosteroids is indicated from the outset. Follow-up radiotherapy to sites of bulk disease and CNS prophylaxis may be necessary. As a general rule, if the disease cannot be eliminated in the first few months of therapy, it is not possible to cure the patient.
- Localized extranodal disease may be treated by surgical resection followed by no therapy, chemotherapy or radiotherapy, depending on the pathology.

Extranodal Non-Hodgkin's Lymphomas

As lymphoid cells are normally located in most tissues of the body it is not surprising that lymphoma may occur as a primary disorder of a nonhemopoietic organ. The gastrointestinal tract is a common site of extranodal lymphoma, followed by lung, skin, liver and brain. Histological classification is generally along the same lines as for nodal disease. As a general rule, in the staging of extranodal lymphoma the patient is not automatically classified as having stage four disease, but rather the primary site is regarded as if it were localized nodal disease and treated as such. Extranodal lymphoma is one of the few hematological malignancies in which surgery may have a primary and definitive role to play.

Summary of Individual Non-Hodgkins Lymphomas

Small Lymphocytic Consistent with CLL (WF Code A, Low Grade, 4% of NHL)

Lymph node histology in this NHL is identical to CLL, males are more frequently affected than females (2.5:1), generalized lymphadenopathy and hepatosplenomegaly are common, the bone marrow is nearly always involved, and 43% of cases are associated with CLL. Some patients may have a significant plasmacytoid component and occasionally a circulating IgM monoclonal protein. This is the histological pattern found in Waldenstrom's macroglobulinemia. The majority are stage IV disease at presentation although 10% may present as I or II or the splenomegalic form of CLL. The median survival is 6 to 8 years for stages I and II and 4 to 6 years for stages III and IV.

Follicular Small Cleaved Cell Lymphoma (WF Code B, Low Grade, 20% of NHL)

This lymphoma, historically known as Brill-Symmers' disease, usually occurs in elderly patients, has an equal sex distribution and is derived from the lymph node follicular center cell (B-lymphocyte), with abnormal clefted lymphoid cells found in the peripheral blood and bone marrow in over 50% of patients. The disease has a median survival of 5 to 7 years with therapy having little effect on long-term outcome. Initial therapy is for symptom relief using low-dose chemother-

apy, or radiotherapy. Spontaneous regression occasionally occurs, but in general the disease undergoes an aggressive large cell, diffuse transformation, commonly in the abdominal nodes.

Follicular Mixed Small Cleaved Cell and Large Cell Lymphoma (WF Code C, Low Grade, 8% of NHL)

This is a similar disease to follicular small cleaved cell lymphoma, but may have a more aggressive course.

Follicular Large Cell Lymphoma (WF Code D, Intermediate Grade, 4% of NHL)

This lymphoma presents as stage III or IV disease in 75% of patients, bone marrow, spleen and liver involvement occurs in approximately 25% of patients. Localized disease is potentially curable, overall median survival is 3 to 6 years.

Diffuse Small Cleaved Cell Lymphoma (WF Code E, Intermediate Grade, 10% of NHL)

This also is a B-lymphocyte disorder probably originating from the follicular center cell disease occurring in the elderly and may transform to more aggressive disease. There is generalized lymphadenopathy and bone marrow involvement is common with progression to major parenchymal involvement. Presentation is as stage III or IV disease in 75% of cases with median survival of 3 to 4 years. Some patients with stage I or II disease may be cured.

Diffuse Mixed Small and Large Cell Lymphoma (WF Code F, Intermediate Grade, 7% of NHL)

Similar to diffuse small cell lymphoma except it is more likely to present as local disease, but may follow a more aggressive course. In this category may also be included some of the T-cell lymphomas having a mixed cellular composition, including Lennert's lymphoma which has a high percentage of epithelioid histiocytes.

Diffuse Large Cell Lymphoma (WF Code G, Intermediate (?High) Grade, 20% of NHL)

This is probably a disorder of B-follicular center cell origin having heterogeneous morphology with cleaved, noncleaved or pleo-morphic cells. It affects all age groups and commonly presents with stage I or II disease (50%). Initially it may respond well to multi-ple agent therapy and does have the potential for cure, but relapse and aggressive clinical course is more common. Prognosis has im-proved considerably in recent years and the disease may be curable in the majority of pa-tients with stage I and II disease and in up to 50% of patients with III or IV disease.

Immunoblastic Lymphoma (WF Code H, High Grade, 8% of NHL)

This type of lymphoma may be of B or T lymphocyte types. The morphology can be variable, but there is not a good correlation with the B or T cell origin of the malignancy and morphology. Some may show marked plasmacytoid features with pyrinophilia whereas others show clear cell or polymor-phous variants. Presentation is with stage I or II disease in 50% of patients, and extranodal presentations of disease are not uncommon. Localized and stage IV disease may occasion-ally be curable, but in general the disease has a poor prognosis. Highly aggressive chemoth-erapeutic regimens are necessary for therapy.

Lymphoblastic Lymphoma (WF Code I, High Grade, 4% of NHL)

Previously known as Sternberg's sarcoma, this aggressive lymphoma typically occurs in children and teenagers, with a male predom-inance of 2.5:1. In the majority of cases the malignant cell is of T-lymphoid origin, al-though null-cell and pre-B cell types have been recognized. Typical morphological ap-pearances show a diffuse or pseudonodular pattern, monomorphous cell population of lymphoblasts, with convoluted nuclei (53%), inconspicuous nucleoli, high mitotic index and T-cell markers. Acid phosphatase is pos-itive (focal staining) as is TdT. A mediastinal mass is present in 60% of patients. Early bone marrow involvement with an acute lympho-blastic peripheral blood picture occurs early in the disease in the majority of patients. The disease normally follows a relentless course with a short survival, with only 15% living more than 2 years, but results are improving each year when more aggressive chemothera-peutic protocols are used. Central nervous system relapse is common.

Small Noncleaved Cell Lymphoma (WF Code J, High Grade, 5% of NHL)

This lymphoma commonly occurs in chil-dren in tropical Africa (Burkitt's type) but may be sporadic in other areas. The geo-graphic distribution is related to climate and the disease is etiologically related to EB virus. There is a male predominance, predilection for jaws, gonads, abdominal viscera and CNS, rarely associated with leukemia and involve-ment of peripheral lymph nodes and spleen is uncommon. The disease has a short survival without treatment, but a good response to chemotherapy. Characteristic histological findings include a starry-sky pattern, histio-cytes with engulfed nuclear debris, uniform, undifferentiated lymphoid cells, small with round and noncleaved nuclei. The non-Burk-itt's form of this disease occurs in adults with gastrointestinal presentation being common.

Cutaneous T-cell Lymphomas (Including Mycosis Fungoides (MF) and Sézary's Syndrome (SCS))

Sézary cell syndrome is essentially the leu-kemic form of mycosis fungoides in which the malignant cell is a helper T-lymphocyte. In both variants there is relative sparing of the bone marrow. The circulating cells have characteristic morphological features with grooved and folded nuclei with a small amount of cytoplasm. MF and SCS are typi-cally indolent diseases of the elderly and cu-taneous involvement is the clinical hallmark, with local lesions in MF or generalized ery-throderma in late disease or in SCS. Periph-eral blood and skin biopsy are the sources of material for diagnosis. Lymph node involve-ment is found in 75% and visceral in 60%. In mycosis fungoides local therapy to the lesions using nitrogen mustard, corticosteroids, psor-alen or electron beam is usually adequate, but visceral disease may require systemic che-motherapy. Systemic chemotherapy or leu-kapheresis is usually necessary for Sézary cell syndrome.

Angioimmunoblastic Lymphadenopathy with Dysproteinemia (AILD)

This condition bridges the gap between a reactive lymphoid disorder and true malig-nancy. It is commonly associated with dys-proteinemia and a positive Coomb's test. The disease typically occurs in the elderly and a past history of allergy (especially drugs) is common. The histological features include effacement of the lymph node with a pleomorphic infiltrate of immunoblasts and plasma cells. Proliferating and arborizing small blood vessels are typical and there may be deposits of amorphous interstitial material. Although the disease may evolve into a more classical immunoblastic sarcoma death from the systemic effects of the disorder and opportunistic infection is more common. There may be an initial response to corticosteroids, but this is rarely sustained.

Malignancies of the Monocyte-Macrophage System

Now that it is possible to definitively identify the origin of hematological malignancies the tumors of the monocyte-macrophage system have been better categorized. Most of the "histiocyte" lymphomas under the Rappaport system turned out to be lymphoid in origin (usually follicular center cell) and fewer than 5% are true histiocytic malignancies.

True Histiocytic Lymphoma (High Grade, 3% to 5% of non-Hodgkin's Lymphomas)

Clinically it is usually difficult to delineate this disease from diffuse large cell lymphomas (WF code G) without the use of specific cell identification techniques. Fever is common with disease activity and histiocytic leukemia may manifest in the terminal stage of the disease.

Malignant Histiocytosis (Histiocytic Medullary Reticulosis)

This condition is one of the most fulminant and dramatic of the hematological malignancies. It has an abrupt onset with systemic symptoms of fever, weight loss, weakness, generalized lymphadenopathy, hepatosplenomegaly, jaundice, pulmonary and pericardial involvement. Lymph node and bone marrow histology is characteristic, but must be differentiated from the recently recognized reactive viral-associated hemophagocytic syndrome (VAHS). In the lymph node the sinuses are predominantly involved with atypical malignant histiocytes, nuclear pleomorphism, multinucleated giant cells and erythrophagocytosis. The bone marrow may reveal marked hemophagocytosis accounting for the pancytopenia and hemolytic anemia. Prognosis is poor and patients rarely survive more than 6 months.

MONOCLONAL IMMUNOGLOBULIN DISORDERS

The term immunoproliferative disease is sometimes used to encompass disorders in which there is an abnormal proliferation of plasma cells with or without monoclonal immunoglobulin production (also called paraproteinemia). However, with a greater understanding of the malignancies of the immune system the term immunoproliferative now has wider connotations and tends to include all malignancies arising from the lymphoid system.

Multiple Myeloma

Pathophysiology

Multiple myeloma is the commonest of the plasma cell dyscrasias. It is characterized by a malignant proliferation of plasma cells in the bone marrow, monoclonal immunoglobulin production and humoral immune paresis (Fig. 9.8). The plasma cells produce bone destruction by direct infiltration and the production of an osteoclast stimulating factor. Bone marrow failure occurs as the disease progresses. Many of the clinical features are secondary to production of a monoclonal immunoglobulin.

Clinical Features

Multiple myeloma may present in the following ways:

- Symptoms of anemia
- Infection: especially pneumonia
- Direct effects of infiltration by malignant plasma cells: bone pain, lytic bone lesion, pathological fractures, spinal cord compression and other compressive effects of a plasmacytoma
- Laboratory abnormalities
- Hyperviscosity syndrome

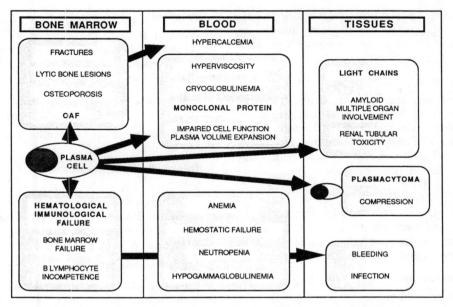

Figure 9.8. The pathophysiology of multiple myeloma—OAF = osteoclast activating factor

- Hemostatic failure
- Uremia
- Peripheral neuropathy
- Amyloid.

Laboratory Features

Hematology

Abnormalities include: Anemia, neutropenia, thrombocytopenia, elevated ESR, coagulation or platelet function defects, rouleaux and background staining on the blood film, abnormal macroscopic appearance of the blood, especially in the blood bank with poor clot formation, gel or cryoprecipitate formation, or the plasma can be difficult to separate on centrifugation. Bone marrow shows plasmacytosis (>15%) with atypical, primitive and multinucleated forms present.

Biochemistry

Abnormalities include: Hypercalcemia, hyperuricemia, hyperglobulinemia, hypoalbuminemia, artifactual anion gap, uremia, and proteinuria. The blood sample may be "difficult" to handle in the laboratory due to "rejection" by autoanalyzers.

Immunology

There is a monoclonal band on serum protein electrophoresis (SPE) in 75% of patients,

IgG in 50%, IgA in 25%. Some 20% of patients secrete only immunoglobulin light chains (Bence-Jones protein) which is filtered in the urine, and only accumulates in the serum in the presence of renal failure. Rare cases of myeloma are nonsecretory, IgD, IgM or IgE. Urine electrophoresis reveals light chains in over 50% of patients. The monoclonal nature of the immunoglobulin is confirmed by immunoelectrophoresis. Normal immunoglobulins are suppressed.

Radiological Features

Abnormalities include: Lytic bone lesions, osteoporosis, pathological fractures, vertebral crush fractures.

Therapy

Chemotherapy

An alkylating agent plus prednisolone is most commonly used. Melphalan (8mg/m^2) and prednisolone (100mg/m^2) for four days each 4 to 6 weeks is the commonest drug therapy, but cyclophosphamide is equally effective. A response with reduction in the monoclonal immunoglobulin and bone marrow infiltrate is achieved in the majority of patients (>70%). The disease may be controlled for several years. There is a wide range of second-line drug combinations, but in general relapsed, drug-resistant disease has a poor out-look. Response to therapy can usually be monitored by following the monoclonal protein level in the blood.

Radiotherapy

This is used where there is identifiable local disease which is causing symptoms or in which there is a high risk of fracture. Myeloma is a radioresponsive disease but widespread use results in considerable bone marrow depression.

General Supportive Measures

Myeloma can be a painful and crippling disease, and there are few hematological malignancies which present the hematologist with such a challenge in palliative care.

Complications

Fractures may present the orthopedic surgeon with difficult fixation problems. The patient should be kept as immobile as possible.

Infections are common, usually bacterial in nature (especially pneumococcal), and require early antibiotic therapy. Immune globulin is indicated in acute infections, but has little role in prophylaxis due to its high catabolic rate.

Hypercalcemia usually responds to rehydration, corticosteroids and chemotherapy.

Renal failure at the time of presentation has generally been regarded as indicating a poor prognosis. Hypercalcemia, hyperuricemia, dehydration, contrast media, antibiotics, sepsis, nephrotoxic drugs, amyloid, hyperviscosity and plasma cell infiltration may be important in some cases, but tubular dysfunction secondary to paraprotein nephrotoxicity is the most important factor. Immunoglobulin light chains which are freely filtered by the glomerulus are toxic to renal tubules. With forced alkaline diuresis, and plasma exchange in some patients, it may be possible to improve renal function, and renal failure per se is less of a prognostic indicator than it has been regarded in the past.

Spinal cord compression is an emergency in myeloma and may require urgent surgical intervention, followed by radiotherapy.

Hyperviscosity syndrome is discussed in chapter 4.

Transformation to plasma cell leukemia or the development of acute leukemia may occasionally occur.

Prognosis

Without therapy the median survival of patients with myeloma is 12 months. With present therapy this has been extended to a median survival of 30 to 36 months.

Uncommon Variants of Myeloma

There are several uncommon pictures in the clinical spectrum of myeloma including the following:

Indolent Multiple Myeloma

The patient has a clear diagnosis of myeloma, but may only be progressing slowly and not require immediate therapy. Some evidence would suggest that these patients are presenting in plateau phase of the disease.

Solitary Plasmacytoma

This is an isolated plasma cell tumor which may occur as a solitary lesion of bone or extramedullary tissue. It usually has a good prognosis and may be cured with excision and radiotherapy.

Nonsecretory Myeloma

Plasma Cell Leukemia.

This is a highly aggressive disease with plasmablasts circulating in the peripheral blood. High protein levels are usually associated with marked extramedullary tumor.

Amyloid

In some patients amyloid is responsible for the clinical features of disease and determining prognosis.

Macroglobulinemia (Waldenstrom's Macroglobulinemia (WM))

In this immunoproliferative disease there is a circulating monoclonal macroglobulin (IgM) produced by B-lymphoid cells with partial plasma cell differentiation. In classical Waldenstrom's macroglobulinemia the circulating IgM level may be sufficient to cause the hyperviscosity syndrome and impairment of hemostasis. Lymphadenopathy and hepatosplenomegaly are usually present. Blood examination usually reveals anemia with variable degrees of leukopenia and thrombocytopenia. ESR is >100mm/h, marked rouleaux and background protein staining are present on the blood film. Plasma viscosity is elevated, but the degree of whole blood hy-

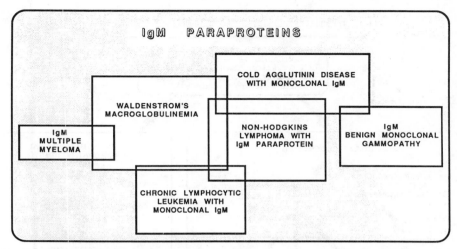

Figure 9.9. The interrelationships between lymphoproliferative disorders which have an IgM monoclonal protein

perviscosity depends on the hemoglobin level. A dense IgM monoclonal protein is present on serum SPE. The morphological appearances in the bone marrow and lymphoid tissue reveal an infiltrate of lymphoid cells ranging from mature lymphocytes through plasmacytoid cells and occasional mature plasma cells. Initial therapy is directed towards reducing the IgM level which may require plasma exchange. Adequate hydration and the avoidance of blood transfusion is important if blood viscosity is high. Long-term therapy with an alkylating agent (cyclophosphamide or chlorambucil) is usually effective in reducing the lymphoid mass and thus the IgM level. Macroglobulinemia has a better prognosis than myeloma with a median survival of 4 to 5 years.

Other Conditions in Which a Macroglobulin May Be Present

The condition described above is classical Waldenstrom's macroglobulinemia. An IgM monoclonal protein may also be found in other lymphoproliferative diseases (Fig. 9.9) including: lymphocytic lymphomas, chronic lymphocytic leukemia, splenic lymphoma, rare cases of myeloma and cold agglutinin syndromes. The IgM level is usually lower and hyperviscosity is not a feature.

Amyloidosis

The term amyloidosis includes a broad group of disorders in which there is a homogeneous tissue infiltrate of eosinophilic material. It can be identified on a congo red stain

by its birefringence under polarized light and by characteristic features on electron microscopy. The classification of amyloidosis is best considered under the following headings:

Primary Amyloid and Amyloid Associated with Plasma Cell Dyscrasias

Primary amyloid has been shown to be derived from immunoglobulin light chain deposition in the tissues (known as amyloid AL). The same type of amyloid may be seen in association with some cases of multiple myeloma. Clinical features may include: peripheral neuropathy, mononeuritis, macroglossia, GIT involvement with malabsorption, cardiac involvement, cutaneous lesions, acquired factor X deficiency and joint involvement. The disease has a poor prognosis but some patients may respond to myeloma-type therapy.

Secondary Reactive Amyloid

Amyloid is seen in association with long-standing chronic inflammatory, infectious and malignant disease. Renal involvement with nephrotic syndrome is common. Hepatosplenomegaly may be present.

Senile Amyloid

This is usually asymptomatic and found at autopsy.

Familial Amyloid

This may be found in hereditary Mediterranean fever or familial peripheral neuropathy.

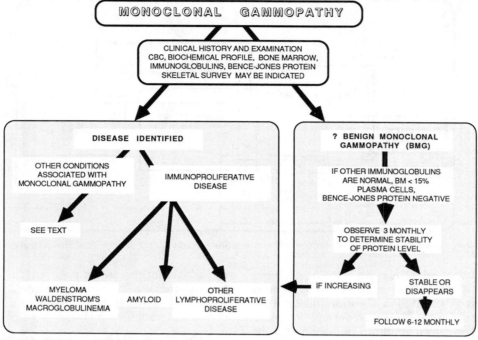

Figure 9.10. Investigation of monoclonal gammopathy

Other Immunoglobulin Disorders

For completeness there are several other conditions in which polyclonal or monoclonal immunoglobulins may be present which warrant passing mention.

Cryoglobulinemia

There are several abnormal plasma proteins which may precipitate with or without fixing complement, resulting in microvascular obstruction and end-organ damage. Cutaneous, digital, renal and cerebral are the microvascular beds usually effected. The cryoglobulin may be a monoclonal or polyclonal immunoglobulin or a combination of both. Treatment should be directed at the underlying disease. Removal of the cryoglobulin with plasma exchange may be indicated.

Benign Monoclonal Gammopathy (BMG)

This is the term used when a monoclonal immunoglobulin is present in the peripheral blood in a concentration of less than 2g/L, normal levels of other immunoglobulins, absence of Bence-Jones protein in the urine, bone marrow plasma cells <20% without significant atypia of the cells and no evidence of an underlying immunoproliferative disease.

BMG increases in incidence with age, reaching levels of 8% in people over the age of 70 years. Figure 9.10 outlines an approach to the finding of an isolated monoclonal gammopathy. It is important that patients with BMG be followed as evolution to myeloma may occur.

Benign Hyperglobulinemia Purpura

This is classically seen in women who present with gravity-dependent purpura in the lower limbs which may be precipitated by exercise and alcohol (explaining the term Saturday night purpura). Some patients have an underlying autoimmune disease such as SLE or Sjögren's syndrome.

Heavy Chain Diseases

A rare group of disorders in which there is a serum monoclonal globulin consisting of one of the heavy chains of an immunoglobulin molecule (M, G, or A). Alpha chain disease is the commonest heavy chain disease. It occurs in Mediterranean countries and presents with malabsorption.

Light Chain Nephropathy

This presents with glomerulonephritis or proximal renal tubular acidosis (Fanconi's syndrome) due to nephrotoxicity of light chains. Follow-up of this disease may reveal an underlying myeloma.

Monoclonal Immunoglobulins in Association with Benign Disorders

These may be found in association with the following disorders:

- Infectious disease
- Liver disease
- Some drug reactions
- Autoimmune disorders (e.g., SLE, pernicious anemia)
- Gaucher's disease.

MYELOPROLIFERATIVE DISEASE

General Concepts

The myeloproliferative disorders are characterized by a panmyelosis with excessive production of erythroid, myeloid or megakaryocytic cell lines, although one cell line is predominantly affected. There may also be excessive proliferation of fibroblasts and reticulum in the bone marrow resulting in myelofibrosis. Some of the myeloproliferative disorders are frankly malignant, such as acute and chronic granulocytic leukemia. In conditions such as polycythemia rubra vera, myeloid metaplasia and essential thrombocythemia, there appears to be an autonomous proliferation of one or more cell lines. For whatever reason, normal growth regulation appears to be lost. In some cases autonomous

productions of growth factors such as interleukin 3 may be responsible. As a general rule, the morphological development of the cells may be dysplastic and the end cells may manifest varying degrees of qualitative abnormality.

Figure 9.11 outlines the relationship between the various myeloproliferative disorders. The natural history of many of the myeloproliferative disorders is to evolve into a more frankly leukemic disorder or to enter a "burnt out" phase with progressive marrow fibrosis. The autonomous myeloproliferation is not only confined to the marrow, but may also occur in sites where hemopoietic development occurred during fetal life, such as the liver and spleen. This occurrence is referred to as myeloid metaplasia or when it occurs as a primary disorder and is not classifiable as one of the disorders mentioned above the term agnogenic myeloid metaplasia is used. There are several common features that may be found in all the myeloproliferative disorders.

Peripheral Blood

Abnormalities are always present in the peripheral blood count and film. Except for myelofibrosis and agnogenic myeloid metaplasia each myeloproliferative disorder has a characteristic excess of one or more of the blood cell lines. As a result of dysplasia, characteristic red cell changes with teardrop poikilocytes, nucleated red cells and the leukoerythroblastic blood film may typically be seen

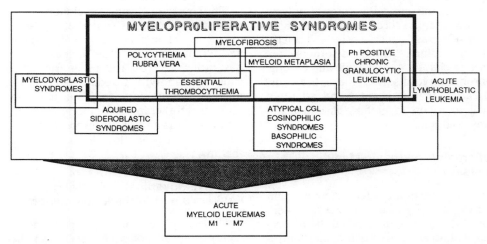

Figure 9.11. The myeloproliferative spectrum. CGL = Chronic granulocytic leukemia; Ph = Philadelphia chromosome

in myelofibrosis. Such changes are suggestive of bone marrow fibrosis.

Fibroblastic Proliferation

The myeloproliferative disorders show an excess proliferation of fibroblastic tissue in the bone marrow and sometimes the other hemopoietic organs. There has been much debate as to whether this is a primary or secondary event, but recent evidence would suggest that platelet-derived growth factors are being released by hematogenous cells and fibrosis is secondary.

Biochemical Abnormalities

Various biochemical abnormalities including hyperuricemia, elevated LDH, elevated B12 binding proteins, and neutrophil alkaline phosphatase.

Hepatosplenomegaly

Except for the finding of the Philadelphia chromosome in chronic granulocytic leukemia, there are no specific markers for any of the myeloproliferative disorders. The diagnosis is usually made from a combination of features outlined above. These findings are usually interpreted after excluding all disorders which are likely to produce reactive hematological changes. It can also be difficult on occasions to classify patients within the myeloproliferative spectrum. Some patients clearly fulfill the criteria for one of the myeloproliferative disorders, but others tend to "fence sit" with features of two or more of the myeloproliferative syndromes.

As many of the clinical features of polycythemia and essential thrombocythemia manifest themselves as hyperviscosity and microcirculatory failure, these disorders are discussed in chapter 4. The acute and chronic myeloproliferative disorders have been discussed earlier in this chapter and attention now will focus on myelofibrosis and agnogenic myeloid metaplasia.

Myelofibrosis/Agnogenic Myeloid Metaplasia

In this disorder of the elderly there is a generalized overactivity of the *hemopoietic* stem cells, but the *hemopoiesis* tends to be ineffective. As well as ineffective hemopoiesis myeloid metaplasia is found in fetal sites of blood cell production, the liver and spleen. The onset is usually insidious with symptoms of anemia and hemostatic failure, or symptoms relating to splenomegaly or infarction. Splenomegaly is almost universal and occasionally of massive proportions. Hepatomegaly is common, especially in advanced disease. As the disease progresses pancytopenia may worsen. This is due to a combination of ineffective hemopoiesis, marrow fibrosis and hypersplenism. In 10% of patients the disease transforms into acute myeloblastic leukemia, and in the majority, death results from narrow failure.

The peripheral blood changes are variable, ranging from various cytophilias to pancytopenia with a leukoerythroblastic blood film usually present; associated folate deficiency may occur. The red cells may demonstrate bizarre morphological alterations with marked anisocytosis, teardrop poikilocytes and irregularly shaped cells. Attempts at bone marrow aspiration are usually unsuccessful ("dry tap"). A trephine biopsy is essential for diagnosis, confirming the presence of increased reticulin and fibrosis. The extent of hemopoietic activity in the marrow is variable, megakaryocytes usually being prominent. There is an acute variant of myelofibrosis which presents with pancytopenia, minimal morphological red cell changes and slight or no splenomegaly and has a fatal outcome within 6 months. This disorder commonly terminates in acute myeloblastic leukemia and in many patients is probably a variant of leukemia from the outset.

The course of chronic myelofibrosis is variable with a median survival of 3 years from diagnosis. Therapy is essentially supportive and symptomatic in nature as specific therapy has little effect on the prognosis. Therapy should be individualized. In some patients massive symptomatic splenomegaly may require chemotherapy, radiotherapy or splenectomy. Anemia and/or thrombocytopenia may be an indication for blood component therapy.

The Myelodysplastic, Evolving Leukemia and Preleukemic Syndromes

Under this heading is grouped a heterogeneous group of potentially malignant hematological disorders which may be the harbin-

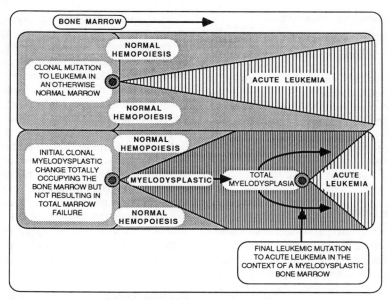

Figure 9.12. The myelodysplastic syndrome and the evolution of leukemia

gers of more classical leukemic states or may behave as slowly evolving marrow failure syndromes (Fig. 9.12). They usually occur in the elderly, have an insidious onset and may manifest in a wide variety of ways. Drugs (especially chlorambucil), ionizing radiation and chemicals have been incriminated in some patients. Late diagnosis and confusion with more common hematological disorders is common. Diagnosis that a particular patient falls within this spectrum of disorders is relatively simple, if a person skilled in hematological diagnosis is consulted. The main difficulties arise when it comes to detailed classification of the disorders. Included within this spectrum of disorders are the following:

- Refractory anemia with excess bone marrow blast cells
- Primary myelodysplasia of the bone marrow
- Acquired sideroblastosis with dysplastic bone marrow
- Aplastic or hypoplastic bone marrow with dysplastic features
- Evolving or smouldering leukemia.

Various peripheral blood findings may be associated with these syndromes: pancytopenia, refractory anemia, unresponsive macrocytic anemia, neutropenia, thrombocytopenia, qualitative granulocyte or platelet defects. Diagnosis is usually made from the combination of the peripheral blood and bone marrow findings. In the majority of patients no specific therapy is warranted and unnecessarily "meddlesome therapy" should be studiously avoided. Regular blood transfusion is indicated in some patients. These patients are in a delicate balance with their environment and while they remain free of infection and bleeding may remain well for long periods of time. However, their host defense reserves are virtually nonexistent and they are unable to mount an appropriate response in time of stress and early attention should be given to infections or hemostatic failure. With patients in whom leukemia becomes progressively manifest, corticosteroids and/or low dose chemotherapy may have a part to play, but it tends to be palliative in most patients and only rarely does the patient show significant hematological improvement.

Hypereosinophilic Syndromes

The finding of blood and/or tissue eosinophilia is a common hematological finding and the causes are listed in chapter 11. However there are some gross reactive eosinophilic syndromes and primary eosinophilias which warrant separate consideration.

Reactive Eosinophilic Syndromes

These may occur in a spectrum of diseases and are initiated by an exogenous infectious agent or antigen, which may or may not be identifiable. Tropical eosinophilia is caused by a filarial organism. Loeffler's syndrome is a transient pulmonary eosinophilia syndrome of unknown cause and there is a potentially fatal multisystem syndrome with asthma, pulmonary infiltrates, central nervous system involvement, peripheral neuropathy and polyarteritis nodosa in which the cause is also unknown.

The Primary Eosinophilic Syndromes

An ill-defined group of disorders, some cases are clearly of a malignant nature, eosinophilic leukemia and Philadelphia chromosome positive cases being clearly recognized. In other cases the gross eosinophilia ($>100 \times 10^9$/L) is associated with a multisystem tissue eosinophilia involving liver, spleen, nervous system, lung and heart with systemic features of fever, weight loss, anemia and thrombosis. Fibrosis may complicate the tissue eosinophilia and patients commonly die from cardiac failure.

Basophilia and Mastocytosis

The reactive causes of basophilia are listed in chapter 11. A primary basophilia may be seen in the myeloproliferative diseases, including chronic granulocytic leukemia, myelofibrosis and polycythemia rubra vera. Basophilic leukemia is a rare entity. There are several rare mast cell malignancies which may present as a localized mastocytoma and urticaria pigmentosa is usually a self-limiting cutaneous syndrome seen in children. Systemic mastocytosis is a disease of the elderly in which bone marrow, liver, spleen, skin and lymph nodes bcome infiltrated and may develop fibrosis. The disorder commonly has a malignant progression with short survival (less than 2 years in many patients). Mast cell leukemia may occur *de novo* or as the progression of other mast cell neoplasias. Many of the distressing clinical features of pruritus, flushing and anaphylactoid reactions are due to the biogenic amine released from the tumor cells. H1 and H2 receptor antagonists may help. Chemotherapeutic attacks on the malignant cells give disappointing results.

Further Reading

Gunz, FW and Henderson, ES *Leukaemia.* 4th ed. New York: Grune and Stratton, 1983.

International Workshop on CLL: Chronic lymphocytic leukaemia: Proposals for a revised prognostic staging system. Br. J. Haematol. 48:365, 1981.

Jaffe, ES *Surgical pathology of the lymph nodes and related organs.* Major problems in pathology Vol. 16. Philadelphia: WB Saunders and Company, 1985.

Kaplan, HS *Hodgkin's disease.* 2nd ed. Massachusettes: Harvard University Press, 1980.

Polliack, A *Human leukaemias: cytochemical and ultrastructural features in diagnosis and research.* Boston: Martinus Nijoff Publishers, 1984.

Schiffer, CA. ed. *Clinics in oncology: transfusion support therapy.* Nov. 1983. Vol. 2 No. 3. Philadelphia: WB Saunders Company Ltd.

Wiernik, PH, Cannellos, GC, Kyle, RA and Schiffer, CA. eds. *Neoplastic diseases of the blood.* Vols 1 and 2, New York: Churchill Livingstone, 1985.

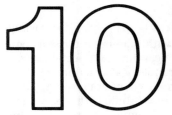

Hematological Aspects of Infection and Systemic Disease

I don't know what I am looking for. That's what makes the search so exciting

Ashleigh Britliant (1933–   )

In Chapter 1 a summary of the body's defense systems is presented and the problems of failure are addressed in chapters 5, 6 and 7. In this chapter the hematological responses to various infectious, traumatic, toxic and undefined insults will be presented. The body has a limited number of ways to respond to exogenous stimuli and there tends to be a final common pathway of response, depending on the nature of the insult. This host defense response may be a major factor in determining the prognosis for the patient. Underactivity or overactivity of the system may be responsible for disease, in the first instance from the disease gaining a hold in the body, in the second from pathological effects on the host from excessive or inappropriate defense system activation. This "Yin and Yang" of host defense functions is an important concept as appropriate modulation, with or without therapeutic intervention, may be crucial to the patient's survival. In this context the role of the circulatory system, especially the microcirculation, is paramount and any threat to its integrity may jeopardize the whole response to disease. Although the bone marrow and liver can tolerate substantial degrees of hypoxia, function will ultimately be impaired if adequate oxygenation is not maintained. The host defense system mediates most of its actions at a microcirculatory level where the interface between the delivery of host defense factors and the site of tissue damage or invasion exists.

From the host defense response it may be possible to predict the nature of the insult and thus establish a specific diagnosis of underlying disease or at least to speculate as to its basic nature. In some of the conditions to be discussed, the history and clinical findings may point to a specific diagnosis in which circumstance the appropriate laboratory investigations will serve to confirm the provisional diagnosis. However, in many other conditions the clinical presentation may be nonspecific leaving the clinician with a long list of possible diagnoses. In such circumstances it may not be possible to consider all potential disease states, and there is a temptation to approach laboratory investigation in a "poker machine pathology" fashion. To avoid such a scenario selective requesting of basic hematological, biochemical, immunological and microbiological investigations, followed by careful and informed interpretation, can provide important clues to assist the clinician in further clinical assessment and specific laboratory and organ imaging investigations.

A complete hematological blood examination (usually referred to as a CBC), including red cell indices, leukocyte count and differential, platelet count, film examination and erythrocyte sedimentation rate, in conjunction with a biochemical profile (12 or 20 analytes) will usually provide sufficient clues as to the presence or absence of organic systemic disease in a patient with the recent onset of nonspecific symptoms and/or signs. A completely normal result on a complete blood examination and biochemical profile makes the presence of infections or inflammatory disease unlikely. By the same token, the presence of occult malignant disease which is responsible for systemic symptoms will nearly always produce reactive hematological changes.

Nonspecific Hematological Reactions to Systemic Disease

THE ACUTE AND CHRONIC PHASE REACTIONS

The well-orchestrated reaction of the hemopoietic and hepatic systems, involving numerous plasma proteins and all the cellular components of the blood, is referred to as the acute phase reaction or chronic phase if the stimulus persists (Fig. 10.1, Table 10.1). The reaction occurs within hours or days of acute physical or chemical trauma, infection, tissue infarction, immunological reactions or pregnancy. If the stimulus does not resolve, the reaction may become chronic with a polyclonal hypergammaglobulinemia. In the reaction, certain cells and plasma proteins are seen to rise and others to fall. The functions of many of these acute phase proteins remain unclear, but presumably they subserve beneficial ef-

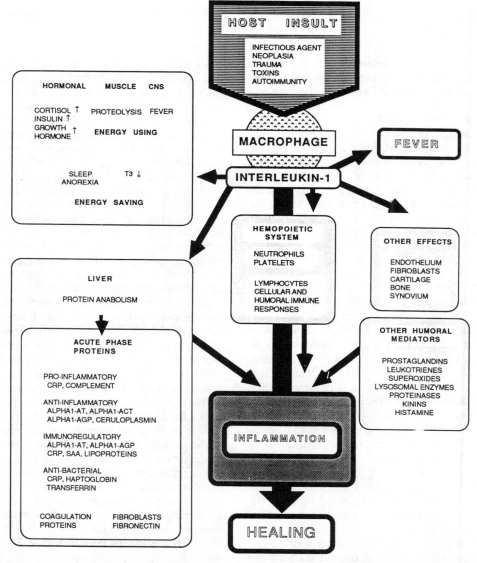

Figure 10.1. The acute phase response—CRP = C reactive protein; SAA = Serum amyloid A Alpha1—antitrypsin; Alpha1—antichymotrypsin; Alpha1—acid glycoprotein.

Table 10.1
The Acute Phase Reaction

Cells rise
Neutrophils
Platelets
fall
Hemoglobin
Lymphocytes

Plasma proteins rise
Fibrinogen and factor VIII
Complement, haptoglobins
C-reactive protein, alpha-2 macroglobulin
Alpha-1 chymotrypsin, orosomucoid
Alpha-1 antitrypsin, ceruloplasmin
Plasminogen
Plasma proteins
fall
Albumin, serum iron and TIBC
Alpha and beta lipoproteins

fects for the patient and should not be "tampered" with unless there is good reason. The fall in hemoglobin, serum iron and albumin are all typical of the acute phase reaction and there are compelling reasons why nature meant this to occur. Most of the proteins that are altered are inflammatory mediators, inhibitors or transport proteins.

Fibrinogen is one of the plasma proteins to show the greatest rise in the acute phase reaction and is responsible for the elevation in the erythrocyte sedimentation rate. The reason for the rise in haptoglobins remains unclear, but they may be important in having a bacteriostatic action by binding hemoglobin in the tissues which would normally be an ideal culture medium for bacteria. The complement proteins are important mediators in the inflammatory response. When such a potent system as the acute phase response is activated the result has the potential to be a two-edged sword. Fluidity of the blood may be threatened and a well-tuned parallel response in the control proteins is necessary to avoid overactivity. The fall in albumin is due to both a redistribution and decreased synthesis. It is a normal response, possibly to compensate for the rise in other plasma proteins. No attempt should be made to "correct" hypoalbuminemia unless a specific adverse clinical feature can be established which is directly attributable to the low oncotic pressure.

From the clinical point of view the essential features of the reaction include some or all of the following:

- The anemia of chronic disease—a mild normocytic normochromic anemia (discussed in Chapter 3).
- Elevation of the ESR due to hyperfibrinogenemia (or polyclonal hypergammaglobulinemia in chronic antigenic stimulation).
- Neutrophilia.
- Lymphopenia.
- Thrombocytosis.
- Biochemical changes—mild hypoalbuminemia and hyponatremia, low serum iron, elevated globulins, C reactive protein.
Protein electrophoresis—elevated alpha-2 and beta globulins, polyclonal hypergammaglobulinemia in persisting antigenic stimulation.

If any or all of these changes are found, a diligent search for infectious, inflammatory or malignant disease should be instigated (Fig. 10.2). This will involve reassessment of the history and physical examination and consideration of the conditions listed in Table 10.2. In many of these diseases fever may be a feature and the list of disorders to consider in a patient with pyrexia of unknown origin will be similar.

REACTION TO VIRAL INFECTIONS

A patient suffering from systemic viral illness will not normally have the acute phase response as outlined above, unless secondary infection has supervened. The ESR is usually normal, neutropenia is commonly present and sometimes mild thrombocytopenia. The lymphocyte count is usually normal, but variable numbers are activated and seen in the peripheral blood as atypical mononuclear cells. Unless hepatitis is an accompaniment of the infection the biochemical profile is usually normal.

REACTION TO PARASITIC INFECTIONS

Patients with parasitic infections are likely to show features of the acute or chronic phase response outlined above, but a prominent feature is likely to be an eosinophilia. If malaria is a possibility a careful examination of the red cells for the presence of parasites is essential.

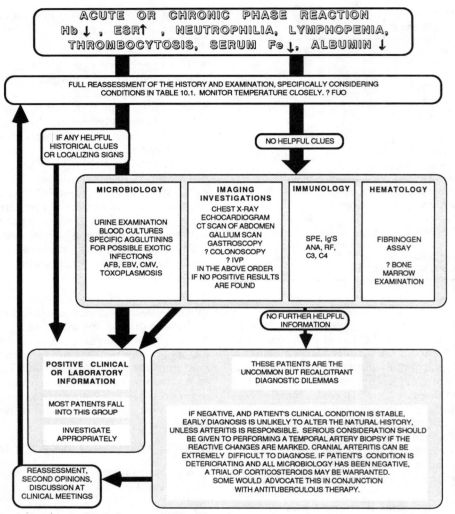

Figure 10.2. Approach to patients with evidence of the acute or chronic phase reaction with or without fever—FUO = fever of unknown origin; EPG = electropheretogram; ANA = antinuclear antibody; AFB = acid fast bacilli; EBV = Epstein-Barr virus; IVP = intravenous pyelogram; CMV = cytomegalovirus; RF = rheumatic fever; SPE = serum protein electrophoresis.

Infections of Particular Hematological Significance

THE ATYPICAL MONONUCLEOSIS SYNDROMES

Any viral infection may induce varying degrees of mononucleosis in the peripheral blood. The atypical mononuclear cells were previously thought to be monocytes but it has been clearly established that the cells are activated T-lymphocytes. The cells are larger lymphocytes than normal with variable morphology of the individual cells. The cytoplasm is prominent and basophilic in appearance and tends to adhere to red cells by wrapping around in a "Dutch skirt" fashion. When the cells are scant in number their presence must be carefully sought by examination of the blood film. They will commonly be missed on a superficial screening of the film or on an automated leukocyte differential.

There are some viral infections which are classically associated with an atypical mono-

Table 10.2
Conditions to Be Considered in the Investigation of a Patient with Hematological Evidence of the Acute or Chronic Phase Reaction

Infections

Bacterial:
- Urinary tract infection
- Occult abscess—Perinephric
  - Hepatic
  - Subphrenic
  - Diverticulitis
  - Pelvic
- Bacterial endocarditis
- Tuberculosis
- Brucellosis
- Osteomyelitis
- Infected intravenous cannula

Protozoal:
- Amoebiasis
- Toxoplasmosis

Viral:
- Virus associated hemophagocytic syndrome

Inflammatory

Autoimmune disorders:
- SLE, arteritis, temporal arteritis
- Polymyalgia rheumatica
- Rheumatoid arthritis, seronegative arthritis
- Juvenile rheumatoid arthritis

Allergic:
- Extrinsic allergic alveolitis
- Drug reactions
- Serum sickness

Granulomatous disease:
- Sarcoidosis
- Granulomatous hepatitis
- Crohn's disease

Malignant

Hematological:
- Hodgkin's disease
- Non-Hodgkin's lymphoma (uncommon)
- Histiocytic malignancies

Solid tumors:
- Gastrointestinal (especially stomach and cecum)
- Pancreatic
- Hepatoma
- Hypernephroma
- Lung
- Gynecological

Miscellaneous
- Atrial myxoma
- Hereditary mediterranean fever
- Venous thromboembolism (especially with pulmonary infarction)

nucleosis such as infectious mononucleosis (glandular fever), cytomegalovirus infection (CMV), acute ARV (AIDS-related virus) infection, herpes zoster and infectious hepatitis. The diagnosis of these conditions is usually confirmed without difficulty; however, there are other clinical conditions which are clearly infectious in nature in which there may be a significant, and sometimes marked, peripheral blood atypical mononucleosis, but an etiological agent cannot be identified. The clinical picture in such patients may be indistinguishable from classical glandular fever, including the prolonged postviral lethargy syndrome and recurrent lymphadenopathy syndrome (see below).

The presence of atypical lymphocytes in the peripheral blood is common in children under the age of seven, particularly during the usual childhood infections. This is the time during which the immune system is being "educated" to protect against the common community infections. The presence of recurrent lymphadenopathy and peripheral blood atypical lymphocytosis in children should rarely be a matter of concern. However, the chronic recurrent glandular fever like syndrome is a constant problem for family physicians and a worry for parents.

INFECTIOUS MONONUCLEOSIS (IM, GLANDULAR FEVER) AND EBV INFECTIONS

Infectious mononucleosis is the clinical manifestation of Epstein-Barr virus (EBV) infection in teenagers and young adults. Infection during childhood results in an acute viral illness indistinguishable from other common childhood viral infections. In adults (>30 years) and the elderly, an atypical glandular fever or pseudolymphoma syndrome may occur and cause a diagnostic dilemma.

Epidemiology and Pathogenesis

The EBV is a lymphotrophic virus transmitted via saliva (thus the origin of the label, the "kissing disease") which specifically infects host epithelial cells and B-lymphocytes, initially of the oropharynx. The host response to this invasion will depend on the state of the immune system at the time. The infected B-lymphocytes may be contained or dissemination may occur and a generalized T-lymphocyte reaction is stimulated, manifested as atypical lymphocytosis in the peripheral blood. In low socioeconomic societies and in third world countries EBV is usually contracted before the age of 5 years and it is only in developed countries in the high socioeconomic classes that infection is delayed into the teenage and adult years, resulting in IM being a common clinical problem. The incubation period and factors that determine the clinical presentation remain unclear, and do not usually follow the classical sequence of other viral infections.

The clinical spectrum of EBV infection is continuing to increase and the identification of this virus as having oncogenic potential under certain circumstances has been of major research interest. The disorders in which the EBV has been implicated as either causal, a potentiator or an associated factor are:

Infectious mononucleosis
Subclinical infection in children
Chronic malaise and lethargy syndrome
Atypical lymphoid hyperplasia
Pseudolymphoma syndromes in adults
B cell lymphomas
Burkitt's lymphoma
Nasopharyngeal carcinoma
X-linked lymphoproliferative syndrome
Lymphoproliferative syndromes in immunodepressed subjects
? Birth defects
Virus associated hemophagocytic syndrome
Bone marrow aplasia
Various cytopenias—Red cell aplasia
              Neutropenia
              Thrombocytopenia
Hypogammaglobulinemia.

Of interest is the observation that proliferation of the EB virus is responsible for lymphocyte ability to enter continuous in vitro culture.

The Clinical Syndrome

IM is characterized by fever, pharyngitis, profound malaise, lymphadenopathy and splenomegaly. Anorexia, nausea, abdominal pain, headache, myalgia, ocular pain and cough are also frequent symptoms. Other physical signs which may be observed include bradycardia, periorbital edema, palatal enanthema, hepatomegaly, jaundice and skin rash (especially if exposed to ampicillin or amoxicillin).

Less common clinical manifestations and complications include hepatitis, splenic pain and spontaneous rupture, pharyngeal obstruction, pericarditis, myocarditis, pancreatitis, pulmonary infiltrates, glomerulonephritis, hemolytic anemia and arthritis. The neurological complications warrant special mention as a wide range of syndromes may occur including meningitis, encephalitis, transverse myelitis, Guillain-Barré syndrome, and various cranial and peripheral neuropathies. The etiology of many of these clinical syndromes is not related to actual viral replication, but

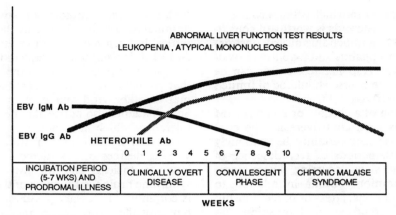

Figure 10.3. Clinicopathological course of infectious mononucleosis

rather the lymphoid or autoimmune reactions, explaining why corticosteroids are sometimes indicated in the management of the severe complications.

Laboratory Features

There are typical hematological and serological features in classical glandular fever which are diagnostic (see Fig. 10.3).

Hematological Features

During the first week of the illness the total leukocyte count is usually normal and it is not until the second week that the atypical mononucleosis appears. The total leukocyte count is usually between 15 and 25 $\times$ 10^9/L, most of the cells being the reactive T-lymphocytes. Mild neutropenia and thrombocytopenia are common. The degree and morphological variability of the lymphocytes helps to differentiate IM from other infections which may cause atypical mononucleosis.

Serological Features

A remarkable feature of IM is the humoral responses seen in which a wide range of antibodies are produced. The best known and most constant is the heterophile antibody (Paul-Bunnell-Davidson antibody) but others are commonly produced including anti-i cold agglutinins, anti-smooth muscle, antinuclear, antimitochondria and other autoantibodies, false positive WR and lymphocytotoxins. The Paul-Bunnell-Davidson antibody is an IgM heterophile antibody which reacts against a variety of animal cells. In most commercial

kits (e.g., monospot) horse cells are used following absorption with guinea pig kidney or bovine red cells. This latter step in the reaction adsorbs the Forssmann heterophile antibodies and makes the test reasonably specific for IM, although it should be emphasized that it is not a specific test for EBV infection. The test is usually negative in childhood EBV infections which do not have the classical IM clinical syndrome. Approximately 90% to 95% of IM patients have a positive test, the remainder are confirmed by specific EBV serology. The heterophile antibodies usually appear during the first or second week of the illness with the titer rising during the acute phase of the illness and falling during the convalescent phase and ultimately disappearing between 3 and 6 months. Reappearance is extremely rare.

Specific EB virus serology can also be performed with examination for IgM antibody responses to confirm the current nature of the infection. Antibody to various EB viral antigens have been demonstrated, but these are more of specialized interest to the virologist.

Clinical Course and Management

Classical IM is a self-limiting disease with most patients making a complete recovery within a few weeks, but the convalescent phase can be frustratingly prolonged in some patients. There is no known specific therapy for the disease, with rest and symptomatic therapy being the best approach, but occasionally intervention may be necessary when specific complications occur. There are several circumstances in which a short course of high-dose corticosteroids is worthy of consideration, including impending airway obstruction, severe encephalitis and inability to swallow or eat. The response to steroids can be dramatic, but the course should be of limited duration (7 to 10 days).

The question of a chronic or recurrent IM syndrome has been controversial. The convalescent phase can certainly be extremely prolonged with periods of recrudescence of symptoms and signs occurring. These recrudescences commonly occur in relation to physical or emotional stress or in relationship to another intercurrent viral infection. No specific therapy has ever been shown to hasten recovery and sympathetic symptomatic and psychological support are essential if secondary functional disorders are to be prevented.

OTHER ATYPICAL MONONUCLEOSIS SYNDROMES

CMV, Infectious Hepatitis, ARV and Toxoplasmosis

As mentioned above there are several identifiable infections which are associated with an atypical mononucleosis. Most of these are ubiquitous in most communities and, except for hepatitis, their diagnosis may be difficult unless rising titers or IgM antibodies are identified. CMV and toxoplasmosis are two conditions which may be difficult and occasionally impossible to diagnose as current or recent infection. It is easy to blame these organisms because antibodies are detectable in the peripheral blood. In the case of toxoplasmosis it can be tempting to treat the patient with antimicrobial therapy, but this is usually without effect and exposes the patient to potentially dangerous adverse effects.

Atypical Mononucleosis of Undetermined Etiology

It has been the author's experience that glandular fever-like atypical mononuclear syndromes are common in the community in which an infecting agent cannot be identified. The clinical presentation is usually one of a viral-like illness with lymphadenopathy, lethargy, somnolence, headache and mild upper

gastrointestinal symptoms of nausea and abdominal discomfort. The acute illness usually settles, but a prolonged convalescence, similar to IM, is common. In association with the convalescent phase has been the observation that patients are more susceptible than normal to other viral and bacterial infections. Some patients also notice allergies or food intolerances which have not been present previously. Whether these features represent varying degrees of disordered immunoregulation is unclear. Like the IM convalescent syndrome prolonged support of these patients is commonly necessary. As these syndromes typically affect adolescents and young adults the repercussions may be considerable in terms of affecting career and social life.

Posttransfusion Atypical Mononucleosis Syndromes

The development of a swinging pyrexia with or without associated atypical mononucleosis 7 to 10 days after transfusion can be a source of great diagnostic confusion, leading to numerous investigations and potentially hazardous invasive procedures or even surgery to identify a site of infection. The temperature may fluctuate markedly with associated rigors and drenching sweats. Occult sepsis, particularly in the surgical patient is frequently suspected. It is important that clinicians be aware of this syndrome which is most commonly caused by cytomegalovirus (CMV), but EB virus, *Toxoplasma gondii,* ARV or unidentifiable agents may be responsible. CMV infection appears to be more common in patients who have undergone splenectomy. Differentiation from posttransfusion hepatitis may sometimes be difficult, as liver function abnormalities commonly occur in the mononucleosis syndromes.

The syndrome can usually be suspected when the triad of pyrexia, atypical mononucleosis and mildly abnormal liver function occurs 7 to 10 days after blood component therapy. In immunocompromised patients (especially transplant patients) these syndromes may present serious overwhelming infection and the patient is unable to mount a satisfactory immune response. CMV infection, in particular, is becoming an increasing problem in relation to marrow transplantation and ways are being sought to prevent and treat the infection, including the provision of blood and blood components from donors negative for CMV antibodies.

Infectious Lymphocytosis

Infectious lymphocytosis is an epidemic illness affecting young children. A marked lymphocytosis of small round lymphocytes averaging 20 to 30×10^9/L is seen. The condition has an incubation period of 12 to 21 days and is a clinically mild or asymptomatic disorder. *Bordetella pertussis* infection may also cause a marked lymphocytosis.

VIRUS-ASSOCIATED HEMOPHAGOCYTIC SYNDROME (VAHS)

This fulminant and potentially lethal syndrome has only recently been identified as an entity in its own right. In the past it has probably been confused with histiocytic malignancies. Accurate definition, pathophysiology and etiology of VAHS remains to be fully elucidated and there may be milder or more chronic forms of the disease and viruses may not always be the etiological agent. It is likely that the syndrome is related more to an inappropriate and excessive monocyte/macrophage system reaction to common viral or other antigenic agents. CMV, EBV and herpes simplex are viruses which have been identified in some patients.

The syndrome usually has a fulminant febrile presentation with rigors and sweats, there is evidence of multiorgan involvement manifested by rash, lymphadenopathy, hepatosplenomegaly, pulmonary infiltrates, jaundice, abnormal liver function, varying degrees of cytopenia or pancytopenia, confusion and pericarditis. The condition is more common in severely immunocompromised hosts (renal transplants and lymphoid malignancies) and may prove fatal. The multisystem nature of the disease makes differential diagnosis difficult. Exclusion of identifiable infectious causes and histiocytic malignancy is important. Diagnosis is usually made on the basis of the clinical findings, peripheral blood abnormalities and bone marrow or lymph node evidence of hemophagocytosis by the histiocytic cells. Therapy of VAHS is empirical at present, but the author has found high-dose corticosteroid therapy controls the condition in most patients, although recrudescence is not uncommon.

PARVOVIRUS INFECTION

It has recently been recognized that parvovirus infection, the agent responsible for erythema infectiosum, may cause bone marrow suppression causing aplastic anemia or aplastic crisis in patients with congenital hemolytic anemia.

INFECTIONS IN WHICH THERE MAY BE PROMINENT HEMATOLOGICAL MANIFESTATIONS

There are a number of infections which may have clinical manifestations indicative of hematological complications or the possibility of an underlying hematological disease. The hematologist is commonly involved in such patients to assist in diagnosis and/or therapy. For brevity conditions falling into this category are listed in Table 10.3.

Table 10.3
Infectious Conditions Which May Have Hematological Manifestations or Complications

Infection	Hematological Features
Bacterial	
Meningococcal septicemia	Vasculitis and DIC
Pseudomonas	Purpura fulminans and DIC
Clostridium perfringens	Intravascular hemolysis
Other septicemias	DIC
Cat scratch disease	Lymphadenopathy
Brucellosis, typhoid, TB	Monocytosis
Viral	
EBV, CMV, ARV, parvovirus, Hepatitis and others	Discussed in the text
Dengue fever	Hemorrhage
Rickettsial	
Rocky Mountain spotted fever	Purpura
Protozoal	
Toxoplasmosis	Mononucleosis syndrome
Malaria	Hemolysis, splenomegaly
Schistosomiasis	Splenomegaly
Leishmaniasis	Splenomegaly
Parasitic	
Worm infestation	Eosinophilia
Hookworm	Iron deficiency
Fish tape worm	Vitamin B12 deficiency

Hematological Aspects of Noninfectious Multisystem Disorders

In this section the hematological features or complications of a wide range of disorders affecting other systems of the body will be summarized. It would be inappropriate to discuss the disorders in detail and most of the presentation will be in tabular form for reference purposes. Most of the hematological features are discussed elsewhere in the text. The purpose of this section is to assist in the integration of hematology with other specialities.

METABOLIC DISORDERS

Hemochromatosis and Other Iron Overload Disorders

Pathophysiology

Hemochromatosis is an autosomal recessive disorder, carried on chromosome 6, in which there is inappropriately excessive iron absorption. The exact defect remains to be elucidated. The multisystem clinical features of the disease are due to the relentless accumulation of iron in most of the body tissues. As the condition is insidious diagnosis has usually been delayed until the fifth or sixth decade of life, but awareness of the disorder is now greater and diagnostic methods more advanced. The hemochromatosis gene is being recognized as probably one of the commonest abnormal genes in the community. Prevention and arresting tissue damage from iron overload is of paramount importance, therefore early diagnosis is essential, considering that hemochromatosis is a preventable disease.

The relationship between idiopathic hemochromatosis and other disorders associated with iron overload remains controversial. The current state of knowledge can be summarized as follows:

- Tissue damage may occur as a result of iron overload in the following conditions:
    Sideroblastic anemia
    Transfusion siderosis
    Thalassemic syndromes (usually with transfusion)
    Alcoholic liver disease
    Excess dietary intake
    Some chronic hemolytic anemias
    Porphyria cutanea tarda.

- Chronic increase in erythropoiesis or ineffective erythropoiesis is a common feature in many patients.
- It is likely that patients who develop severe tissue damage syndromes are heterozygous or homozygous for the hemochromatosis gene.

Clinical Features

The classicial bronze diabetes picture of the past is rare nowadays as the diagnosis is made earlier and therapy instituted. The clinical manifestations of the disease are legion and every patient is likely to have different features. The commonest presentations are rheumatological, abnormal liver function, incidental detection or as a result of family studies.

Clinical features include:

- Slate-grey skin pigmentation.
- Abnormal liver function, cirrhosis, hepatoma.
- Endocrine dysfunction—diabetes, hypopituitarism, hypogonadism.
- Peripheral neuropathy.
- Cardiomyopathy.
- Arthritis—pseudogout or classical radiological changes in the hands or knees.

Laboratory Features

- The serum iron is raised above twice the upper limit of normal, transferrin saturation (or TIBC) is 75% to 100%.
- Ferritin is a good test of iron stores and is usually well over 1000ng/ml. 1 ng/ml = approx 8mg iron.
- It is generally held that a liver biopsy should be performed for definitive diagnosis, but in some patients the clinical and laboratory evidence may be so strong that this invasive procedure can be avoided.
- Histocompatibility studies—as the hemochromatosis gene is closely linked to the HLA complex on chromosome 6, it is possible to carry out detailed family studies to identify homozygous and carrier states. In some circumstances the disease can be diagnosed years or decades before it is likely to become manifest.

Therapy

Regular venesection is necessary until the excess iron is removed. This can usually be carried out weekly or more if tolerated until the ferritin is in the normal range. To maintain control of the disease second monthly venesection is then necessary. Removal of iron will prevent progression of the tissue damage, but damage already present cannot always be reversed. Liver function will usually improve and pigmentation resolve, but improvements in arthritis, cardiac function or portal hypertension are less likely.

OTHER METABOLIC DISORDERS

The following metabolic disorders may have hematological features.

Lipid Storage Diseases

Gaucher's and Niemann-Pick disease have hepatosplenomegaly as a prominent feature.

Porphyria

Erythropoietic porphyria.

Abetalipoproteinemia

Red cell acanthocytosis and malabsorption.

Autoimmune Disorders

Systemic Lupus Erythematosus

- Anemia of chronic disease
- Autoimmune hemolytic anemia
- Neutropenia
- Immune thrombocytopenia
- Autoimmune marrow suppression
- Qualitative platelet dysfunction
- Lupus anticoagulant
- Recurrent venous thrombosis.

Rheumatoid Arthritis

- Anemia of chronic disease
- Iron deficiency anemia
- Sideroblastic anemia

- Aplastic anemia secondary to therapy
- Chronic neutropenia
- Felty's syndrome
- Thrombocytopenia, usually therapy related.
- Qualitative platelet defects secondary to nonsteroidal antiinflammatory drugs.

Alcoholism

Red Cells

- Macrocytosis
- Direct toxic suppression of hemopoiesis
- Folate deficiency
- Reversible sideroblastic anemia
- Blood loss with or without iron deficiency
- Hemolytic anemia associated with liver disease or severe hypophosphatemia.

Leukocytes and Host Defenses

- Mild neutropenia, but poor granulocyte response to infection.
- Impaired granulocytic function
- Direct immune suppressive effects of alcohol.

Hemostasis

- Thrombocytopenia
- Qualitative platelet defects, especially if alcohol is combined with aspirin.
- Coagulopathies associated with liver disease or vitamin K deficiency.

Hypersplenism

Further Reading

Gordon-Smith, EC and Torrigiani, G. eds. *Seminars in haematology* Vol. 19 No. 2. Tropical Disease. New York: Grune and Stratton Inc., 1982.

Hardisty, RM and Weatherall, DJ. *Blood and its disorders* 2nd ed. Oxford: Blackwell Scientific Publications, 1978.

Schlossberg, D. ed. *Infectious mononucleosis*. Praeger monographs in infectious disease. New York: Praeger Scientific, 1983.

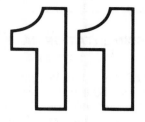

The Interpretation and Investigation of Abnormal Laboratory Results

Oh, how fallacious sometimes are diagnostics.

J. J. Vicarius (1664–   )

The relatively inexpensive nature and wide availability of simple investigations such as a complete blood count and biochemical profile, results in the intentional or incidental finding of abnormalities which require further explanation. There is no denying that the routine performance of a complete blood count and biochemical profile may provide valuable information in the pursuit of disease diagnosis or therapeutic monitoring. Even so, considerable caution must be exercised to avoid overinterpretation and unnecessary investigations and at the same time to ensure that all valuable clues are noted. It is important that the abnormalities are interpreted in their clinical context and relevance to the problem at hand determined. The following question should be addressed when an abnormality is detected on a profile investigation.

Why Was the Investigation Performed and What Is the Likelihood of the Abnormality Being Significant in Relation to This Particular Patient?

The likelihood of an abnormal laboratory finding being insignificant increases or decreases when interpreted in the light of the clinical information. Tests may be ordered for the following reasons:

For Diagnosis in Symptomatic Patients

The clinical history and physical findings will direct the clinician in test ordering. If an initial abnormality is found consistent with the clinical findings, the probability of this being the cause of the patient's problems is high.

Tests Ordered for Screening in Symptomatic Patients

It is common that patients present with symptoms, and possibly signs, which are not specific enough to make a provisional diagnosis or indeed direct the clinician towards the likely diseased system. Under these circumstances, ordering the inexpensive screening hematological and biochemical investigations is justified. If abnormalities are detected, the significance must be carefully interpreted in retrospect. Under some circumstances, the laboratory findings are likely to be nonspecific, but confirm that the patient probably has organic disease which requires further investigation.

Tests Ordered for Screening in Asymptomatic Patients

Clinical and laboratory health screening is becoming more common to assist in the early detection of disease. Health screening can be a two-edged sword if not carried out with due attention to the likelihood of detected abnormalities being significant. Remembering that 5% of "normal people" will lie outside the normal range when any particular parameter is measured, there is a high likelihood of insignificant abnormalities being detected in screening an asymptomatic population. The predictive value of any investigation is much lower when the test is used as a health screening procedure rather than a diagnostic procedure in a high probability population (see chapter 2). The clinican must decide whether the abnormality warrants further, possibly invasive, investigations. Unfortunately this cannot always be done with purely medical considerations in mind. The increasing influence of medicolegal considerations in the management of patients is of concern. Unfortunately, many investigations are performed for legal reasons rather than on a sound clinical basis. When an abnormality is detected during health screening, it is important to consider the following questions:

- Is the abnormality diagnostic of a specific disease requiring further investigation?
- Is early diagnosis of the disease important?
- Is the abnormality a risk factor for disease rather than a specific cause and would correction of this risk factor improve the outlook for the patient?
- If further investigation is not warranted at present, should the abnormality be followed up?

Investigations Performed for the Monitoring of Disease or Risk Factors

When an abnormality or underlying disease has been identified, laboratory investigations may be valuable in the monitoring of disease progress or therapy. Such an approach is important in clinical medicine and the main question relates to the frequency of monitoring.

An Approach to Abnormal Results of Laboratory Investigations

In the earlier chapters of this book individual clinical and laboratory problems have been addressed. Under these circumstances the clinician normally has a problem-orientated deductive approach in order to achieve a diagnosis. In contrast, in this chapter, the emphasis will be on laboratory abnormalities detected in asymptomatic patients, in patients in whom the clinical history is nonspecific or unexpected abnormalities have appeared when investigating for specific problems.

ERYTHROCYTE SEDIMENTATION RATE (ESR)

The ESR is one of the oldest laboratory tests in clinical medicine and is truly a broad-spectrum, nonspecific indicator of disease and a useful monitor for the progress of disease. Despite its antiquity the basic phenomena underlying the ESR are not well understood. Attempts to dislodge the ESR as a standard laboratory test have been unsuccessful, and if correctly performed and interpreted; it will retain its foothold as an economical, simple and useful investigation. For practical purposes elevation of the ESR is due to increased aggregation of the red cells due to alteration in plasma proteins. The commonest reason for elevation of the ESR is an increase in plasma fibrinogen level associated with the acute or chronic phase reaction, but increases in other macromolecules in the plasma will increase the level, especially immunoglobulins. The ESR is age, sex and pregnancy dependent (see appendix) and mild elevations are relatively unhelpful. In general elevation over 50mm/h will usually have an explanation and should be pursued. If greater than 100mm/h the possibilities are more limited (see Fig. 11.1). Figure 11.1 presents a practical approach to the investigation of an elevated ESR, when the cause is not obvious from the clinical story. A low ESR may be seen in polycythemia, hypofibrinogenemia (e.g., DIC or partially clotted specimen), severe plasma hyperviscosity, cryoproteinemia and an old blood specimen.

CYTOPHILIAS

Polycythemia

See chapter 4.

Neutrophilia

Neutrophilia is usually a reactive condition readily explained as part of the acute or chronic phase reaction to clinically evident disease. If neutrophilia is not explained by the clinical condition of the patient, the following should be considered:

Occult infectious, inflammatory or malignant disease

Cigarette smoking

Early myeloproliferative disease

Stress-related syndromes, exercise, recent surgery

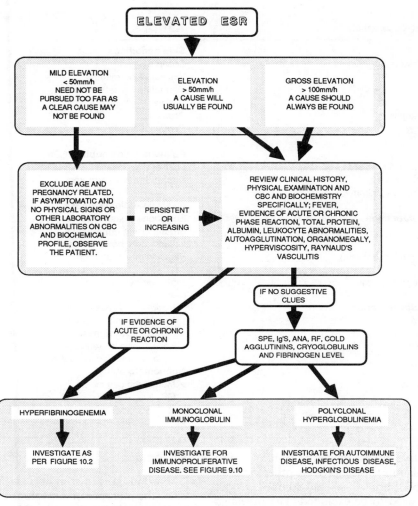

Figure 11.1. An approach to an elevated erythrocyte sedimentation rate (ESR); SPE = serum protein electrophoresis; ANA = antinuclear antibody; RF = rheumatoid factor

Corticosteroids
Pregnancy

In each of these conditions there are likely to be other laboratory features to assist in diagnosis.

The Leukocyte Differential

Differential analysis of the leukocyte count is one of the oldest hematological investigations. With automated differential blood counts becoming more readily available, the performance of tedious manual differentials is becoming less of a demand on the laboratory services. The differential leukocyte count al-

lows determination of the absolute numbers of each of the peripheral blood leukocytes which is the key information rather than the relative percentages of each cell type.

Lymphocytosis

An absolute lymphocytosis requires explanation, especially in an adult. If the lymphocytes have atypical "reactive" morphology there is usually an underlying viral infection, although a mature lymphocytosis may be seen in several childhood infections (see chapter 8). A mature lymphocytosis in an adult must be assumed to be due to lympho-

Table 11.1
Causes of Eosinophilia

Allergic	**Skin conditions**
Atopic subjects	Eczema
Asthma	Exfoliative dermatitis
Urticaria	Dermatitis herpetiformis
Hay fever	Scabies
Serum sickness	Psoriasis
Food allergy	Pemphigus
Drugs	
	Pulmonary eosinophilia
Autoimmune disorders	Loeffler's syndrome
Polyarteritis nodosa	Sturge-Strauss syndrome
Goodpasture's syndrome	
	Gastrointestinal disease
Parasitic infections	Eosinophilic gastroenteritis
Hookworm	Protein losing enteropathy
Filariasis	Inflammatory bowel disease
Bilharzia (Schistosomiasis)	Parasitic infestations
Hydatid	
Toxocara and Trichuris	**Malignancy**
	Hematological
Nonparasitic infection	Hodgkin's disease
Scarlet fever	Non-Hodgkin's lymphomas
Tuberculosis	Histiocytic malignancies (esp. T-cell)
Aspergillosis	Eosinophilic leukemia
	Chronic granulocytic leukemia
Drugs	**Nonhematological**
Sulfonamides	Metastatic carcinoma
Penicillins	GIT, lung, kidney

proliferative disease (usually chronic lymphocytic leukemia) until proven otherwise, but tuberculosis, brucellosis and secondary syphilis may need to be excluded. The investigation of lymphoproliferative lymphocytosis is discussed in chapter 9.

Eosinophilia

Eosinophilia can be one of the most "frustrating" cytophilias to investigate. If an allergic, drug or parasitic cause is not apparent and there are no other clinical clues present the search can be a long and frequently fruitless one. It is unlikely that any serious disease is being missed and the patient can usually be followed as long as an adequate history and full clinical examination, complete blood count, biochemical profile, chest x-ray and stool examination have been performed. Table 11.1 lists possible causes of eosinophilia. The primary eosinophilic syndromes are discussed in chapter 9.

Basophilia

Basophilia is uncommon and usually indicates the presence of a myeloproliferative disease, e.g., chronic granulocytic leukemia, polycythemia rubra vera, myelofibrosis or basophilic leukemia. Other less common causes include hypothyroidism, recovery from infection, postsplenectomy and hepatic cirrhosis.

Monocytosis

Many conditions said in the past to be associated with monocytosis, the cytophilia has now been identified as being an atypical lymphocytosis. A true monocytosis may be seen in conjunction with chronic infections such as tuberculosis, brucellosis, bacterial endocarditis or protozoal infections or in inflammatory bowel disease and sarcoidosis. Occasionally it may be seen in association with solid tumors but most malignant causes are usually hema-

Table 11.2
Causes of Thrombocytosis

Reactive

Acute or chronic phase reaction
  Infectious, inflammatory or malignant disease
Bleeding and iron deficiency
Recovery phase from megaloblastic anemia
Marrow recovery post chemotherapy (esp. cytosine arabinoside)
Vinca alkaloids
Stress related disorders, exercise
Corticosteroids
Postsplenectomy
Hemolytic anemia
Malignancy: Hodgkin's disease
                Solid tumors

Primary

Myeloproliferative disease
  Essential thrombocythemia
  Polycythemia rubra vera
  Chronic granulocytic leukemia
  Myelofibrosis/myeloid metaplasia

tological in nature (see chapter 9). Unexplained monocytosis should be followed as the cause will eventually become apparent in most patients.

Leukemoid Reactions

The term leukemoid is used when there is a marked reactive cytophilia suggesting the diagnosis of leukemia. The peripheral leukocyte count is usually $>50 \times 10^9$/L to be classified as leukemoid.

Lymphoid Leukemoid Reactions

These may be seen in viral infections, especially in children, e.g., infectious lymphocytosis and infectious mononucleosis. Whooping cough and tuberculosis may also occasionally be responsible.

Granulocytic Leukemoid Reactions

These may be seen in severe bacterial infection, hemolysis, burns, eclampsia, toxic reaction to chemicals, after hypoxia (e.g., cardiac arrest), nonhematological malignancy, Hodgkin's disease and bone marrow infiltration. Extremely marked neutrophilia may be seen in toxic megacolon, bacilliary dysentry and pseudomembranous colitis. In these two conditions massive numbers of neutrophils are sequestered into the colon. If the patient suddenly becomes shocked or the colon is resected the neutrophil count may suddenly rise as the cells formed by the marrow are unable to reach their intended destination. In such circumstances it is essential that hydration and tissue perfusion be maintained or fatal leukostasis may ensue.

Eosinophilic Leukemoid Reactions

These may be seen in some of the conditions outlined in Table 11.1.

Thrombocytosis

Thrombocytosis is a common cytophilia (Table 11.2) and usually occurs on a reactive basis in association with the acute or chronic phase reaction. If no cause is found on clinical or laboratory investigation and the patient is a nonsmoker, early myeloproliferative disease is likely.

Abnormal Blood Count and Film (CBC)

A complete blood count is a most valuable and inexpensive investigation and can reasonably be regarded as a justifiable screening investigation along with such investigations as a biochemical profile, chest x-ray and cardiograph. If abnormal, the CBC in conjunction with an ESR is generally a good indicator of organic disease. The cytophilias, cytopenias, abnormal indices and ESR have been discussed elsewhere, and in this section attention will be addressed to abnormal red cell morphology.

Abnormal Red Cell Morphology

On blood film examination this may give important clues to disease. In general, there are changes in the red cell indices to indicate that hematological disease is present or hematological abnormalities secondary to disease of other systems. Most red cell changes are discussed in the appropriate sections in chapter 3 in relation to anemia; however there are several morphological (anisocytosis and poikilocytosis) alterations in the blood film which may be the main clue to disease.

Table 11.3
Red Cell Morphology and Disease

Liver disease	Macrocytes and target cells
Alcoholism	Macrocytes, stomatocytes
Uremia	Burr cells
Hyposplenism	See chapter 8
Marrow dysplasia	Anisocytosis + +, macrocytes, tear drops, fragments
Abetalipoproteinemia	Acanthocytosis
Hereditary spherocytosis	Regular spherocytes
Hypothyroidism	Irregularly contracted cells, anisocytosis, poikilocytosis
Microangiopathy (MAHA)	Irregular fragmented cells, schistocytes, helmet cells
Heinz body damage (? drugs)	Fragmented spherocytes, bite cells
Hemoglobinopathies	Target cells, stippling, hypochromia, sickle cells, stomatocytes
Sideroblastosis	Hypochromic cells, Pappenheimer bodies
Malaria	Intracellular parasites
Abnormal blood groups	Variety of red cell changes
Lead poisoning	Basophilic stippling
Bone marrow infiltration	Leukoerythroblastic changes

Table 11.4
Biochemical Abnormalities in Hematological Disease

Hyperkalemia	Hemolyzed sample, marked leukocytosis
Hypercalcemia	Hematological malignancy, esp. lymphoma, myeloma
Hyperuricemia	Hematological malignancy, myeloproliferative disease
Hyperproteinemia	Monoclonal protein: myeloma, benign monoclonal gammopathy, polyclonal hyperglobulinemia
Hypoalbuminemia	Myeloma
	Nephrotic: amyloid, renal vein thrombosis
Elevated LDH	Hemolysis
	Ineffective erythropoiesis
	Myeloproliferative disease
	Megaloblastosis
	Sideroblastosis
Hyperbilirubinemia	Hemolysis
(unconjugated)	Hemolytic anemias
	Post transfusion of stored blood
Abnormal liver	Hematological malignancy
enzymes	Atypical mononucleosis syndromes
Elevated serum iron	Hemochromatosis
	Sideroblastosis
	Thalassemias
Reduced serum iron	Acute or chronic disease
	Iron deficiency
Abnormal renal	Hemolytic uremic syndrome
function	Secondary to hypercalcemia
	Secondary to hyperuricemia
	Myeloma kidney
	DIC
	Obstructive uropathy
	Amyloid
Abnormal blood gases	Spurious hypoxemia secondary to leukocytosis
Increased anion gap	Hyperproteinemic disorders, especially multiple myeloma
Discolored plasma	Hemoglobinemia
	Methemalbuminemia
	Myoglobinemia plus uremia
	After iron infusion

Table 11.3 lists conditions in which the red cell morphology may be helpful.

Abnormal Leukocyte Morphology

Hypersegmentation

Hypersegmentation of the neutrophil nuclei is seen in megaloblastic anemias, liver disease, sepsis, oral contraceptive use, as a hereditary defect and occasionally in severe iron deficiency.

Left Shift in the Neutrophils with Band Forms Present

This is seen in infections, toxic states, acute hemolysis or hemorrhage and in some neutropenic states.

Toxic Granulation

This is seen in bacterial infections, various acute stressful or toxic states and liver disease.

The Leukoerythroblastic Blood Film

Primitive leukocyte and red cell precursors may be released into the peripheral blood whenever there is a breakdown in the marrow-blood barrier. The peripheral blood film is polychromatic, nucleated red cells are present, granulopoiesis shows a left shift with myelocytes, metamyelocytes and occasionally more primitive cells and the red cells show marked anisocytosis and poikilocytosis with characteristic teardrop cells present. The possible causes of a leukoerythroblastic blood film are:

Marrow infiltration
  Fibrosis
  Carcinoma
  Hematological malignancy (myeloma, lymphoma)
  Tuberculosis
  Storage diseases

Primary myelofibrosis and myeloid metaplasia
Severe hemorrhage
Severe hemolysis
Marble bone disease (osteopetrosis)
After severe hypoxia (cardiac arrest)

Abnormal Results of Biochemical Investigations Relevant to Hematological Disease

Table 11.4 summarizes abnormalities which may be detected in a biochemical profile which may be indicative of underlying hematological disease which may not have been apparent on initial clinical assessment.

Abnormalities Detected in the Blood Transfusion Laboratory

The blood transfusion laboratory commonly detects abnormalities in blood samples during compatibility tests for the provision of blood for transfusion. These findings may be important clues to diagnosis and are summarized in Table 11.5.

Laboratory Artifacts and Other Spurious Laboratory Results

During the performance of in vitro laboratory investigations abnormalities in the cellular or plasma components of the blood may result in spurious results. This particularly applies with the wide use of automated ma-

Table 11.5
Hematological Abnormalities Which May Be Incidentally Detected by the Blood Transfusion Laboratory during Compatibility Testing

Positive Coombs' test result	Autoimmune hemolysis
	Drug reaction
	Transfusion reaction
Autoagglutination	Cold agglutinins
Serum autoantibodies	Autoimmune hemolysis
Serum alloantibodies	Transfusion reaction
	Fetal immunization of mother
Clotting abnormalities	Coagulopathy
Plasma protein abnormalities	Myeloma, cryoglobulinemia
Abnormally colored serum	See under biochemistry

Table 11.6
Possible Reasons for Spurious Results with Automated Cell Counters

Parameter	Spurious Increase	Spurious decrease
Leukocytes	Cryoproteins	Clotted sample
	Heparin	Smudge cells
	Nucleated red cells	
	Platelet clumping	
Red cell count	Cryoproteins	Clotted sample
	Giant platelets	Autoagglutination
	Marked leukocytosis	In-vitro hemolysis
		Microcytic red cell
Hemoglobin	Carboxyhemoglobin	Clotted sample
	Cryoproteins	
	In-vivo hemolysis	
	Heparin	
	Marked leukocytosis	
	Hyperbilirubinemia	
	Hyperlipidemia	
	Monoclonal proteins	
Hematocrit	Cryoproteins	Autoagglutination
	Marked leukocytosis	In-vitro hemolysis
	Giant platelets	Clotted sample
	Hyperglycemia	Microcytic red cells
MCV	Marked leukocytosis	Cryoproteins
	Autoagglutination	Giant platelets
	Hyperglycemia	In-vitro hemolysis
	Rigid red cells	Microcytic red cells
MCHC	Autoagglutination	Marked leukocytosis
	Clotting	Spuriously low Hb
	In-vitro hemolysis	Spuriously high Hct
	In-vivo hemolysis	
	Spuriously high Hb	
	Spuriously low Hct	
Platelets	Cryoproteins	Clotting
	Hemolysis	Heparin
	Microcytic cells	Giant platelets
	Red cell inclusions	Platelet clumping
	Leukocyte fragments	Platelet satellitism

chines for most of the commonly performed investigations.

Cell Counting and Indices

There are numerous problems which may occur in the automated measurement of hematological cell indices. These problems are usually detected by the laboratory staff or the blood sample is rejected or "voted out" by the cell counter. Either way the spurious result may be a clue to diagnosis. Such problems are listed in Table 11.6.

12 Preventive Medicine Aspects of Hematology

Disease often tells its secrets in a casual parenthesis.

Wilfred Trotter (1872–1939)

There are three important clinical contexts in which proper clinical and laboratory assessment of the hemopoietic system is important for the early diagnosis or prevention of disease or complications. In most circumstances the essential screening information can be obtained from the historical and clinical findings, in combination with a low-cost blood count and biochemical profile. In specific disease states awareness of the potential hematological abnormalities or complications is necessary, or should be sought, in order that the appropriate investigation can be requested. Having identified the "clinical ball park" further analysis of the problem can be found in the appropriate section of the text by referring to the index.

Preoperative Assessment

Careful preoperative assessment of hemopoietic function may be repaid several times over if major complications are avoided.

Screening for Disease and Risk Factor Assessment in Asymptomatic Patients

The early detection of certain hematological abnormalities may not only lead to the early diagnosis of disease, but also the identification of important risk factors.

The Identification of Incidental or Associated Hematological Abnormalities Which May Affect the Management and Outcome of the Primary Disease

With the hemopoietic system's central role in host defenses and healing any impairment may have major implications in relation to the patient's therapy and the natural history of the disease in question.

Preoperative Assessment

Whenever surgery or other invasive procedures are being contemplated, it is important to establish that the hemopoietic system will respond appropriately. It is also essential that if any defects are detected, appropriate therapeutic and blood component therapy decisions are made in advance to ensure a coordinated approach to the surgery. The following areas warrant consideration.

OXYGEN TRANSPORT

Recognition and appropriate therapy for anemia seems obvious. However, it is all too common to see "top-up" transfusions prior to elective surgery when an anemia could have been clearly corrected if surgery was delayed for a brief period. Under other circumstances, depending on the degree of urgency or the reversibility of the anemia, preoperative transfusion may be essential. Any abnormalities in the blood suggestive of a hyperviscosity or microvascular type disease as outlined in chapter 4 should be identified and appropriate steps taken if time permits. As a general rule polycythemia and thrombocytosis should be corrected if time permits.

There has been much discussion about the optimal hemoglobin for safe anesthesia and surgery. There is good physiological evidence confirming the hemoglobin level of 10.0g/dL which has been accepted by anesthetists for decades. All other things being equal, a hemoglobin of 10.0g/dL seems an optimal level for safe anesthesia. In patients with respiratory disease, a higher level is probably desirable.

HEMOSTASIS

As already pointed out in chapter 6, historical assessment of hemostasis has the highest predictive value in determining whether a patient will bleed in association with elective surgery or invasive procedures.

HOST DEFENSES

As discussed in chapter 7, optimal functioning of the nonspecific and specific host defenses is essential for healing and control of infection. Under most circumstances, host defense function can be assessed clinically and by the performance of certain simple laboratory investigations.

RISK OF VENOUS THROMBOEMBOLISM

As outlined in chapter 5, prevention of venous thrombosis depends on early and constant assessment of risk factors.

BLOOD TRANSFUSION REQUIREMENTS

Careful attention should be given to elective assessment of requirements for blood and blood components. This particularly applies if there are specific hemostatic or host defense defects, if large blood loss is expected or there are serological difficulties leading to limited availability of blood of the appropriate group. For further information the reader is referred to major texts on the subject in the list of references.

Hematological Disorders of Relevance to the Surgeon and Anesthetist

Aside from obvious hematological disease, some of the important hematological conditions which may be relevant to the anesthetist and surgeon for the anticipation and prevention of complications are:

Anemia
Hemostatic disorders
Antiplatelet therapy
The anticoagulated patient
The compromised host
The hypercoagulable patient
Past transfusion reactions
Porphyria
Hepatitis B and AIDS-related virus infection
Various hemolytic disorders
Sickle cell disease
Enzyme deficiencies
Hemoglobinopathies
Hyperviscosity syndromes

Screening for Disease and Risk Factors

In order to justify expenditure on health screening for the early identification of disease or risk factors, it is important that it can be justified on a cost-benefit analysis. Unfortunately, many health screening programs have failed in this respect. From the hematological point of view, there are certain diseases in which the patient may be asymptomatic, but early diagnosis or knowledge of the disorder is beneficial. Most screening in hematology should be on selected patients as referred to above.

When mass screening is considered as a public health measure, the ultimate cost benefit is of paramount importance. In general it is only possible to justify screening specific high-risk populations. A complete blood examination is the only hematological investigation which can be advocated for use in nonselective mass health screening. In the complete blood count most of the hematological risk factors for common diseases can be detected at a reasonable cost to the individual or community. It is possible to identify the following abnormalities on a CBC and blood film which may be important for identifying risk factors or asymptomatic disease.

Hemoglobin

Anemia, polycythemia

Table 12.1
Specific Populations Who May Have Hematological Abnormalities Requiring Investigation

Population	Potential Problems
Pregnancy	Anemia: Iron and folate
	Smoking and alcohol
	Autoimmune disease: ITP, SLE
	Venous thromboembolism
	Serological incompatibilities and fetus
	Red cell: especially ABO and rhesus
	Rarely platelets and leukocytes
	Hemostatic defects
	Recurrent abortion
Smoking	Polycythemia
	Thrombocytosis and neutrophilia
	Hyperaggregable platelets
	Macrocytosis
Stress related syndromes	Stress polycthemia
Smoking	Reduced red cell deformability
Obesity	Thrombocytosis and hyperaggregability
Alcohol	Hyperfibrinogenemia, elevated ESR
Type A personalities	Leukocytosis
Hypertension	
Diabetes	

Red Cell Indices

Iron deficiency, macrocytosis, alcohol-related changes, hemoglobinopathies

Morphology

Rouleaux, hemoglobinopathies, hyposplenism

Platelet Count

Thrombocytosis, thrombocytopenia

Leukocyte Differential

Cytopenias, cytophilias and abnormal morphology

Specific Populations in Which Early Diagnosis and Therapy Is Appropriate

Certain people are susceptible to specific problems which may require intervention in the asymptomatic phase. These conditions are outlined in Table 12.1.

Further Reading

Wilson, RE *Surgical problems in immuno-depressed patients.* Major problems in clinical surgery. Vol. 30. Philadelphia: WB Saunders Company, 1984.

Normal Values

Normal hematological values are expressed as mean ± 2 SD (95% range).*

Red-cell count

Men	$5.5 \pm 1.0 \times 10^{12}/L$
Women	$4.8 \pm 1.0 \times 10^{12}/L$
Infants (full-term, cord blood)	$5.0 \pm 1.0 \times 10^{12}/L$
Children, 3 months	$4.0 \pm 0.8 \times 10^{12}/L$
Children, 1 year	$4.4 \pm 0.8 \times 10^{12}/L$
Children, 3 to 6 years	$4.8 \pm 0.7 \times 10^{12}/L$
Children, 10 to 12 years	$4.7 \pm 0.7 \times 10^{12}/L$

Hemoglobin

Men	15.5 ± 2.5g/dL
Women	14.0 ± 2.5g/dL
Infants (full-term, cord blood)	16.5 ± 3.0g/dL
Children, 3 months	11.5 ± 2.0g/dL
Children, 1 year	12.0 ± 1.5g/dL
Children, 3 to 6 years	13.0 ± 1.0g/dL
Children 10 to 12 years	13.0 ± 1.5g/dL

Packed cell volume (PCV; hematocrit value)

Men	47 ± 7%
Women	42 ± 5%
Infants (full-term, cord blood)	54 ± 10%
Children, 3 months	38 ± 6%
Children, 3 to 6 years	40 ± 4%
Children, 10 to 12 years	41 ± 4%

Mean cell volume (MCV)

Adults	86 ± 10fl
Infants (full-term, cord blood)	106fl (mean)
Children, 3 months	95fl (mean)
Children, 1 year	78 ± 8fl
Children, 3 to 6 years	81 ± 8fl
Children, 10 to 12 years	84 ± 7fl

Mean cell hemoglobin (MCH)

Adults	29.5 ± 2.5pg
Children, 3 months	29 ± 5pg

*Modified from Dacie, J. V. and Lewis, S. M. *Practical Haematology.* 6th ed. London: Churchill Livingstone, 1984.

Children, 1 year	27 ± 4pg
Children, 3 to 6 years	27 ± 3pg
Children, 10 to 12 years	27 ± 3pg

Mean cell hemoglobin concentration (MCHC)

Adults and children 325 ± 25g/L $32.5 \pm 2.5\%$

Reticulocytes

Adults and children	0.2–2.0% (c. 25–85 $\times 10^9$/L)
Infants (full-term, cord blood)	2–6% (mean 150 $\times 10^9$/L)

Blood volume

Red-cell volume, men	30 ± 5ml/kg
women	25 ± 5ml/kg
Plasma volume	45 ± 5ml/kg
Total blood volume	70 ± 10ml/kg

Red-cell life-span 20 ± 30 days

Leucocyte count

Adults	$7.5 \pm 3.5 \times 10^9$/L
Infants (full-term, 1st day)	$18 \pm 8 \times 10^9$/L
Infants, 1 year	$12 \pm 6 \times 10^9$/L
Children, 4 to 7 years	$10 \pm 5 \times 10^9$/L
Children, 8 to 12 years	$9 \pm 4.5 \times 10^9$/L

Differential leucocyte count

Adults:
Neutrophils	2.0 to 7.5 $\times 10^9$/L (40% to 75%)
Lymphocytes	1.5 to 4.0 $\times 10^9$/L (20% to 45%)
Monocytes	0.2 to 0.8 $\times 10^9$/L (2% to 10%)
Eosinophils	0.04 to 0.4 $\times 10^9$/L (1% to 6%)
Basophils	<0.01 to 0.1 $\times 10^9$/L ($<1\%$)

Infants (1st day):
Neutrophils	5.0 to 13.0 $\times 10^9$/L
Lymphocytes	3.5 to 8.5 $\times 10^9$/L
Monocytes	0.5 to 1.5 $\times 10^9$/L
Eosinophils	0.1 to 2.5 $\times 10^9$/L
Basophils	<0.01 to 0.1 $\times 10^9$/L

Infants (3 days):
Neutrophils	1.5 to 7.0 $\times 10^9$/L
Lymphocytes	2.0 to 5.0 $\times 10^9$/L
Monocytes	0.3 to 1.1 $\times 10^9$/L
Eosinophils	0.2 to 2.0 $\times 10^9$/L
Basophils	<0.01 to 0.1 $\times 10^9$/L

Children (6 years):
Neutrophils	2.0 to 6.0 $\times 10^9$/L
Lymphocytes	5.5 to 8.5 $\times 10^9$/L
Monocytes	0.7 to 1.5 $\times 10^9$/L
Eosinophils	0.3 to 0.8 $\times 10^9$/L
Basophils	<0.01 to 0.1 $\times 10^9$/L

Platelet count	150 to 400 $\times 10^9$/L
Bleeding time (Ivy's method)	2 to 7 min
(Template method)	2.5 to 9.5 min

Prothrombin time   10 to 14 s
Partial thromboplastin time (PTTK)   35 to 43 s
Prothrombin-consumption index   0 to 30%
Plasma fibrinogen   200 to 400mg/dL
Osmotic fragility (at 20° C and pH 7.4)   0.4 to 0.45g/dL

Percent NaCl	**Percent hemolysis**
0.30	97 to 100
0.40	50 to 90
0.45	5 to 45
0.50	0 to 5
0.55	0

		Ref Range	Ref Range International Units
Serum iron	13 to 32μmol/L	67–179μg/dl	
Total iron-binding capacity	45 to 70μmol/L	251–391μg/dl	
% saturation		20–55%	0.20–0.55
Transferrin	1.2 to 2.0g/L	120–200mg/dl	
Serum vitamin B12	160 to 925ng/L	169–425pg/ml	118–682pmol/L
Serum folate	3 to 20μg/L	3–210ng/ml	6.8–45nmol/L
Red-cell folate	160 to 640μg/L	160–640ng/ml	362–1450nmol/L
Plasma hemoglobin	10 to 40mg/L	1.0–4.0ng/dl	0.16–0.62μmol/L
Serum haptoglobin (Hb-binding)	0.3 to 2.0g/L	30–200mg Hb/dl	4.6–31.0μmol/L

Sedimentation rate (Westergren, 1 hour) (at 20° ± 3°C)
Men	17 to 50 years	1 to 7mm
	>50 years	2 to 10mm
Women	17 to 50 years	3 to 9mm
	>50 years	5 to 15mm

Plasma viscosity (at 25°C)   1.61 ± 0.05 cP

Heterophile (anti-sheep red-cell)
  agglutinin titer   <80
  after absorption with guinea-pig kidney   <10

Cold agglutinin titre (4°C)   <64

Appendix 2 Drug Associations

Sometimes the best medicine is to stop taking something.

Ashleigh Brilliant (1933–   )

Drugs that have been reported to cause a positive result on direct antiglobulin test and hemolytic anemia

Acetaminophen
Amidopyrine
P-aminosalicylic acid (PAS)
Antihistamines
Carbromal
Cephalosporins
Chlorinated hydrocarbon insecticides
Chlorpromazine
Dipyrone
Fenfluramine
Hydralazine
Hydrochlorothiazide
Ibuprofen
Insulin
Isoniazid
Levodopa
Mefenamic acid
Melphalan
Methadone
Methyldopa
Methysergide
Nomifensine
Penicillins
Phenacetin
Probenecid
Procainamide
Quinidine
Quinine
Rifampicin
Stibophen
Streptomycin
Sulfonamides
Sulfonylurea derivatives (oral hypoglycemic agents)
Tetracycline
Tiamterene
Trimellitic anhydride

Drugs which have been associated with agranulocytosis

Acetazolamide
Acetylsalicylic acid
Ajmaline
Allopurinol
Amidopyrines
Amodiaquine
Ampicillin
Antipyrine
Aprindine
Brompheniramine
Bumetanide
Captopril
Carbamazepine
Carbenicillin
Carbimazole
Cephalexin
Cephalothin
Chloramphenicol
Chlordiazepoxide
Chlorothiazide
Chlorpromazine
Chlorpropamide
Chlorthalidone
Cimetidine
Clindamycin
Clomipramine
Cloxacillin
Clozapine
Colchicine
Dapsone
Desipramine
Diazepam

Diazoxide
Di-isopyramide
Doxycycline
Ethacrynic acid
Ethosuximide
Fenoprofen
Flucytosine
Fluphenazine
Fumagillin
Gentamicin
Gold Salts
Griseofulvin
Hydralazine
Hydrochlorothiazide
Hydroxychloroquine
Ibuprofen
Imipramine
Indomethacin
Isoniazid
Levodopa
Levamisole
Lincomycin
Mepazine
Mephenytoin
Meprobamate
Mercurials
Methazolamide
Methicillin
Methimazole
Methyldopa
Methylpromazine
Methylthiouracil
Metiamide
Metronidazole
Nafcillin
Nitrofurantoin
Novobiocin

Oxacillin
Oxophenarsine
Para-aminosalicylic acid
Paracetamol
Penicillamine
Penicillin
Pentazoline
Phenindione
Phenylbutazone
Phenytoin
Primidone
Procainamide
Prochlorperazine
Promazine
Promethazine
Propranolol
Propylthiouracil
Pyrimethamine
Quinidine
Quinine
Rifampicin
Ristocetin
Salicylazosulphapyridine
Streptomycin
Sulfadiazene
Sulfafurazole
Sulfamethoxazole-trimethoprim
Sulfamethoxypyridazine
Sulfapyridine
Sulfathiazole
Thenalidine
Thiacetazone
Thioridazine
Thiouracil
Tolbutamide
Trimepazine
Trimethadione

Drugs which have been associated with thrombocytopenia

Acetaminophen
Acetazolamide
Acetylsalicylic acid
Allylamid
Allylisopropylcarbamide
Aminosalicylic acid (PAS)
Antazoline
Carbamazepine
Cephalothin
Chloroquine
Chlorothiazide
Chlorpromazine
Chlorpropamide
Clonazepam

DDT
Desipramine
Diazepam
Digitoxin
Diphenylhydantoin
Fenoprofen
Gold salts
Heparin
Hydrochlorothiazide
Hydroxychloroquine
Isoniazid
Levodopa
Meprobamate
Methicillin

Methyldopa
Novobiocin
Organic arsenicals
Oxyphenbutazone
Penicillin
Phenothiazine
Phensuximide
Phenylbutazone
Potassium perchlorate
Prochlorperazine
Propylthiouracil
Quinidine
Quinine
Refampicin

Ristocetin
Sodium valproate
Stibophen
Streptomycin
Sulphadiazine
Sulphafurazole
Sulphamethazine
Sulphamethoxypyridiazine
Sulphathiazole
Sulphonamides
Tetracyclines
Tolbutamide
Trimethadione
Trimethoprim

Drugs which may be associated with eosinophilia

Allopurinol
Amiloride
Amphotericin B
Ascorbic Acid
Aspirin
Barbiturates
Benzocaine
Bleomycin
Capreomycin
Cephalosporins
Chloramphenicol
Chlorimpramine
Chloroquine
Chlorpropamide
Dapsone
Diazoxide
Dimercaprol
Diphenylhydantoin
Erythromycin estolate
Fluctosine
Gold salts
Indanedione derivatives
Iron dextran
Isoniazid
Menadiol
Methotrexate

Methyldopa
Methylene blue
Niridazole
Nitrites
Nitrofurantoin
Nitrofurazone
Para-aminosalicylic acid
D-Penicillamine
Penicillins
Pentazocine
Phenacetin
Phenazopyridine
Phenothiazines
Potassium iodide
Prilocaine
Primaquine
Procarbazine
Rifampicin (rifampin)
Salazosulphapyridine
Sodium cromoglycate
Sulphafurazole
Sulphamethizole
Sulphamethoxypyridazine
Sulfonamides
Tartrazine
Tetracyclines
Tolbutamide

Drugs which induce megaloblastic change

Alcohol (chronic)
p-Aminosalicylate
Analgesics
Arsenic
Azathioprine
Azauridine
Benzene

Chlordane
Colchicine
Cyclophosphamide
Cytosine arabinoside
5-Fluorodeoxyuridine
5-Flurouracil
Hydroxyurea

6-Mercaptopurine	Phenytoin
Metformin	Primidone
Methotrexate	Pyrimethamine
Neomycin	Sulphasalazine
Nitrofurantoin	Tetracycline
Nitrous oxide	Triamterene
Oral contraceptives	Trimethoprim
Phenobarbitone	Vinblastine

Drugs which have been associated with aplastic anemia

Acetazolamide, chlorothiazide and related diuretics
Anticonvulsive agents
Antihistaminics
Chloramphenicol
Chloroquine
Gold
Mepacrine
Oral antidiabetics
Organic arsenicals
Penicillamine
Phenothiazines
Phenylbutazone, oxyphenbutazone
Quinidine
Sulphonamides
Thyrostatic agents
Various nonsteroid antirheumatics (NSA)

Appendix 3 General References

Please don't supply any more information, I'm already too well informed.

Ashleigh Brilliant (1933–   )

Further Reading

Alberts B, Bray D, Lewis, JM, Raff M, Roberts K and Watson JD *Molecular biology of the cell.* New York: Garland Publishing, Inc., 1983.

Babior BM, Stossel TP *Hematology: a pathophysiological approach.* New York: Churchill Livingstone, 1984.

Beal RW, Isbister, JP *Blood component therapy in clinical medicine.* Melbourne: Blackwell Scientific Publications, 1985.

Dacie JV and Lewis SM *Practical haematology* 6th ed. London: Churchill Livingstone, 1984.

DeGruchy GC In: Penington D, Rush B, Castaldi P eds. *Clinical haematology in medical practice.* 4th ed. Oxford: Blackwell Scientific Publications, 1978.

Eastham RD *Clinical haematology.* 6th ed. Bristol: Wright, 1984.

Hall R and Malia RG *Medical laboratory haematology.* London: Butterworths, 1984.

Hardisty RM and Weatherall DJ *Blood and its disorders* 2nd ed. Oxford: Blackwell Scientific Publications, 1978.

Hoffbrand AV and Lewis SM *Postgraduate haematology.* 2nd ed. London: William Heinemann Medical Books Limited, 1981.

Hoffbrand AV and Pettit JE. *Essential haematology.* 2nd ed. Oxford: Blackwell Scientific Publications, 1984.

King DW, Fenoglio CM, Lefkowitch JH *General pathology: principles and dynamics.* Philadelphia: Lea and Febiger, 1983.

Koepke JA ed. *Laboratory haematology.* New York: Churchill Livingstone, 1984.

Miller DR ed. *Blood diseases of infancy and childhood.* 5th ed. St Louis: CV Moseby Co., 1984.

Mollison PL *Blood transfusion in clinical medicine.* 7th ed. Oxford: Blackwell Scientific Publications, 1982.

Nathan DG, Oski FA. *Haematology of infancy and childhood.* 2nd ed. Vol. 1 and 2 Philadelphia: WB Saunders Company, 1981.

Oski FA, Naiman, JL *Haematologic problems in the newborn.* Major problems in clinical paediatrics, Vol. 4. 3rd ed. Philadelphia: WB Saunders Company, 1982.

Stites DP, Stobo JD, and Wells JV. *Basic and clinical immunology.* 6th ed. Norwalk, Connecticut/Los Altos, California: Appleton & Lange, 1987.

Trubowitz S and Davis S *The human bone marrow: anatomy, physiology and pathophysiology* Vol. 1 and 2. Florida: CR Press Inc., 1982.

Williams WJ, Beutler E, Erslev AL, Lichtman MA *Hematology* 3rd ed. New York: McGraw-Hill Book Company, 1983.

Wintrobe MM *Clinical haematology.* 8th ed. Philadelphia: Lea and Febiger, 1980.

Zipursky A ed. *Perinatal haematology. Clinics in perinatology,* Vol. 11 No. 2, 1984.

Index

Page numbers in *italics* denote figures; those followed by "t" denote tables.